The Essential Guide to Hysterectomy

The Essential Guide to Hysterectomy

A Gynecologist's Advice on Your Choices
Before, During, and After Surgery—
Including Alternatives to Hysterectomy

Lauren F. Streicher, M.D.

M. EVANS
Lanham • New York • Boulder • Toronto • Oxford

Illustrations prepared by Janet Abercrombie. Figure 4-3 on page 55 is reprinted with permission of the American College of Obstetricians and Gynacologists from Laparoscopy, ACOG Patient Education Pamphlet AP061. Washington, D.C. © ACOG, 1998.

Published by M. Evans
An imprint of The Rowman & Littlefield Publishing Group, Inc.
4501 Forbes Boulevard, Suite 200, Lanham, Maryland 20706
www.rlpgtrade.com

Estover Road
Plymouth PL6 7PY
United Kingdom

Distributed by NATIONAL BOOK NETWORK

Library of Congress Cataloging-in-Publication Data
Streicher, Lauren F.
    The essential guide to hysterectomy : a gynecologist's advice on your choices before, during, and after surgery, including alternatives to hysterectomy / Lauren F. Streicher ; illustrations, Janet Abercrombie
    p. cm.
    ISBN-10: 1-59077-057-9 ISBN-13: 978-1-59077-057-3 (pbk. : alk. paper)
    1. Hysterectomy—Popular works. 2. Patient education. I. Title.
RG391.S83 2004
618.1'453—dc22   2004015377

Book design by Rik Lain Schell
⊖™ The paper used in this publication meets the minimum requirements of American National Standard for Information Sciences—Permanence of Paper for Printed Library Materials, ANSI/NISO Z39.48-1992.

Manufactured in the United States of America.

This book is dedicated to the memory of

My dad, Dr. Daniel Streicher, who never would have predicted that his daughter, the doctor, would read the gynecologic textbook he used as a medical student as a reference to write her own book. I miss him every day.

Mary Donnellon, who said she wanted to dance at my publishing party. You are dancing in my heart and in my memories.

Contents

Acknowledgments

The following colleagues reviewed chapters and were instrumental in assuring accuracy of information on the following topics:

Dr. Shireen Ahmed	*Anesthesia*
Dr. Laura Berman	*Sex after hysterectomy*
Dr. Nehama Dresner	*Depression*
Dr. Brian Kaplan	*Pregnancy after hysterectomy*
Dr. Louis Keith	*History and politics*
Dr. Tom Mustoe	*Plastic surgery*
Dr. Eugene Pergament	*Genetics*
Dr. Janet Rader	*Prophylactic hysterectomy*
Dr. Janet Tomesko	*The cervix decision*
Dr. Robert Vogelzang	*Uterine artery embolization*
Dr. Fred Zar	*Medical complications*
Judith Florendo, PT	*Pelvic physical therapy*
Jim Karas	*Exercise after hysterectomy*
Paul Streicher	*Power of attorney, living wills*

I would also like to thank:

My partners, Jane Blumenthal, Shari Goldman, Bonnie Wise, and Kim McMahon. Not only the best doctors I know (and awesome surgeons) but my dearest friends.

My brother, Paul, who saved me from computer emergencies too numerous to count. If not for Paul, I would have written the whole book longhand with carbon paper for backup.

Ann Hawkins, my agent, for agreeing to look at a manuscript from a gynecologist with no writing experience.

Enrica Gadler, my editor, for putting up with a gynecologist with no writing experience.

My mom, Lyle Streicher, for everything.

My daughters, Rachel and Danielle, who make it all worthwhile.

Introduction

Performing hysterectomies for twenty years has given me a unique perspective regarding its impact on women's lives. What has really influenced my views, however, is twenty years of talking to women before and after their surgery. One thing is consistent. The more information a woman has prior to surgery, the better the choices she will make, and the better her long-term outcome will be.

I decided to write this book when I realized that there is just too much information to cover during the course of a typical pre-operative consultation. I often meet with patients who are scheduled to have a hysterectomy and try to discuss possible removal of the ovaries, removal of the cervix, anesthesia options, post-operative hormone replacement, and potential complications, all in thirty minutes. It is frustrating to me and my patient to cover such huge amounts of complicated information in such a short period of time. Many things are only superficially discussed, or the thirty-minute consultation turns into a ninety-minute marathon, with my patient furiously scribbling notes and me talking in fast-forward.

My decision to write this book also stemmed from the fact that there were no books on the subject that I could comfortably recommend. My patients often find the books directed to the general public overly simplistic and frequently turn to technical, hard-to-understand medical books for more in-depth information. With *The Essential Guide to Hysterectomy*,

I have sought to bridge that gap by presenting thorough, up-to-date medical knowledge in an accessible, conversational way.

Any discussion of hysterectomy must also acknowledge that the procedure has become politicized. The backlash against past over-utilization of hysterectomy has unfortunately resulted in women being led to believe that avoiding hysterectomy is always in their best interest, when in fact it is not. Most books on hysterectomy reflect this controversy and are extremely one-sided. The message is either, "never have a hysterectomy under any circumstances, your life will be ruined," or, "you're having a hysterectomy . . . here's what to bring to the hospital!"

While most hysterectomies *are* appropriate and beneficial, there are still women who have unnecessary surgery or who are not offered less invasive alternatives. Surgical technology has exploded in the last five years, and I've written this book as the source women can turn to in order to learn about uterus-sparing alternatives to hysterectomy, such as thermal ablation and uterine artery embolization, and new surgical innovations such as laparoscopic outpatient hysterectomy. We've come a long way since I did my first hysterectomy twenty years ago, and my fellow residents and I laughed at the notion that a uterus could be removed through a one-inch laparoscopic incision. Little did I know that one day I would perform most of my hysterectomies using that technique.

If you have been advised to have a hysterectomy, this book will serve as a comprehensive guide to the choices you should be aware of and discuss with your surgeon. Topics not typically covered in other books about hysterectomy are also addressed, such as pregnancy after hysterectomy, prophylactic surgery for women genetically at risk for gynecologic cancers, plastic surgery at the time of hysterectomy, sex, and exercise after surgery.

The following pages present treatment options in a balanced, objective, and scientific manner so that women looking for alternatives won't feel that they are being sold a procedure they are trying to avoid, and women who desire a hysterectomy will know what to expect. It is time to take the "hysteria" out of hysterectomy and empower women with accurate, unbiased information, so they can make appropriate decisions regarding the health issues that affect themselves and their families.

Part I

Hysterectomy Past and Present

Chapter 1

The History and Politics of Hysterectomy

Hysterectomy. The very word evokes emotions and reactions unlike any other surgical procedure. For many women, hysterectomy symbolizes the end to fertility, femininity, sexuality, and even their very identity. The negative connotation is troublesome, as hysterectomy also represents the potential to liberate women from pain, bleeding, and cancer. Our ancestors could only have wished for the ability to eliminate the gynecologic problems that made many women's lives horrific and the inevitability of another menstrual cycle a constant shadow.

THE UTERUS—WHERE IT ALL BEGINS

The uterus, where life originates, has long been identified as a possible source of disease. Galen, an ancient Greek physician (second century A.D.), attributed most female problems to the uterus. Hippocrates, famous for his oath, was of the opinion that a uterus, if not fed with sperm, would go wild. Even philosophers got involved. Plato wrote, "when it [the uterus] stays barren too long after puberty, it is distressed and sorely disturbed, and straying about in the body and cutting off the passages of the breath, it impedes respiration and brings the sufferer into the extremest anguish and provokes all manner of disease besides."

Hystera, the Greek word for uterus, eventually became the root word for many medical terms describing conditions that plague women. Whereas the origin of the word hysteria dates back to ancient Greece, the modern concept of hysteria as a negative psychological state did not emerge until the late nineteenth century. It was during the 1800s that an American gynecologist theorized that a "wandering, sick womb" could cause both physical as well as psychological disturbances such as anxiety, depression, an inability to perform the dual roles of wife and mother, and in particular, insanity. This concept continued well into the late 1800s when nearly every ailment that might befall a woman, including tuberculosis and stomach, liver, heart, and lung disease, was at some point blamed on a "sick, wandering" uterus.

Women were advised to placate their "angry" uterus by having babies, being submissive, not educating themselves, keeping quiet, not expressing their opinions, and most important, letting the men run the show. Hysteria, with all its negative connotations, was born. At that time, surgically removing the source of the problem was not a practical option and gynecologic treatments to "restore" uterine health proliferated.

HISTORICAL ALTERNATIVES TO HYSTERECTOMY

Alternatives to hysterectomy are not only a phenomenon of the twentieth century. This wasn't because particular value was placed on keeping one's uterus, or because historical feminist factions advocated the avoidance of unnecessary surgery. It was simply that hysterectomy wasn't available as a safe or reasonable option. In the early days of hysterectomy, only a truly desperate woman would agree to the operation, which was performed without anesthesia and all too frequently lead to the patient's demise. Those who did survive were destined to endure extraordinary pain and years of recuperation. The sad fact is that when hysterectomies were performed before the mid-1940s, they were an infrequent and perilous undertaking. Since our ancestors did not have the option of hysterectomy, they tried to deal with unpleasant or life-threatening gynecologic conditions in other ways.

Ancient Alternatives

The ancient Egyptians first described uterine prolapse, a condition in which the uterus drops down and hangs outside the vagina. Treatment consisted of ingesting a mixture of grain, fruit, and cow's milk. Roman documents dating from 30 A.D. note that astringent washes and medicated pessaries (vaginal inserts) were used to put the uterus back in proper position.

Abnormal uterine bleeding, resulting in anemia and poor health, has also plagued women since the beginning of time. The medical word for heavy bleeding, *menorrhagia*, is derived from the Greek *men* (month), and *rhegyai* (to burst forth). Ancient healers tried many remedies to decrease the flow and the subsequent weakness that resulted.

Hippocrates (460–377 B.C.) advocated the use of cupping (applied to the breasts, of all places!) to decrease bleeding. Beaver oil, calves' gall (bile), and dried snake were also used as remedies. A woman who suffered from heavy menstrual flow in the first century A.D. would have undergone a treatment regimen that consisted of applying ligatures to the armpits and groin in an attempt to reduce blood flow to the body and thus the uterus. This was followed by the intravaginal application of burnt cork and liquid pitch. To complete the treatment, pessaries soaked with the yolks of roasted eggs, alum, or manna were then inserted.

"Modern" Options

In the 1800s, innovative physicians came up with equally creative remedies for treating gynecologic problems. Uterine prolapse in particular continued to be common due to multiple pregnancies and protracted labors. Women who suffered from prolapse frequently also suffered from urinary and fecal incontinence. It was a tragic condition since not only would the uterus hang outside the vagina, but it often became infected and emitted a horrible stench. The treatment? In 1870, it was standard therapy to apply leeches to the vulva or directly to the cervix to coax the uterus back into place. Occasionally, a curious leech would actually crawl *into* the uterus, creating excruciating pain. Physicians were cautioned to carefully count the leeches since errant annelids were known to get lost in the vagina.

The nineteenth-century woman who suffered from a prolapsed uterus had few choices. She could be bedridden and shunned by her husband, her family, and society. She could endure regular bleedings and application of leeches to her genitals. Or she could face excruciating pain and possible death from hysterectomy. It was no wonder that some women chose the almost certain mortality of surgery as their most appealing option.

During that same era, women who suffered from heavy bleeding due to uterine fibroids, hormonal imbalance, or cancer often became severely weakened or died from the resultant anemia. Attempts to destroy the lining of the uterine wall to reduce heavy flow were standard therapy in addition to bloodletting and leech application. The 1883 version of endometrial ablation (see chapter 8) consisted of irrigating the uterine cavity with carbolic acid, silver nitrate, or nitric acid. Other methods included the use of ionizing radiation or electrocautery.

The early twentieth century wasn't much better. By the early 1940s, the use of X rays and radium to decrease excessive menstrual bleeding was popular. It was soon discovered that while those treatments were effective, they resulted in a much higher rate of uterine and cervical cancer than ordinarily seen.

Hurray? for Hysterectomy—Alternatives Abandoned

During the 1940s, advances in surgical technology and anesthesia made hysterectomy a reasonable option, and mercifully, most alternative treatments were abandoned. Between 1950 and 1980, few new alternatives to hysterectomy were introduced as hysterectomy seemed to have such clear advantages over other available options.

It was during the late 1970s and early 1980s that women became aware that increasing numbers of unnecessary hysterectomies were being performed. Many women were coerced into having hysterectomies they didn't want or need. What happened? How was it that a life-saving, life-enhancing operation became overutilized and/or inappropriately performed? As usual, politics and social structure, rather than medicine, were the overriding forces. In this regard, it's important to know where we came from in order to know where we are going.

A Brief History of Hysterectomy

The first documented hysterectomy was performed in the second century A.D. by Soranus of Ephesus, who solved the problem of a prolapsed uterus by simply cutting it off. Little information is available about that operation, and there is minimal information about other early attempts to remove the uterus.

During the nineteenth century, the time of the Civil War and increasing industrialization, hysterectomy was attempted by a number of brave physicians and their even braver patients. Modern women have little or no concept of the suffering women of that era endured.

Severe cases of uterine prolapse were common after multiple protracted and often unattended births. Cancers were invariably diagnosed at late stages. Hysterectomy was a valiant, and final, attempt to aid only the most miserable, suffering women who agreed to the procedure out of total desperation. Anesthesia as we know it didn't exist, so alcoholic stupefaction was used to induce loss of senses. Up to six men would hold the woman down so the surgeon, who was probably as terrified as the woman, could wield the knife. Fortunately for all, antiseptic technique and anesthesia (chloroform) were introduced in the mid to late 1800s, and although pain, complications, and mortality were still extremely high, at least death after hysterectomy wasn't a near-certainty.

An overview of the evolution of hysterectomy is helpful in understanding how far we've come:

1812—Dr. G. B. Paletta inadvertently performed the first vaginal hysterectomy. He amputated what he thought was a cancerous cervix, but in reality, it was the entire uterus that had prolapsed. His unfortunate patient died of infection three days later.

1822—The first *deliberate* vaginal hysterectomy was performed. The woman survived the operation in spite of the fact that her intestines came out of her vagina with her uterus. A gauze pack was used to push them back inside until she healed. Although she survived, the poor woman had to contend with stool coming out of her vagina for her remaining days.

1843—Dr. Walter Burnham of Massachusetts was in the process of removing an ovarian mass. During the surgery, the patient vomited, a common scenario with an unanesthetized patient who had likely eaten just prior to surgery. As the mass came out and could not be replaced, Dr. Burnham was forced to remove what turned out to be the upper part of her uterus, thus performing the first subtotal hysterectomy. He repeated the operation fifteen times. Three of his patients survived.

1843—Around the same time that Dr. Burnham was attempting to get the uterus back into the open abdomen, the first intentional, successful abdominal hysterectomy was performed in England. There was no attempt to remove the cervix, as it was felt to be too dangerous.

1853—Dr. G. Kimball of Boston, Massachusetts, performed the first successful abdominal hysterectomy, including the removal of the cervix, for treatment of fibroids. Heady with success, he repeated the operation forty-two times over the next twenty-three years. Nine patients survived.

1861—A successful, intentional, uncomplicated vaginal hysterectomy for prolapse was performed by Dr. S. Choppin of New Orleans, Louisiana.

1900s to 1940s—Subtotal abdominal hysterectomy became a standard operation in the United States. Removing the cervix was generally regarded as being too dangerous, unnecessary, and a cause of prolonged surgery.

1940s—The availability of antibiotics, anesthesia, and sterile technique, all pushed by the surgical advances that came out of military needs in World War II, made total hysterectomy a reasonable option. In addition, total hysterectomy, as opposed to subtotal abdominal hysterectomy, came into vogue due to an increased awareness that cervical cancer was a major cause of mortality, preventable by removal of the cervix at the time of surgery.

1970—Over half a million hysterectomies were performed in the United States.

1989—The first laparoscopic hysterectomy was successfully completed.

Hysterectomy—Forties' Style

The 1940s was the first time that hysterectomy became a routine procedure, as most women were expected to, and usually did, make a full recovery. Despite the use of sterile technique, antibiotics, and anesthesia, our grandmothers' experience of hysterectomy was very different from that of her modern counterparts.

The 1941 edition of Crossen and Crossen's *Diseases of Women*, a standard gynecologic textbook, gives an accurate rendition of what a woman undergoing hysterectomy in the 1940s would experience.

Women were generally admitted to the hospital two days prior to surgery. Sleep was an important part of the preoperative preparation and a bromide or other sedative was administered to "quiet the nervous system." Enemas the night before and the morning of surgery were mandatory and were cited as a modern improvement over the dieting and purging that had formerly been recommended.

Following the morning enema, the patient's abdomen was lathered, shaved, and bound with sterile dressings. The pubic region, vulva, and perineum were shaved and a douche was administered. One hour before surgery, the patient was placed in a quiet, dark room and given morphine. The purpose of this was to alleviate pre-operation "anxiety," which was "troublesome," and to decrease the amount of anesthesia needed. In addition, the patient would not know when she would be on the way to the operating room.

Anesthesia was administered with an ether mask. The abdominal incision was always vertical, either in the center of the abdomen or off to one side. It was not unusual for the incision to extend well above the belly button. During surgery, hot water bottles were placed under the blankets to "diminish the risk of shock."

Following surgery, the patient was immediately given small amounts of water. Vomiting was felt to be a positive thing since it helped clear out ether-saturated mucous from the nose and oral cavities. Persistent vomiting, however, was problematic, because occasionally the patient inhaled her stomach contents and died.

On the second postoperative day, the woman would be given an enema to "secure a bowel movement." By the fourth day after surgery, it was time to prop the woman up in bed and start solid food. Daily bladder catheterization was recommended, even if the woman appeared to be urinating without difficulty, to assure emptying of the bladder and irrigate the bladder with antiseptic to decrease the risk of infection. Nurses were instructed to massage the patient daily and carry out an evening alcohol rub.

By day five, the woman was permitted to sit straight up in bed! Only on the eighth or ninth day was actual sitting on the edge of the bed permitted. The dressing over the incision was left undisturbed for ten days, at which time the bandages and the stitches were removed. (We're still in the hospital here.) Adhesive strips and a new dressing were placed for an additional week. The tenth day was also when it was permissible to get out of bed, but only if the patient was felt to be doing exceedingly well. It was encouraged to keep women who were "worn out" by ill health or heroic work for their children "in bed for two or more weeks before attempting ambulation." Total hospital time for an *uncomplicated* hysterectomy averaged three to four weeks.

Once discharged from the hospital, women were encouraged to limit their activity and take tonics for three to six months, or until fully recovered. The above scenario, of course, only applied to uncomplicated cases. One can only imagine the recuperation involved if there were significant problems such as bleeding or infection. Quite the contrast to today's patient, who checks in for her laparoscopic hysterectomy at 6:00 A.M., is home with Band-Aids and possibly a few stitches on her belly by dinner time, and is back at work within two weeks.

Risks? Death was no stranger, and the surgeon was warned to only operate on women if absolutely indicated. Infection, anesthetic complications, and hemorrhage were still common, daunting complications. Surgical sponges were small, not routinely counted as they are today, and were sometimes left in the patient's abdomen with disastrous complications. One quarter of patients with retained sponges died; the remainder had protracted recoveries. A full five pages of Crossens' *Diseases of Women* is devoted to various strategies to avoid losing a surgical sponge at the time of surgery.

Largely as a result of advances made during World War II, changes in medicine, surgical technique, and anesthesia were exponential. By the 1950s, a woman could expect to have a much safer surgical experience and a far shorter recuperation. Unfortunately, the ease with which surgery could be performed, combined with a social structure that promoted the idea of "doctor as god," lead to the proliferation of hysterectomies, some of which were unnecessary. The backlash of this phenomenon is still with us.

The Fifties—Paternalism Takes Over

The 1950s and 1960s were a time of paternalism in various social strata, including medicine. The doctor, who was male in 98 percent of cases, decided what was best for his patient and made decisions without consulting patients. Dr. Marcus Welby was the TV prototype of this godlike paragon, and he spoke decisively and with authority in countless American households on a weekly basis. This phenomenon affected both male and female patients, but had a more profound impact on women since they regularly required medical intervention due to childbirth and gynecologic issues. The medical establishment was justifiably proud that women could undergo and recover from hysterectomy in an expedient way. In their defense, most gynecologists of that era lived up to societal expectations of making godlike decisions.

Although misguided by today's thinking, the gynecologist of that time really believed that the large number of hysterectomies being performed was benefiting women who would otherwise have suffered needlessly. This was understandable given the limitations of the alternatives in a time when hormonal treatments and minimally invasive surgery were not yet an option. Neither ultrasound nor other imaging techniques were available to determine whether a pelvic mass was ovarian or uterine, benign or malignant. Indeed, surgery was really the only way to accurately diagnose and manage serious gynecological problems.

At the same time, very little was understood about the origin of the many medical problems for which hysterectomy was performed. Studies from the 1950s through the 1970s show that probably up to one-third of these operations were performed for indications that would appear illogical today. For example, uterine prolapse, other improper positions of the uterus, and uterine infections were believed to cause back pain. Attempts to cure backaches with hysterectomy followed. The operation seemed to help, but of course it was probably not the removal of the uterus, but the four to six weeks of bed rest during recuperation that actually benefited the woman. Had the woman simply been allowed to get off her feet, lie in bed, and recuperate, her backache would likely have resolved just as well.

Of equal importance, women were generally not given explanations as to why surgery was recommended and were often led to believe that they were at risk for developing cancer if they did not submit. In keeping with prefeminist attitudes of what was appropriate, women rarely questioned the recommendations of their doctor. Arming oneself with forty pages of options from the Internet clearly was not an option.

Sterilization accounted for an enormous percentage of hysterectomies. Dr. Ralph Wright, an outspoken 1970s gynecologist, stated, "To keep a useless and potentially lethal organ is incompatible with modern gynecological concepts. Hysterectomy is the only logical approach to surgical sterilization of women." Women went to their doctors requesting contraception and became convinced that hysterectomy was really a better option, with the added bonus that there would be no more troublesome periods! Lucky patients only received sterilization, but that also consisted of a full abdominal operation to remove tubes since laparoscopy had not yet been invented.

A particularly common scenario in which hysterectomy was utilized for sterilization was when a sympathetic gynecologist found a "reason" for his Catholic patient, who was not allowed to get a tubal ligation or use birth control, to have a hysterectomy. Thus, numerous women could legitimately end their yearly pregnancies in a manner that was acceptable to their church.

Of course, not all hysterectomies were inappropriate. Most indications for hysterectomy were performeed to treat the same problems for which women undergo surgery today: abnormal bleeding, uterine prolapse, cancer, and fibroids. Unfortunately, the proliferation of hysterectomies performed for reasons now known to be inappropriate created the subsequent backlash.

The Seventies—Feminism Comes to the Rescue

The 1970s spawned feminism and the realization that women could take control of their own bodies and make appropriate decisions concerning their health, fertility, and sexuality. Books such as *Our Bodies, Ourselves*; *Seizing Our Bodies*; and *The Hidden Malpractice, How American Medicine Mistreats Women* sold millions of copies and created a much-needed awareness of how many women underwent unnecessary and undesired surgery. As a result, women soon demanded to be included in the decision process. The tide began to turn and the flood of automatic, inappropriate hysterectomies dramatically decreased. This, of course, was an appropriate and favorable result of women's heightened awareness in a time when Americans were questioning the established authorities and a patriarchal medical system.

The unfortunate outcome of this chain of events was an overreaction, resulting in the premise that hysterectomies should *never* be done except in life-threatening situations and a movement developed for women to avoid hysterectomy at any cost. Hysterectomy became politicized, with attacks from angry women who felt that their gender was being victimized by profit-motivated physicians. Diatribes against hysterectomy proliferated, asserting that hysterectomies were not only unnecessary and disempowering to women, but were done primarily for financial gain.

A NEW CENTURY—FINDING A BALANCE

As with most extreme reactions, the pendulum swung to the other side. We've gone from an era in which hysterectomies were performed too frequently to an era in which consumers believe that hysterectomies should *never* be performed until every other option has been exhausted. As a result, many patients feel compelled to seek alternative therapies that are not always the best solution to their problems. Indeed, it is an injustice to women to insist that they undergo multiple less effective treatments rather than one definitive treatment that will provide a permanent cure. Ideally, every woman who faces this issue should be provided with information in an unbiased, scientific way so that, in consultation with her doctor, she can make appropriate decisions based on her needs and desires.

Who's Really Profit-Motivated Here?

The image of the profit-motivated physician encouraging unnecessary hysterectomies started in the 1970s, but the insurance industry, which benefits from women avoiding expensive, one-time medical procedures such as hysterectomy, has perpetuated it. Insurance companies currently have the greatest impact on a woman's course of treatment. It is the insurance companies that have taken on the paternalistic role doctors once assumed in granting "permission" as to what procedures a woman can or cannot have, despite her preference, or what her doctor has advised is in her best interest.

If truth be told, a profit-motivated physician has more to gain by offering a *non*definitive therapy. A patient who has multiple small fibroids and undergoes myomectomy, uterine artery embolization, or hysteroscopic resection (in any order) is likely to require multiple office visits, ultrasounds, uterine biopsies, blood counts, and mini-day surgical procedures, yet will still retain her problem. If, on the other hand, that same patient undergoes a laparoscopic hysterectomy, she is done with her problem and will likely require no more than an annual routine visit with her gynecologist. Over time, the physician who performs the hysterectomy will make a lot less money.

At the same time, the insurance company pays less money. Multiple procedures stretched over years ensure that the patient, not the insurer, pays more in the form of co-payments, deductibles, and uncovered costs. Costly one-time hospital fees are avoided, and, given the frequency with which patients change insurers, the burden is frequently divided over multiple companies. Overall, the potential cost to an individual insurance carrier is much lower with years of alternative therapies than with one big-ticket item.

So Who Needs a Hysterectomy?

That depends. Some would say that the only women who need hysterectomies are women who risk death if they forgo the procedure. Using those criteria, hardly *anyone*, unless she has cancer or a life-threatening hemorrhage, absolutely *needs* a hysterectomy.

If one considers "need" in a broader sense, however, people often benefit from things that life itself does not depend on, but that greatly influence the quality of a patient's life. Even if a hysterectomy is not life-saving, it may be one woman's best option. Another woman may be better off with an alternative therapy.

Some women are willing to put up with a lot to avoid losing their uterus or having surgery and are more than willing to have frequent visits to the gynecologist, ultrasounds, endometrial biopsies, and alternative therapies. For those women, this is the right thing to do. Other women immediately say, "Take it out . . . I want to be done with it." Today's woman has choices, and ultimately it is making a good choice based on accurate information that empowers women.

Although many women have convinced themselves, or have been convinced, that they must first submit themselves to painful and sometimes riskier alternatives that may or may not work, women are *not* having significantly fewer hysterectomies. Once they go through with surgery, the overwhelming majority of women are pleased with the result and comment that they wish they had done it sooner. The key is that *they* decided after weighing all options that hysterectomy was the best option. Someone else did not decide for them.

Chapter 2

Anatomy 101

Hysterectomy (like natural childbirth) means different things to different people. Hysterectomy actually refers only to the removal of the uterus, and has nothing to do with the fallopian tubes or the ovaries. Since removal of the tubes and ovaries is frequently done at the time of hysterectomy, many people understandably, but mistakenly, think that they are always part of the procedure. Furthermore, the uterus is divided into the upper part of the uterus (the *fundus,* or body) and the lower part of the uterus, the cervix. Removal of the upper part of the uterus does not always require removal of the cervix. Prior to hysterectomy, it's important to consider and discuss each part separately and then decide what stays and what goes.

THE PELVIC ORGANS

The uterus is a muscular organ, normally the size of a small pear (see Fig. 2-1). During pregnancy, of course, it expands to hold whatever it needs to, whether it's a six-pound baby or quadruplets. It normally weighs about two ounces and sits in the pelvis behind the pubic bone, nestled between the bladder and the rectum.

The *endometrium* is the lining of the uterine cavity. The top part of it sloughs off each month (menstruation) unless a woman becomes pregnant; then it becomes a soft, cushy bed for the developing fetus. As this lining changes throughout the month, a pathologist looking at endometrial tissue under a microscope can determine *to the day* what part of her cycle a woman is in. In a menopausal woman, the lining normally gets really thin and should be totally inactive, which is why postmenopausal bleeding always needs to be evaluated.

Go a little deeper into the uterine wall and you hit the *myometrium*, the muscular part of the uterus. This muscle gets its main workout in labor, but also plays a role in menstruation by controlling blood flow. Fibroid tumors originate in the myometrium before they either push into the cavity or protrude outside the wall of the uterus. The thin outermost layer is known as the *serosa* and covers the entire uterus.

The *cervix* is the opening to the uterus. It lets menstrual blood out and sperm in. It is fused to the bottom of the uterus but is actually a separate structure, both anatomically and functionally. Normally, the

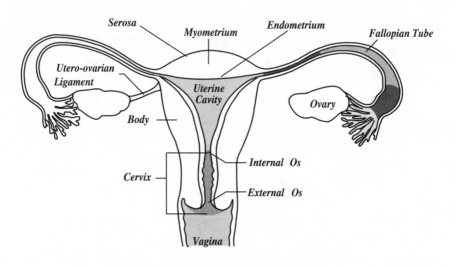

Figure 2-1. Pelvic organs and ligaments.

cervix is a thick-walled tubular structure about three to four inches long; it shortens and thins out in labor to allow the baby to exit the uterus. The *internal os* (opening) is the part that connects to the uterus; the *external os* is at the back of the vagina and is what the gynecologist sees when she uses a speculum during your pelvic exam.

The *fallopian tubes* are the sperm's highway to the egg. They not only connect to the uterus, but also actually burrow through the wall of the uterus and open into the top of the uterine cavity. The egg joins the sperm in the tube, where fertilization occurs. The fertilized egg then travels down the tube, enters the uterus, and implants in the uterine wall until a baby emerges nine months later.

The *ovaries* are next to the uterus. Each is attached to the uterus by a thin structure called the *utero-ovarian ligament.* The important attachment for the ovaries, however, is the infundibulopelvic ligament, which carries the ovarian artery (the ovary's major blood supply) and attaches to the ovary on the side *opposite* the uterus. Therefore, when the uterus is removed but the ovaries are not, the main blood supply and anatomy of the ovary is not disrupted. Ovaries secrete the hormones estrogen and progesterone. Estrogen stimulates receptors in multiple locations throughout a woman's body, including the uterus, breasts, and vaginal walls. Among other things, estrogen is responsible for female sexual maturation, libido, sexual response, and initiation and regulation of the menstrual cycle. Progesterone is responsible for preparing the uterus for pregnancy and maintaining the pregnancy.

Life would be easier for the surgeon if the only structures in the pelvis were the uterus, tubes, and ovaries (and if they came neatly labeled), but that, of course, is not the case (see Figs. 2-1, 2-2, and 2-3). The bladder, ureter, vagina, and bowels are all in the same vicinity and are intimately involved in most gynecologic issues.

The bladder is the highly expandable sac that stores urine that has exited the kidneys. The back part of the bladder is actually fused to the front of the cervix and the lower part of the uterus. That's why women who have an enlarged uterus from pregnancy or fibroids often complain of bladder pressure and have to urinate frequently. This close proximity of the bladder to the uterus is the reason the bladder is vulnerable to injury during pelvic surgery. During a cesarean section, the bladder is actually lifted off the front of the uterus to make the incision through which the baby can be delivered. A hysterectomy also involves moving the bladder away from the front wall of the uterus, which sounds risky but is actually a simple surgical maneuver.

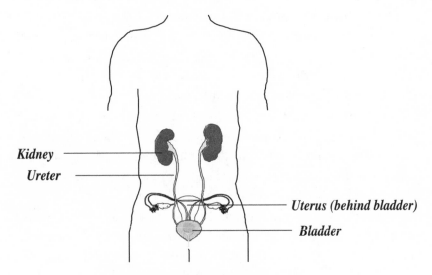

Figure 2-2. Front view of the pelvis.
Figure 2-3. Side view of the pelvis.

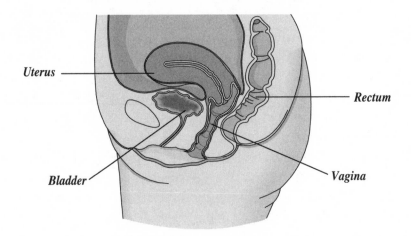

The ureters are the tubes connecting the kidneys to the bladder. They run down the side of the pelvis, but get really close (about half an inch) to the cervix at one point. The ureters are not easily seen at the time of surgery since they are under the pelvic lining. A surgeon needs to know exactly where they are, otherwise an injury to the ureter can occur. The time when the ureter is most vulnerable to injury is during the part of a hysterectomy when the surgeon is working in the area where the cervix and uterus join together. Complications involving the ureter are more likely if the ureter is in an unexpected location, especially if large fibroids or scar tissue distort the usual anatomy. Fortunately, ureteral injuries are rare and the ureter is usually unaffected during surgery.

The vagina is located below the cervix. Hysterectomy (except in the case of some types of cancer) never involves removal of any of the vagina, which is why there is no difference in vaginal length or diameter after surgery. If the cervix is removed, the back of the vagina is sewn shut and the vagina usually feels no different during intercourse (to the man or the woman) than when the cervix was still there.

Right behind the uterus is the rectum, the lowest part of the bowel. This is where stool accumulates, waiting to emerge as a bowel movement. If a uterus tilts backwards (a normal anatomic variant called *retroversion*), the uterus actually rests on the rectum. Unlike the bladder, there is no actual attachment; in fact, there is usually a space between the rectum and the back wall of the uterus. However, if the uterus is enlarged by fibroids, a woman can experience rectal pressure and sometimes constipation. The rectum usually does not present a challenge during hysterectomy unless it is a difficult vaginal procedure, or if the patient's anatomy is distorted from infection or scar tissue. Rectal injury occurs much less frequently than injury to the bladder, but sometimes scarring is so severe that the rectum *is* attached to the back of the uterus, which can increase the risk of injury.

Then there are the intestines. The intestines are approximately sixteen feet long and drape over, under, and on top of all the things that a surgeon needs to see during surgery. Usually the intestines are slippery and mobile, so that when a woman gets tilted head down (yes, you get tilted upside down during surgery after you go to sleep), the intestines fall away from the pelvis where they can be safely tucked out the way. The problem is that sometimes the intestines don't fall out of the way with repositioning; the intestines may be stuck to the uterus, tubes, or ovaries from something like endometriosis, infection, or scar tissue from a prior surgery. Then the surgeon needs to carefully cut the intestines away from the pelvic structures without injuring anything.

THE MENSTRUAL CYCLE

In addition to knowing where everything is, it's important to know what everything does.

Menstruation is not only a female rite of passage, but also a reassuring indication of gynecologic health. The sole purpose of the menstrual cycle is to prepare the uterus for pregnancy. Monthly bleeding caused by the shedding of the lining of the uterus heralds an unproductive cycle and gives the body another chance to become pregnant.

The uterus, ovaries and eggs are present in every girl at birth; hormonal changes that initiate the menstrual cycle do not occur until adolescence. *Follicle-stimulating hormone* (FSH) and *luteinizing hormone* (LH) are hormones known as *gonadotropins*, which are secreted from the pituitary gland. As early as age nine, FSH and LH stimulate the ovary so that a follicle develops. A follicle is a group of cells that form a small ovarian cyst, which surrounds the egg and produces large amounts of estrogen and small amounts of progesterone. Estrogen causes the endometrial lining to thicken and grow. This occurs during the first part of the menstrual cycle, known as the *proliferative phase*.

At the time of *ovulation*, the follicle ruptures and the egg is released. In most women, this occurs mid-cycle, two weeks before menstruation begins. The egg then travels down the fallopian tube, where it may or may not meet up with a sperm. If fertilization does occur, the fertilized egg travels down the tube and implants in the wall of the uterus. One common question is, "What happens to the egg after hysterectomy, when there is no tube or uterus to go to?" Contrary to what you might

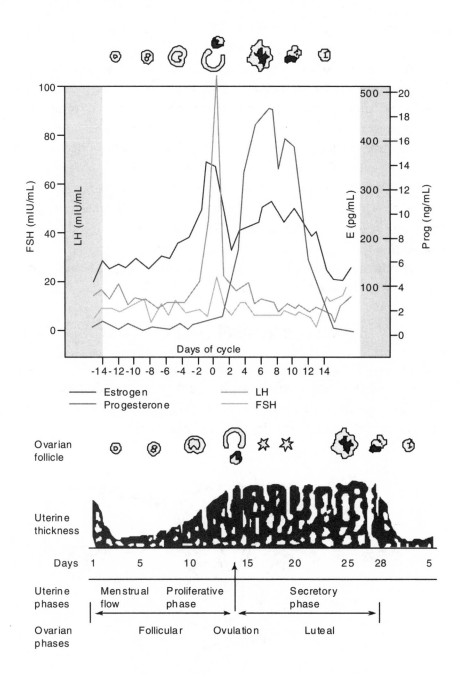

Figure 2-4. Menstrual cycle.

be picturing, the eggs don't pile up on the floor of your pelvis. The body simply absorbs them.

The ruptured follicle is now referred to as a corpus luteum cyst and primarily produces progesterone, as opposed to estrogen. The main function of progesterone is to prepare the lining of the uterus to support a pregnancy in the event that fertilization has occurred. This portion of the menstrual cycle is known as the *luteal phase* and lasts fourteen days.

At the end of the luteal phase, progesterone levels plummet and the lining of the uterus (the endometrium) sloughs off, resulting in menstruation. This cycle repeats itself approximately 450 times during a woman's life until menopause, when the aging ovary no longer produces estrogen.

So now that you know what and where everything is, terminology in respect to types of hysterectomy can be defined.

HYSTERECTOMY NOMENCLATURE

Total abdominal hysterectomy (TAH) refers to removal of the uterus and cervix through an abdominal incision. It can be done with or without removing the tubes or ovaries (Fig. 2-5). *Oophorectomy* is the removal of the ovaries and *salpingectomy* (Fig. 2-6) is the removal of the tubes. If you

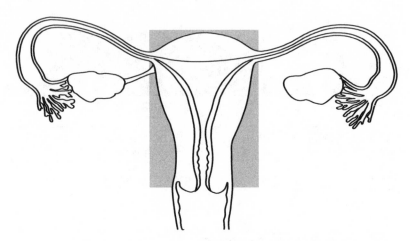

Figure 2-5. Total abdominal hysterectomy (shaded parts removed).

are having a total abdominal hysterectomy, *bilateral* (meaning "two-sided") salpingo-oophorectomy (BSO) (Fig. 2-7), you will have your uterus, cervix, tubes, and ovaries removed. If you are having a total abdominal hysterectomy with *right* salpingo-oophorectomy, you will keep your left tube and ovary. If you have your uterus, cervix, and tubes removed, it is known as a total abdominal hysterectomy with bilateral salpingectomy.

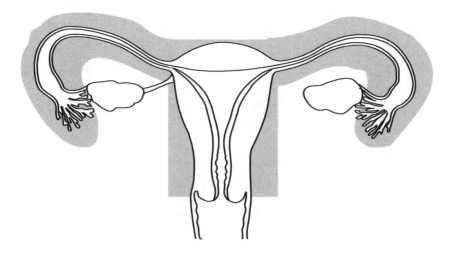

Figure 2-6. Total abdominal hysterectomy, salpingectomy.
Figure 2-7. Total abdominal hysterectomy, bilateral salpingo-oophorectomy (shaded parts removed).

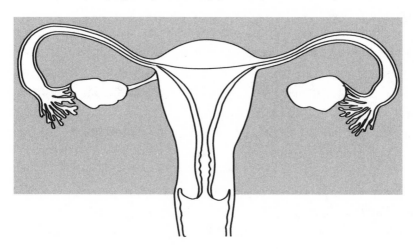

Subtotal hysterectomy (also called *supracervical* hysterectomy) (Fig. 2-8) means that the upper part of the uterus is removed, but not the cervix. If everything is removed but the cervix, you have had a subtotal hysterectomy, bilateral salpingo-oophorectomy. If the tubes and ovaries stay, it is a subtotal hysterectomy.

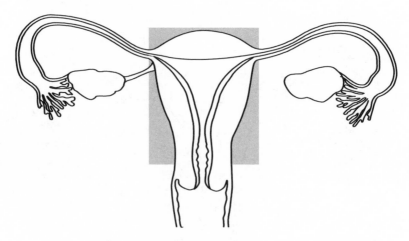

Figure 2-8. Subtotal hysterectomy (shaded parts removed).

Vaginal hysterectomy, in which the uterus is removed through the vagina, always includes removal of the cervix as there is no other way to do the procedure. The operation is officially called a total vaginal hysterectomy. Again, the tubes and ovaries are listed separately.

A salpingectomy is removal of the tubes alone; oophorectomy, removal of the ovaries alone; and salpingo-oophorectomy is where the tubes *and* ovaries are removed.

Radical hysterectomy is done only as staging and treatment of cancer and includes removal of the uterus and cervix along with removal of many lymph nodes. It is usually only done by a gynecologic oncologist, and only if cancer has been diagnosed.

Without a doubt, the most common question about anatomy involves the mystery of the empty space. Women are really concerned about what's going to happen to the void left by the uterus. Picture this. If you have a bowl of spaghetti with a large meatball in the middle and a few smaller meatballs on the side, and then someone removes the large meatball, the space the meatball formerly occupied is replaced by the spaghetti. No one would know that the meatball was ever there. A woman's pelvis is like a bowl, the uterus like a meatball, and the ovaries are like small meatballs. Bowel, of course, is the spaghetti. If the uterus is removed, the bowel falls into the space (which is only the size of a pear) and there is no "empty space."

Usually when one refers to different types of hysterectomies, they are differentiated not only by *what* is removed, but also by *how* it is removed. Twenty years ago, there were only two ways to get a uterus out: through a humongous abdominal incision or through the vagina. Advanced laparoscopic techniques have changed all that. Now in addition to abdominal or vaginal hysterectomies, there are minimally invasive techniques in which the entire uterus can be removed through a one-inch incision. The types of hysterectomies are explained in detail in Part III.

Chapter 3

Who Gets a Hysterectomy? Who Absolutely Needs One?

Over half a million hysterectomies are performed every year. It's an extraordinary number when you realize it means that, if current trends continue, more than one third of American women will eventually lose their uterus. Extraordinary, since it is well established that the majority of gynecologic problems have treatments other than hysterectomy that can be considered before proceeding with surgery. In fact, about ninety percent of hysterectomies are performed for non–life-threatening indications with available alternatives. So who are the more than half a million women a year who undergo hysterectomy, and why do they do it? When can hysterectomy be avoided, and when is it actually the best option? Are these numbers as extraordinary as they seem, or reflective of appropriately done surgery?

According to statistics compiled by the Centers for Disease Control (CDC), hysterectomy is the most frequently performed major operation on non-pregnant women. The CDC generally collects data for five years and reports it three years later. The most recently published data cover 1994–1999 and was reported in 2002.

WHO AND WHERE?

During that five-year period, an average annual rate of 5.5 per 1,000 women resulted in approximately 600,000 hysterectomies each year. The majority of surgeries were performed on women between the ages of forty and forty-four, but by age sixty, thirty-seven percent of women in the United States will have had a hysterectomy.

Where you live has an influence on the probability of having surgery; women who live in southern or midwestern states have consistently higher percentages of hysterectomies than in other areas of the country. It is striking that rates not only vary dramatically from region to region, but also have even been found to vary by as much as five-fold among physicians at the *same* hospital. This implies that physician preference has a large impact on which treatments a woman is offered. In reality, it is more likely that women who choose hysterectomy, either due to personal preference or after failed alternative therapies, seek out experienced gynecologists who do a higher volume of surgery.

Race also impacts on the probability of surgery. African-American women are the most likely women to have a hysterectomy, with a rate of 6.2 per 1,000. One logical explanation for this discrepancy is that African-American women are at the highest risk for developing fibroid tumors, by far the most common reason for hysterectomy. Certainly there are other factors that might influence the disproportionate number of hysterectomies performed on African-American women, such as geographic region.

It's interesting that in spite of the increasing availability of alternatives during the last ten years, the hysterectomy rates have not dramatically decreased. In fact, preliminary data from the 2000 National Hospital Discharge Survey published in June 2002 report an *increase* in hysterectomies over the 1994–1999 period, with 633,000 hysterectomies performed. That either suggests that women are still not offered alternative options, or that the utilization of alternative therapy *delays* but does not decrease the ultimate need for hysterectomy. Since CDC statistics do not document if women tried or were offered alternatives prior to hysterectomy, it is impossible to know.

WHY?

There are eight basic groups of reasons why a woman might have a hysterectomy, but almost seventy-five percent of hysterectomies are done because of the big three: fibroids, endometriosis, and uterine prolapse. The breakdown for reasons that women undergo hysterectomy is as follows:

Fibroids

Fibroids are the most common indication and account for 40 percent of hysterectomies. While only 33 percent of caucasian women identified fibroids as the reason for surgery, 68 percent of African-American women who underwent hysterectomy had the diagnosis of fibroids.

Pelvic Pain

Pelvic pain accounts for almost one third of hysterectomies in some areas of the country. Endometriosis is the most likely diagnosis, and Caucasian women are more likely to be diagnosed with endometriosis than African-American women. Caucasian women are not more likely to *have* endometriosis; they are just more likely to receive that diagnosis.

Pelvic Relaxation

Weakening of the pelvic floor results in conditions such as uterine prolapse (dropped uterus), *cystocele* (dropped bladder), and *rectocele* (dropped rectum). Surgery as a result of pelvic relaxation accounts for roughly one fifth of the hysterectomies performed in the United States. These conditions are even more common in developing countries where women tend to have a greater number of pregnancies.

Bleeding

Bleeding in the absence of fibroids also accounts for a significant number of hysterectomies. This category includes women who bleed heavily due to hormonal problems or blood-clotting disorders. Emergency hysterectomies done at the time of childbirth for postpartum hemorrhage that cannot otherwise be controlled are also in this group.

Ovarian Mass

Benign ovarian growths such as cysts or solid tumors frequently result in hysterectomy, particularly if the diagnosis is uncertain. This used to be a more common reason for hysterectomy in the days before ultrasound was available to help determine the origin of a mass and the likelihood of malignancy.

Precancerous Conditions

Precancerous, or potentially cancerous, conditions that turn out not to be cancer account for roughly 5 percent of hysterectomies. Conditions under this category include endometrial hyperplasia and persistent cervical dysplasia. Also included are women who have abnormal uterine bleeding with the inability to sample the uterine lining to rule out the possibility of cancer.

Cancer

Women diagnosed with cervical, uterine, ovarian, or fallopian-tube cancer account for almost 10 percent of hysterectomies. The majority of women who require a hysterectomy due to cancer are over age fifty-five. The number of hysterectomies done for malignancy has significantly decreased in the last ten years, primarily due to increased detection and treatment of cervical precancer. Hysterectomies due to other types of gynecologic cancers have remained relatively stable.

Prophylactic Hysterectomy

A growing number of women who are at genetic risk for the development of ovarian cancer are choosing to undergo hysterectomy (see chapter 20). The number of women included in this category are difficult to document since the diagnosis listed is often a condition such as fibroids or prolapse, which is used as an excuse to have surgery for insurance purposes.

Planned Hysterectomy After Cesarean Section

There was a time when hysterectomies were "planned" after a last cesarean section in a woman who needed one anyway due to fibroids or other gynecologic problems. Catholic women who were ineligible for tubal ligation also frequently had hysterectomies after multiple cesarean sections. In general, however, planned hysterectomy is no longer performed since complication rates are significantly higher than if the hysterectomy is done at a later time.

The mathematicians among you have already determined that the total number of hysterectomies by indication equal far more than 100 percent. There are a number of reasons for this. Many women have a hysterectomy for more than one indication. The woman who has pelvic pain from endometriosis and bleeding from fibroids will be counted in both categories. In addition, there are regional, age, and ethnic differences that change the numbers depending on the population (more fibroids in the south, more prolapse in the east). The above statistics are simply meant to give a general idea.

Clearly, the vast majority of indications for hysterectomy are for non–life-threatening conditions for which definitive surgery may be the best option, but is not the only option. Details of alternatives for non–life-threatening indications for hysterectomies are discussed in Part II. The rest of this chapter covers those situations in which there is essentially *no* choice. These are the situations in which women died before they had hysterectomy as an option.

PERI- AND POSTPARTUM HEMORRHAGE

If this section pertains to you, chances are you already had an emergency hysterectomy after delivering a baby, and you are gathering information after the fact. No one expects it, plans for it, or learns about it before it happens to her. This type of hysterectomy is rarely predicted or discussed in advance.

Virtually every hysterectomy performed immediately after pregnancy is due to a life-threatening hemorrhage that can't otherwise be controlled. While the loss of your uterus is understandably devastating, there is at least a little comfort in realizing that you live in a time when the capability of emergency hysterectomy is safe and possible. There are a number of situations that can create uncontrollable bleeding after delivery:

Atony

Uterine atony is a condition in which the uterus doesn't contract normally following delivery of the baby. Usually, immediately after delivery of the placenta, the uterus that has been stretched out to accommodate the baby, placenta, and amniotic fluid immediately shrinks so that the cavity is essentially obliterated. If the uterine muscle does not contract properly, heavy bleeding results. There are a number of conditions that predispose to uterine atony, but almost all are related to a uterus that has been either overstretched or is overtired from prolonged contracting. Just as a rubber band that has been stretched too many times, or beyond its capacity, loses its elasticity, a uterus that has been overworked contracts poorly.

Multiple gestations, large babies, prolonged labor, or an infected uterus all predispose to atony. Women who have had multiple pregnancies are also at risk. Uterine atony is also known to occur in women who have no known risk factors. When a woman has heavy bleeding following delivery of the baby and placenta, a number of different drugs and surgical maneuvers are available that usually succeed in making the uterus contract. If those drugs fail, hysterectomy is the last, lifesaving resort.

Abnormal Placental Attachment

Normally, the placenta spontaneously separates from the wall of the uterus and is expelled after a baby is born. If the attachment of the placenta to the uterine wall is abnormal, the placenta can actually burrow into the uterine wall so that normal separation doesn't occur. When this happens, the uterus is unable to contract and it bleeds. Depending on the depth of infiltration into the uterine wall, this condition is identified as a *placenta accreta, placenta increta,* or *placenta percreta.* Women who have had prior cesarean sections are at increased risk for this problem, although it can occur even with a first pregnancy. If the placenta cannot be removed using a number of other techniques, hysterectomy is the final resort.

Uterine Rupture

Hundreds of years ago, uterine rupture was a far more common phenomenon than today. When women labored for a long period of time and the baby did not deliver, either due to its size or position, something eventually had to give. That something used to be the uterus. It was not unusual for a woman (and the baby) to die from a uterine rupture during a protracted labor. Now women undergo cesarean sections when it is clear that the baby won't deliver vaginally so that uterine ruptures are a rare phenomenon, particularly as a result of a prolonged or obstructed labor. Uterine rupture is known to occur at a higher rate in women with prior scars from cesarean sections, or tumultuous labors.

Again, as in the event of a postpartum hemorrhage, multiple steps are taken to stop bleeding before a hysterectomy is contemplated. It's a fine line. No one wants to do a hysterectomy unnecessarily, but if the surgeon waits *too* long, a maternal death might occur, an obviously more catastrophic event than the loss of the uterus. In addition, when someone loses blood quickly, they can develop a *coagulapathy,* or inability to clot blood, which makes a bad situation worse. Even in the best of hands, when everything is done absolutely correctly, the situation may be dire.

Lowering the Risk

Short of avoiding pregnancy, there is no way to eliminate the possibility of atony, accreta, or uterine rupture. The majority of these situations occur with no warning. If you are known to be at increased risk for a postpartum hemorrhage, there are precautions that may decrease the probability of hysterectomy, or at a minimum, decrease complication rates.

It is important to prevent or correct anemia with iron supplementation throughout your pregnancy. Consider having autologous blood or donor-designated blood on hand. (See chapter 15.) A "scheduled" delivery will ensure that a team experienced in obstetric emergencies is available. If you are known or suspected to have a placenta accreta, or if you have had problems with atony in the past, plan to deliver at a tertiary care center with anesthesiologists and personnel who frequently handle obstetric hemorrhage. If possible, have interventional radiology on stand-by, as a uterine artery embolization can sometimes stop uterine hemorrhage. (Uterine artery embolization is discussed in chapter 8.) If you are considering vaginal birth after cesarean section (VBAC), make sure that your physician is experienced in VBAC, can recognize the signs of uterine rupture, and is at a hospital where it can be managed expeditiously.

Recovery and Complications

Due to the difficult circumstances in which most postpartum hysterectomies are done, the complication rates are understandably significantly higher than for every other type of hysterectomy. Virtually every possible complication, including blood loss requiring transfusion, infection, and injury to surrounding structures such as bladder, ureter, and bowel occurs more frequently, and is far more acceptable, than with hysterectomy for other indications. Most women in this category have the advantage of being young, healthy, and able to tolerate significant blood loss and surgical complications better than a seventy-year-old undergoing hysterectomy. The seventy-year-old, however, does *not* have a new infant to take care of!

Not only is the woman who undergoes postpartum hysterectomy anemic and in pain, but she is also a new mother. That means taking care of a newborn, breastfeeding, potentially taking care of other children, *and* recovering from an unexpected hysterectomy. In addition to a higher complication rate, it is not surprising that postpartum hysterectomy results in a higher rate of depression than any other indication for hysterectomy. In these cases, it's difficult to tell if a woman is suffering from postpartum depression because she just had a baby, or post-hysterectomy depression because she'll never have another. This is a situation in which help from a psychiatrist or therapist should be sought sooner rather than later.

ECTOPIC PREGNANCY RESULTING IN HYSTERECTOMY

Ectopic pregnancies are pregnancies that implant in locations other than the uterine cavity where they belong. Normally, conception occurs in the fallopian tube. The fertilized egg then travels down the length of the tube to implant in the wall of the uterus. Sometimes the fertilized egg doesn't quite make the trip and remains in the tube. Ectopic pregnancies that occur in the fallopian tube do not require hysterectomy as part of their treatment. Rarely, the pregnancy implants in the part of the tube that is buried in the uterus, otherwise known as a cornual pregnancy. While it is possible to resect the ectopic pregnancy without removing the uterus in most cases, sometimes bleeding can't be controlled and a hysterectomy becomes necessary.

Another rare form of ectopic pregnancy is a cervical pregnancy in which the pregnancy implants and starts to grow in the cervical canal. When the pregnancy is removed, uncontrollable bleeding can ensue, and again, hysterectomy can save lives. The majority of ectopic pregnancies are managed by tubal surgery or medication to dissolve the abnormal pregnancy tissue. Scenarios that result in hysterectomy are extremely rare. Most gynecologists see only one or two during an entire career.

Gynecologic Hemorrhage

Fibroid tumors are the most common cause of nonobstetric uterine hemorrhage. Alternatives to hysterectomy for women with fibroids are discussed in detail in chapters 4 and 5. Fibroids, however, are not the only reason for heavy bleeding.

Abnormal buildup of tissue or a hormonal imbalance can also cause extremely heavy bleeding. Administering estrogen and/or progesterone usually stops the bleeding and treats the hormonal imbalance. For women who are medically unable to receive even short-term hormone therapy, or for whom the treatment is not successful, hysterectomy is the only choice.

Infection

Prior to the availability of modern antibiotics, pelvic infection was a life-threatening condition. If an abscess of the tube or ovary developed, mortality was a certainty unless surgery was performed to remove the infected tissue. Prior to the 1980s, treatment of a bilateral tubo-ovarian abscess consisted of a total hysterectomy and removal of both tubes and ovaries. Since those women were infertile as a result of the infection and subsequent destruction of the tubes, it was felt that there was no reason to preserve the uterus. The advent of in vitro fertilization (IVF) changed that premise since IVF allows women to become pregnant even in the absence of functional tubes. With the advent of broad-spectrum antibiotics, major surgery for treatment of a tubo-ovarian abscess is rarely necessary. If drainage is needed, it can often be accomplished with the help of an interventional radiologist who can drain the infected area while visualizing it using ultrasound or magnetic resonance imaging (MRI) technology.

In spite of these advances, there are situations when a tubo-ovarian abscess must be treated surgically, and sometimes must involve removal of the uterus, tubes, and ovaries as a life-saving procedure. In a stable patient, it is almost always appropriate to start with medical treatment and only use surgery as a last resort. Equally rare, but possible, is a situation in which a severe uterine infection following childbirth requires hysterectomy.

CANCER

Many gynecologic cancers require hysterectomy. These are discussed in chapter 9. In fact, the diagnosis of cancer is the most common indication for a life-saving hysterectomy for which there are no available alternatives.

NONEMERGENT HYSTERECTOMY

The majority of hysterectomies are done for conditions that are not life-threatening. All of the indications for hysterectomy discussed in the following chapters have alternative therapies that may be acceptable, preferable options for many women. For others, hysterectomy is the best option available to improve quality of life and decrease suffering.

Part II

Uterine Disorders and Alternatives to Hysterectomy

Chapter 4

Fibroids— What, Where, and How

Fibroids, as the most common indication for hysterectomy, get three chapters. For all the trouble they cause, they really deserve their own book, maybe even a movie. What follows is a brief description of what they are, who gets them, and the problems they can cause. The next two chapters delve into the details of what can be done about them.

WHAT ARE THEY?

The official nomenclature for a fibroid tumor is *uterine leiomyoma*. They are also referred to as *myomas*. Fibroids are benign (noncancerous) tumors that arise from the smooth muscle cells of the uterus. They are solid, as opposed to cystic, and vary widely in size. Often they are microscopic. They can also grow to the size of a beach ball.

Often women confuse uterine fibroids with breast fibroadenomas. They are unrelated, and if you or a family member has one, it doesn't mean you are more likely to get the other. Another misconception is that hormones cause fibroids. Though fibroids *respond* to estrogen and progesterone by growing larger, estrogen and progesterone do not cause them.

WHERE ARE THEY?

All fibroids originate from the myometrial (middle) layer of the wall of the uterus. The direction in which fibroids grow determines what type they are and what sort of symptoms they may cause. Hence, all fibroids are described according to their location in the uterus.

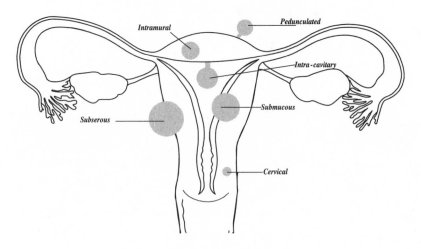

Figure 4-1. Uterus with multiple fibroids.

Subserosal Fibroids

A subserosal fibroid is under the outermost (serosal) layer of the uterus. It generally doesn't protrude through the muscle into the cavity; it goes in the other direction. Women with subserosal fibroids often have no symptoms, and in fact may be unaware of their existence. However, if the fibroid is very large, pressure may be exerted on other pelvic structures. If the fibroid is on the front of the uterus, the woman knows every bathroom within a five-mile radius of her home and work. There is a constant pressure resulting in the feeling of needing to urinate even when her bladder is empty. When the bladder starts to fill . . . well, there's not a whole lot of room.

If the fibroid is on the back of the uterus, constipation and rectal pressure may be the issue. Women who have had a baby know that incredible feeling of pressure on the rectum as the baby's head moves down the vagina right before delivery. Women with large fibroids sitting on their rectum experience that sensation on a regular basis.

Sometimes subserosal fibroids actually hang outside the uterus, attached only by a stem or stalk. They are then referred to as *pedunculated* fibroids. Occasionally, a pedunculated fibroid is mistaken for an enlarged ovary on pelvic examination or ultrasound. Another subtype of subserosal fibroids is the intraligamentary fibroid, which is off the side of the uterus in the area where the uterine arteries run. Intraligamentary fibroids are particularly difficult to remove.

The woman with large subserosal fibroids is the one who looks five months pregnant despite her normal weight and the three hundred sit-ups she does every night. It is not unheard of to have to buy an entire new wardrobe after surgery, an expense generally not covered by most insurance companies.

Submucosal Fibroids

Submucosal fibroids originate in the layer closest to the cavity of the uterus. Sometimes they are primarily in the wall of the uterus and only cause a small hill in the uterine cavity, but they can fill the uterine cavity completely. A submucosal fibroid entirely in the cavity of the uterus is referred to as an *intracavitary* fibroid.

Sometimes an intracavitary fibroid is on a stalk. Those are the fibroids that can emerge through the cervix and end up in the vagina. The uterus essentially goes through labor in order to dilate the cervix and deliver the fibroid into the vagina. This can be *really* painful. Once the fibroid is in the vagina, it's usually quite easy to remove.

Submucosal fibroids cause more trouble than any other type of fibroid. It is the submucosal fibroid that is usually responsible for heavy bleeding, miscarriage, and infertility, ultimately leading some women to the operating room.

Intramural Fibroids

Intramural fibroids start, and hopefully stay, within the uterine wall. If they grow towards the cavity, they become submucosal. If they grow outside the wall, they become subserosal. As long as they stay small and stay put, they rarely cause trouble.

Cervical Fibroids

Cervical fibroids are, yes, in the cervix. They tend to cause bleeding and can impact on pregnancy just as submucosal fibroids do. Women who prefer not to remove their cervix at the time of hysterectomy often don't have that option if they are unlucky enough to have a cervical fibroid.

Can a fibroid be both submucosal and subserosal? Sure. If a fibroid starts in the muscle, gets really big, and grows in both directions, it can both protrude outside the uterus and into the cavity of the uterus. It's actually quite common, particularly in very large fibroids. Women who have these bleed heavily and look pregnant.

WHO GETS THEM?

Any woman can get fibroids, but some women are more likely candidates than others. Fibroids most commonly appear during the years in which women produce estrogen and progesterone; in other words, the reproductive years. Most women develop symptoms as a result of their fibroids during their thirties and forties, but some women continue to have problems even after menopause. Many women assume (and bank on the assumption that) their fibroids will disappear after their periods stop. They generally don't, but usually stop growing and eventually shrink over time.

Twenty-five percent of women in the reproductive years have fibroids that they are aware of, due to either symptoms or discovery at the time of a routine gynecologic examination. Far more often, small, asymptomatic tumors exist in the uteruses of women who are totally oblivious to their presence. Often they are identified serendipitously on an ultrasound done for another reason.

Multiple factors are associated with an increased likelihood that someone will have fibroids. These include:

▼ **Family history.** There is definitely a genetic pre-disposition for fibroids. If your mother, sister, aunt, or grandmother had them, you are likely to have them as well.

▼ **African-American heritage.** African-American women are not only more likely to have fibroids, but their fibroids tend to be bigger and more symptomatic. They also develop problems at a much younger age than their Caucasian counter-parts.

▼ **Pregnancy history.** Women who have never been pregnant are at increased risk for develop-ing fibroids. The reason for this is unclear.

▼ **Diet.** Eating red meat is known to increase the likelihood of developing fibroids. Once someone is diagnosed with fibroids, eliminating meat from the diet makes no difference in symptoms or growth.

Certain factors are known to decrease the risk of fibroid develop-ment. These include:

▼ **Pregnancy.** Women who have had at least one pregnancy beyond twenty weeks are at decreased risk of fibroid development.

▼ **Oral contraceptive pill use.** One would think that blasting potential fibroid cells with estrogen and progesterone would increase their propen-sity for growth. In truth, the opposite is usually seen. Once you have fibroids, the pill does not make them shrink.

▼ **Smoking.** The reason is unclear why smokers have less fibroids; not a reason to start.

▼ **Eating green vegetables.** Your mother was right.

What Kind of Symptoms?

Symptoms are related much more to the location of fibroids than to the size of the fibroid. A subserosal plum-sized fibroid will most likely be totally asymptomatic. The same size fibroid in the cavity of your uterus can create a floodlike monthly bleed.

Speaking of size, there are many ways to describe the size of a fibroid. The most accurate way to describe the size is by an actual measurement. Ultrasound measures fibroids in terms of centimeters. There are 2.54 centimeters in every inch. Therefore, a 5-centimeter fibroid is roughly 2 inches in diameter. Sometimes the entire uterus (with fibroids) is measured rather than individual fibroids. A normal uterus is about 7 centimeters long. Therefore, if a uterus and fibroid together measure 15 centimeters, it means the uterus has roughly doubled in size. It's not unusual for a fibroid to be substantially bigger than the uterus.

Traditionally, gynecologists describe a fibroid uterus as if it were a pregnant uterus. This dates back to a time before ultrasound when exact measurements weren't available and this was simply the easiest way to communicate size to other gynecologists. If your gynecologist says your uterus is fourteen-week size, it means that the fibroids have enlarged your uterus to the size it would be if you were fourteen weeks pregnant.

Today, most gynecologists try to describe fibroids in a way that is easy for you to visualize. Here comes a politically incorrect, sweeping sexist generalization. Male gynecologists describe fibroids in terms of balls used in various sports. "Mrs. Jones, you have a fibroid the size of a softball!" Women gynecologists seem partial to fruit, "Mrs. Jones, you have a Florida grapefruit sitting on your bladder!"

Symptoms from fibroids vary widely, from women who have no symptoms at all (the majority), to women who feel the fibroid is controlling their life. Typical problems in symptomatic women include:

▼ **Bleeding.** Bleeding can be a subjective problem that is difficult to quantify. Sometimes a woman says she is hemorrhaging, yet another woman with double the blood loss reports "normal periods." What's really important is that a woman subjectively realizes that her periods are heavier and longer than they were in the past. Most gynecologists (and insurance companies) rely on anemia to validate a woman's heavy bleeding. This is unfair since it often takes months of heavy bleeding before someone's blood count drops, particularly if she is taking supplemental iron. Suffice it to say that women with fibroids can bleed a lot. It's also important to note that bleeding from fibroids is almost always at the time of menstruation. Bleeding that occurs at other times is usually from another cause.

▼ **Pelvic pressure.** Large fibroids can push on the bladder, rectum, or cause abdominal distention. Many women can feel their own fibroids just by resting their hand on their belly. Many women are unaware of pressure symptoms due to their gradual onset.

▼ **Pain.** Pain can result from degeneration of a large fibroid in which a portion of the fibroid outgrows its blood supply and dies. This is more common during pregnancy when fibroids grow quickly. Heavy menstrual bleeding also causes pain. The uterus contracts (cramps) in an attempt to expel the clots the heavy bleeding causes.

▼ **Pregnancy problems.** One third of women with fibroids who become pregnant experience significant growth, particularly in the first trimester. This is actually when many women first become aware that they have fibroids. Most women sail through their pregnancy without a problem, other than the fact that their belly gets a lot bigger, a lot faster. Both miscarriage and preterm delivery are increased by the presence of submucosal fibroids. Large fibroids can occasionally cause premature separation of the placenta resulting in heavy bleeding, fetal compromise, and rarely, stillbirth. Delivery can also be complicated since the distorted shape of the uterus leads to an increased rate of breech and transverse (lying sideways) babies, requiring cesarean section. Sometimes, even if the baby is head-down, a vaginal delivery is impossible due to a large fibroid blocking the path of the baby out of the uterus. Postpartum hemorrhage is more common in women with fibroids since the uterine muscle is unable to contract normally after the baby delivers. This occurs whether the baby is delivered vaginally or by cesarean section.

▼ **Infertility.** Infertility issues are always problematic since so many factors can influence one's ability to conceive. Many women who don't become pregnant are in their late thirties or forties and may also have age-related problems such as ovulatory dysfunction. Fibroids can certainly impact on fertility, particularly if their location blocks the fallopian tube or prevents implantation from submucosal fibroids impinging on the uterine cavity. This is a problem that has increased in magnitude due to the number of women who delay pregnancy until their thirties or forties, giving their fibroids extra time to grow. Fibroids should be removed in a woman who is trying to become pregnant only in the absence of other infertility factors or if the fibroid is significantly distorting the uterine cavity.

Do Fibroids Ever Become Cancerous?

No, fibroids *never* turn into cancer, and don't let anyone tell you otherwise. There is an entity called *leiomyosarcoma* in which a tumor that resembles a fibroid is actually a cancerous growth that originates from the same location that fibroids come from. Leiomyosarcomas, however, are not fibroids that turned bad. They were *never* fibroids. They started as leiomyosarcomas from their very beginnings. The problem is that it is difficult to tell from an ultrasound if a uterine tumor is a benign fibroid or a malignant leiomyosarcoma. Since leiomyosarcomas grow quickly, it is always advisable to remove any rapidly growing uterine tumor, even though it usually turns out to be just a benign fibroid. This is particularly true in a postmenopausal woman, in whom malignancies are more likely to occur and rapid growth of a benign tumor is less likely.

DIAGNOSTIC PROCEDURES TO EVALUATE FIBROIDS

Virtually every treatment option for fibroids depends on knowing the precise location and size of the fibroids. Prior to any treatment plan, some sort of diagnostic imaging is critical to forming an appropriate course of action. The following diagnostic tools are commonly used to determine what options are possible and appropriate.

Ultrasound

Ultrasound uses high-frequency sound waves rather than X rays to take pictures of the uterus, ovaries, and other abdominal organs. Most women are familiar with ultrasound due to its widespread use in pregnancy to evaluate a developing fetus. Ultrasound is commonly available and frequently done in the gynecologist's office. Images are seen (or *visualized*, in medical terminology) on the computer monitor and can also be printed as a permanent record.

Transabdominal ultrasound requires a full bladder. While you lie on a table, a transducer is gently pressed to your lower abdomen over your uterus and ovaries. A gel is placed between the transducer and your skin to improve contact and transmission of sound waves. Ultrasounds are painless if you can ignore the discomfort of pressure against a very full bladder.

Transvaginal ultrasound involves a thin condom-covered wand (probe) that is inserted in the vagina. The gel is placed in the condom, not in your vagina. Transvaginal ultrasound has the advantage of not requiring a full bladder and gives a better image of the cavity of the uterus. It is also generally more useful to evaluate endometrial thickness. Generally you can place the probe yourself with the help of the technician.

A full evaluation usually includes both transvaginal and transabdominal ultrasounds.

Saline-Infused Sonography

Saline-infused sonography (SIS) is also known as a sonohysterogram. A sonohysterogram is an ultrasound that goes one step further by using sterile water to distend the uterine cavity. Normally, the uterine cavity is only a potential space. If a fibroid is protruding from the wall into the cavity, it's not obvious since the walls are collapsed together. Picture a deflated balloon with a pebble stuck in one of its walls. If you took a picture of the balloon, you wouldn't know if the pebble was right in the middle of the wall, protruding into the balloon, or poking outside the balloon. If you filled the balloon with air and looked again, the direction in which the pebble was protruding would be quite obvious. On a standard ultrasound, you would see the fibroid, but until you fill the cavity with water, you can't tell how much of the fibroid is in the cavity of the uterus versus in the wall of the uterus. By doing a sonohysterogram, usually in the office, one can determine with great accuracy how much of the fibroid is protruding into the cavity of the uterus. In short, a sonohysterogram allows a two-dimensional image to be seen in three dimensions.

SIS starts like a simple ultrasound. The gynecologist then places a speculum in the vagina and slips a narrow catheter (tube) into the cervical os. The speculum is removed and the transvaginal probe placed in the vagina. Sterile water is then injected into the catheter to distend the uterus while the ultrasound is done. Most women experience mild cramping. Occasionally, cramping is severe but generally lasts less than a minute. The entire procedure takes less than five minutes and gives a great deal more information than a standard ultrasound regarding the shape of the uterine cavity and possible distortion by submucosal or intracavitary fibroids. It is also an excellent technique to diagnose uterine polyps.

Hysterosalpingogram

A hysterosalpingogram (HSG) is another imaging technique that gives information similar to an SIS. To do an HSG, contrast dye is injected into the uterine cavity with a small catheter, using essentially the same technique as in the sonohysterogram. Once the dye fills the uterine cavity and outlines the contour of the fibroid, an X ray is taken. Like sonohysterography, the procedure takes about five to ten minutes and can cause cramping, which quickly dissipates. Ibuprofen will help alleviate the discomfort and should be taken thirty minutes prior to the test. The disadvantage of an HSG is that it must be done in an X ray department rather than a gynecologist's office. Also, cramping is sometimes more severe in HSG than in SIS. Since no ultrasound is involved, no information is obtained regarding the ovaries or outer contour of the uterus. HSG is useful for imaging the shape of the cavity of the uterus and identifying submucosal or intracavitary fibroids. It is also useful to determine if fallopian tubes are open or blocked. HSG has been available longer than SIS and many gynecologists are more experienced and comfortable with this procedure.

Magnetic Resonance Imaging

Magnetic resonance imaging (MRI) is another way of taking a picture of the pelvic organs. During an MRI, you lie on a table that slides into a tunnel-shaped magnetic field. Images are interpreted by a computer that can generate cross-sections of organs to be visualized. The test takes about thirty to sixty minutes, and although painless, is uncomfortable for the claustrophobic. MRIs give excellent images of fibroids, but are not done routinely because they are quite expensive and, in most circumstances, are not necessary to formulate a treatment plan.

Hysteroscopy

Hysteroscopy (Fig. 4-2) is a surgical procedure that utilizes a scope with a light and a camera to look inside the uterus and evaluate the cavity for the presence of benign polyps and fibroids. After a speculum is placed in the vagina, the scope is passed through the cervical opening and into the uterine cavity, allowing the surgeon to directly visualize any fibroids that are distorting or protruding into the uterine cavity. The size of the scope varies. For diagnostic hysteroscopy, the scope is very slender since the purpose is only to look and diagnose what the problem may be. This can be done in an office setting or in an outpatient facility with either local or general anesthesia. Operative hysteroscopy requires a larger scope since in addition to looking, instruments are passed through the scope that can be used to biopsy, cut, or burn polyps and fibroids. In order to accomplish this, the cervix must be dilated (widened) to accommodate a scope with a larger diameter. This is generally done using anesthesia as an outpatient procedure.

Laparoscopy

Laparoscopy (Fig. 4-3) is a surgical procedure that requires general anesthesia. A small incision is made in the fold of the belly button and a scope attached to a light and camera is inserted into the abdomen in order to visualize the outside of the uterus and other pelvic structures. Gas is placed through the laparoscope into the abdominal cavity to expand the space so that all structures can be clearly seen. Depending on what procedures are to be performed using the laparoscope, two or three other tiny (5-mm) incisions may be placed elsewhere in the lower abdomen in order to introduce instruments to grasp, cut, or suture tissue. Laparoscopy is usually performed on an outpatient basis and has a minimal recovery period.

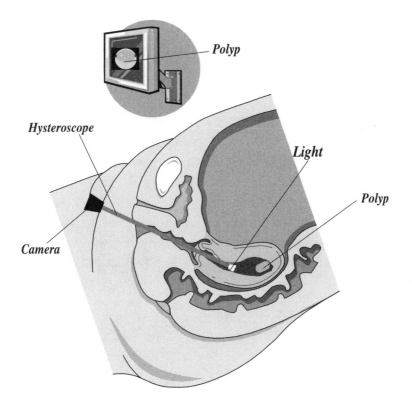

Figure 4-2. Hysteroscopy.

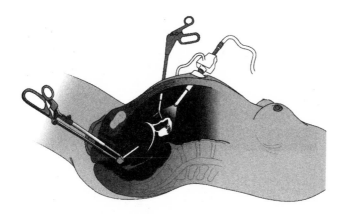

Figure 4-3. Laparoscopic setup.

DECISION TIME

So you know you have fibroids, you know where they are, and you know you have to do *something*. What are your options? That depends on your age, pregnancy plans, location of fibroid(s), and availability of various alternatives. It also depends on your willingness to have potentially multiple procedures and continued gynecologic surveillance. The alternatives fall into two categories: surgical and medical. A third option, of course, is to do nothing, which is totally reasonable if your fibroids aren't causing problems and are not growing. Assuming that you've already determined that you need to do something, and you don't necessarily want a hysterectomy, here's what's out there.

Chapter 5

Nonsurgical Treatment of Fibroids

Many women who seek alternatives to hysterectomy are trying to avoid the loss of their uterus. Some women really aren't trying to avoid losing their uterus; they are trying to avoid surgery of any kind. Nonsurgical options for women with symptomatic fibroids exist and the expectation is that many more alternatives will become available in the near future.

Uterine Artery Embolization

The call usually comes about a week before the surgery is scheduled. "What about uterine artery embolization? I heard from (the Internet/my girlfriend/a magazine) that there is this procedure that will make my fibroids disappear and I won't need a hysterectomy!" Then the accusing tone, *"Why didn't you tell me about it!"*

For women who are looking for a nonsurgical treatment for their fibroids, uterine artery embolization (UAE) sounds almost too good to be true. Even in women with very large fibroids, small synthetic pellets can be injected into the uterine artery, which then block the blood supply to the fibroids. The offending fibroids shrivel up and die and the lucky woman lives happily ever after. Sometimes.

Interventional radiology is a remarkable specialty that came into being only during the last twenty years. Basically, noninterventional radiologists are physicians who interpret X rays and other images such as computerized tomography (CT) scans, MRIs, and ultrasounds. Interventional radiologists also interpret images, but then take it one step further by doing procedures on patients while the imaging is occurring, using the image to guide them. A familiar example of interventional radiology would be amniocentesis, in which fluid is withdrawn from the amniotic sac while the physician watches the image on ultrasound.

Uterine artery embolization has actually been around for more than twenty years as an emergency treatment for life-threatening hemorrhage, which occasionally occurs postpartum or from uterine cancer. It works by blocking off the major blood supply to the uterus, resulting in decreased blood flow and therefore less bleeding. Essentially, it's the same concept used when damming a river.

In 1995, an innovative physician came up with the idea of using the same technique to treat heavy bleeding in a small group of women with fibroids prior to their scheduled hysterectomy. To everyone's surprise, the women who were pretreated with UAE no longer needed hysterectomies since blocking their uterine arteries resulted in shrinkage of fibroids and eliminated their symptoms. A new procedure was born. By 2003, 40,000 uterine artery embolizations for the treatment of fibroids had been done throughout the world, and the numbers continue to rise.

Here's how it works. The sedated woman lies on an X ray table and a catheter is inserted into the groin using a needle. Using fluoroscopy (a "live X ray"), the radiologist threads the catheter into the woman's pelvic arteries until it reaches the uterine artery. During the entire procedure, the radiologist is able to watch exactly where the catheter is going to assure that it gets into the right place.

Once the catheter is in the uterine artery, little beads or particles are injected until the blood flow is blocked (Fig. 5-1). The procedure is most commonly done using sedation and local anesthesia. Some centers

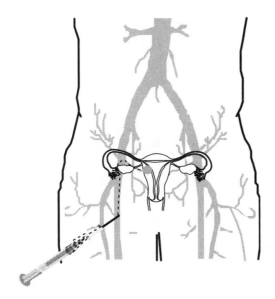

Figure 5-1. Uterine artery embolization.

now offer epidural anesthesia to further assure a pain-free procedure. The embolization itself usually only takes between sixty and ninety minutes, depending on the experience of the person doing it and the difficulty of the case. Once the blood supply is cut off, the fibroids no longer receive oxygen and essentially die.

First the good news. Seventy to ninety percent of women who undergo uterine artery embolization have a significant decrease in the heavy bleeding their fibroids cause. Ninety percent report a dramatic change in pressure symptoms, with up to a 60 percent decrease in documented uterine size. Eighty percent of women note much less menstrual cramping and a high percentage of women report satisfaction with the procedure. Most women are in the hospital for twenty-four hours or less, with an average total recovery of eight days.

Uterine artery embolization is a particularly good alternative for a woman who is a risky surgical candidate due to a medical condition like obesity or severe lung disease. It's also the ideal option in someone who is known to have lots of scar tissue from prior procedures, yet requires treatment of severe bleeding or pressure from large fibroids.

Another scenario in which this procedure is valuable is in the woman who would benefit from, and desires, a laparoscopic hysterectomy, but is not a good candidate due to the size of her fibroids. Sometimes a woman who is anemic from prolonged heavy bleeding needs to build up her blood count before surgery. Pretreatment with UAE may decrease the size of her uterus and stop heavy bleeding so that she can then undergo a laparoscopic procedure instead of major surgery (see chapter 12).

Now, the not very good news. Ideally, the goal of any procedure, surgical or alternative, is to be definitive. That is, the goal is to eliminate the problem so that future procedures will be unnecessary. Unfortunately, women who have UAEs need a subsequent procedure such as myomectomy, hysteroscopy, or hysterectomy at least 10 percent of the time due to continued symptoms. Of course, the same can be said for myomectomy and other uterus-sparing procedures.

The big seller, of course, is that you avoid recovery from surgery. The big secret is the pain. When blood supply is cut off to an organ, significant pain can result. A person having a heart attack has chest pain because the heart muscle suddenly loses part of its blood supply. When the blood supply is cut off to a fibroid, *necrosis* (tissue death) occurs and major pain can ensue, especially if the fibroid is large.

Certainly, there is a wide range of what a woman can expect to experience. Centers that do a larger number of embolizations are much better at pain control than facilities where only a small number are done. Like anything else, the doctor's experience, especially in a newer procedure, greatly influences the patient's experience. Most women can expect to have moderate to very heavy cramping for about six to eight hours after the embolization. Intravenous narcotics are required for pain control. Many interventional radiologists are now using epidural anesthesia that will completely eliminate severe postprocedure pain. During the week following the procedure, most women can expect mild to moderate pain controlled by oral narcotics.

If pain lasts more than a week, re-evaluation by the interventional radiologist is appropriate to check for problems or complications. Sometimes the pain is severe enough to require days of narcotics, but in rare cases the pain continues for months as tissue dies and sloughs off. Two percent of women experience the passage of a necrotic fibroid, in which case hospitalization is almost always required. Some women who've had a hysterectomy following a uterine artery embolization report that the pain and debilitation from the UAE was *much* greater than from surgery, particularly if they ultimately had a laparoscopic hysterectomy.

Not every woman is a good candidate for successful relief of symptoms. The best results are seen in a uterus that is small enough to still be below the level of the umbilicus. Pedunculated fibroids also do not embolize as successfully as intramural or subserosal fibroids. Pretreatment evaluation with an MRI is essential to determine the exact type and size of the fibroid. It is also important to make sure that what you are dealing with is a fibroid as opposed to some other kind of pelvic mass.

Because there are very limited data, most interventional radiologists feel that women who wish to preserve fertility are not candidates for UAE. Interestingly, some postprocedure pregnancies have occurred. While most of these pregnancies are healthy, some studies have demonstrated that miscarriage rate, postdelivery hemorrhage, and premature births occur at a higher rate in women after myomectomy. Fertility may also be diminished. Therefore, women who potentially desire pregnancy are not candidates.

There have been many reports of premature menopause after UAE. The likelihood of this seems to be directly related to age and usually occurs in women over age forty-five. It is most likely caused by particles getting into the ovarian artery and causing early failure of ovarian tissue. Very rarely, particles have gotten other places they're not supposed to be, such as the bladder, buttocks, and labia, resulting in damage to those tissues.

If the procedure is prolonged, there is ongoing diagnostic radiation for up to two or more hours. There have also been reports of serious allergic reaction to the dye, or infection resulting in necessary hysterectomy. Death from complications of the procedure is rare, but has been reported in 4 of the 40,000 patients. Women should expect to experience some degree of postembolization syndrome in which there is fever, pain, nausea, and vomiting after the procedure. This can be quite mild and tolerable or, occasionally, it can be quite severe and require days of hospitalization and testing to assure that a more serious infection has not occurred. One in two hundred patients who have UAE will require hysterectomy due to a uterine infection.

Complications of Uterine Artery Embolization

Infection resulting in hysterectomy	<1%
Premature menopause	2.5% – 15%
Passage of fibroid	4%
Severe postembolization syndrome	2% – 7%
Damage to other structures	<1%
Death (pulmonary embolus, sepsis)	<1%

While complications do exist, keep in mind that every procedure has the potential for a problem to occur. In this case, the complication rate is very low and UAE should be considered to be a safe procedure.

So why don't more gynecologists recommend this procedure?

There's no question that while most gynecologists are somewhat familiar with UAE, it's not something that is done commonly enough for everyone to be well informed about. Up to this point, most articles about the procedure have been in journals directed at radiologists, not gynecologists, so information has rarely shown up in publications that your gynecologist would have seen.

Uterine artery embolization is also not yet as widely available or performed as commonly as hysterectomy or myomectomy. Certainly most major medical centers and large hospitals can do it, but at this point, smaller hospitals generally don't have physicians available who are adept at the procedure, and just as importantly, are not experienced at post-procedure management of pain and complications. With time, that will change, as the number of experienced interventional radiologists continues to increase. At this point, a patient should be wary of having an embolization procedure in a facility in which it is not done regularly.

Dr. Robert Vogelzang, Professor of Radiology and Chief of Vascular and Interventional Radiology at Northwestern Memorial Hospital in Chicago, has performed over six hundred UAEs. He feels that "the procedure produces excellent results in properly selected patients because this method treats all your fibroids regardless of how many you have." He agrees that a good outcome depends on care from an experienced interventional radiologist who works collaboratively with a gynecologist.

Critics often say your gynecologist is not offering the procedure because there is no economic advantage for doing so. Unquestionably, no gynecologist wants to lose their patient to another physician for a problem they feel is in "their turf," but it's not about losing the money. Gynecologists familiar with the procedure are aware that women who have UAE will continue to need gynecologic follow-up, often requiring additional revenue-producing procedures. There really is no financial disincentive to referring the patient for an alternative procedure when that patient is likely to return with income-generating gynecologic needs. If anything, it is the woman who has a hysterectomy who needs little in the way of expensive gynecologic care in subsequent years. In reality, a gynecologist most likely doesn't mention the procedure because there is no experienced center readily available, they are not familiar with it, or they simply don't think it's the best option.

Many gynecologists are also reluctant to jump on the bandwagon of a new procedure until large numbers and studies have established long-term safety and efficacy. Forty thousand patients and five to seven years of experience may seem like a lot, but it's not the same as looking at that same group of women twenty years later to see how they're doing and to determine what problems, if any, develop. More cancer? Less cancer? Early menopause? High re-operation rate? Sexual response issues? No one knows. Your gynecologist may be waiting to find out.

EXPECTANT MANAGEMENT

Expectant management means doing nothing and hoping the problem will go away. Sometimes this is wishful thinking; sometimes this is a reasonable option. Expectant management is based on two factors: how fast the fibroids are growing and when they stop growing.

A typical candidate for expectant management is the woman who is forty-nine years old, with heavy but manageable menstrual cycles. If she goes through menopause at the average time (age fifty-one) and if her fibroids are not growing rapidly (ruling out a leiomyosarcoma), and if she is willing to put up with her symptoms for a few years, she can certainly wait it out. The trick is figuring out how long it will be until she goes through menopause. The average age may be fifty-one, but just as there are women who go through menopause at forty-five, there are women who menstruate until they are fifty-five, or older. An FSH (follicle-stimulating hormone) blood level gives some idea of when the ovaries are getting ready to close shop, but is no guarantee. A woman might be willing to put up with something for one or two years to avoid surgery, but not seven or eight years. It's anyone's guess.

Rate of growth is also a factor. Often women can tolerate their symptoms at a certain size, but are not willing to put up with more pressure, bleeding, or abdominal distention than they already are experiencing. A wait-and-see approach may be reasonable since fibroid growth patterns are unpredictable. Just because a fibroid went through a growth spurt doesn't mean it's going to continue to grow. The real dilemma involves the woman who doesn't want to lose an opportunity for a vaginal or laparoscopic procedure just because she has waited too long. If she waits and they don't grow, she wins. If she waits and they do grow, they may ultimately be too big to be removed laparoscopically or hysteroscopically. She may be stuck with bigger surgery than she would have needed two years earlier. It's a gamble many women are willing to take.

GnRH Analogues

Women are always excited to hear that there is a drug that consistently and dramatically shrinks fibroids. They are less excited when they learn the shrinkage is only temporary. There are a number of different GnRH analogues; the best known one is depot leuprolide, manufactured under the trade name Lupron.

GnRH stands for gonadotropin-releasing hormone. It works by suppressing hormone secretion from the pituitary gland, which in turn shuts down ovarian estrogen production. In short, GnRH causes an instant menopause. It is usually administered by a monthly injection, but is also available as a nasal spray.

Since fibroids are dependent on estrogen for growth, the sudden absence of estrogen makes most fibroids shrink. Multiple studies have shown that fibroids can reduce in size by 35 to 60 percent over a four-to-six-month treatment course. As soon as the treatment is over, the fibroids grow back to their original size. If that were not the case, there would be no need for this chapter.

Why would anyone take a drug that only works for a few months? There are actually many situations in which treatment with GnRH is useful.

First of all, GnRH buys you time. There is never a good time to have surgery, but some times are better than others. If a teacher needs to wait for summer before she can take time off for surgery, a course of Lupron will stop her monthly hemorrhage so she can make it through the school year.

It goes way beyond convenience for most women. If heavy bleeding has resulted in anemia, treatment will allow someone to replenish her iron stores so that she can go into surgery with a normal blood count. This not only makes surgery safer and recovery easier, but also significantly decreases the chance that a transfusion will be needed.

If a woman is not a candidate for a vaginal hysterectomy or a laparoscopic hysterectomy because her fibroids are too big, shrinkage will enable her to have a minimally invasive procedure and avoid an abdominal hysterectomy. A woman close to menopause can use GnRH until she goes through a natural menopause and avoid having to do anything about her fibroids. Women who are attempting to conceive but are unable due to fibroids often conceive easily after treatment with GnRH. Women who are scheduled to have a hysteroscopic resection of a fibroid require GnRH to decrease fibroid size and uterine vascularity.

The bottom line is that there are many circumstances in which GnRH is useful as an adjunct to other treatment options or to buy time. The list above includes only a few examples.

Why stop GnRH? Why not just continue treatment for years? The answer is that using GnRH for more than six months can result in severe osteoporosis. Most women are also less than crazy about the hot flashes, vaginal dryness, insomnia, breast tenderness, depression, headaches, and decreased libido that are common during treatment.

If things get really intolerable, side effects can be minimized by add-back therapy with estrogen and progesterone. Sometimes the most painful part of the treatment is the cost, since Lupron can run a few hundred dollars a month. For all these reasons, GnRH is really most useful as preparation for surgery, rather a treatment by itself.

ANTIPROGESTATIONAL AGENTS

Another medical option for the treatment of fibroids are antiprogesta-tional agents. Mifepristone, also known as RU-486, is an antiproges-terone pill, commonly used for early pregnancy termination. The anti-abortion rights movement to limit the availability of mifepristone has had the unfortunate consequence that its many other useful appli-cations have been limited as well. The many potential health benefits of this medication have essentially been controlled by special-interest groups with their own agenda. Politics aside, mefepristone successfully shrinks fibroids as well as Lupron, but with the advantage that it does not result in bone loss or cause hot flashes. As with Lupron, fibroids return to their original size once therapy is withdrawn. In addition to its unavailability, mifepristone is prohibitively expensive, making long-term use impractical. Currently, many other antiprogestational agents are under investigation.

DANAZOL

Danazol, a derivative of testosterone, was used commonly in the 1980s for treatment of endometriosis until better things came along. Danazol doesn't shrink fibroids, but it can stop bleeding due to fibroids. If you thought the side effects of GnRH sounded bad . . . well, add hair growth, acne, weight gain, muscle cramps, decreased breast size, oily skin, and mood swings to the list. For these reasons, Danazol is almost never prescribed today.

COMMONLY RECOMMENDED THINGS THAT DON'T WORK

Hormone Therapy

Many women are treated using combinations of estrogen and proges-terone in the form of oral contraceptive pills, or progesterone alone. Given that estrogen is to fibroids like fertilizer is to grass, it's no sur-prise that hormones don't shrink fibroids. Having said that, every gynecologist has patients with fibroids who have a significant decrease in monthly bleeding when they take birth control pills. The reason that happens is simple. The fibroids weren't the only thing causing the bleeding. Not every woman who has fibroids has abnormal bleeding. Women who have fibroids can have heavy bleeding for reasons totally unrelated to their fibroids, most commonly anovulatory cycles (see chapter 8). Birth control pills and monthly progesterone treatment work like a charm in those women, many of whom also happen to have fibroids. If the bleeding is solely from a large intracavitary fibroid, the bleeding will likely continue in spite of the pills. There is also the concern that the hormones will only make the fibroids grow quicker. It is reasonable to give hormone therapy a try if your doctor recommends it, but be sure and have a follow-up ultrasound to check for growth.

Nonsteroidal Anti-Inflammatory Drugs

Nonsteroidal anti-inflammatory drugs (NSAIDs) include ibuprofen and naproxen, among others. They are certainly useful to manage pain in women with fibroids, but no study has shown that they decrease the amount of bleeding or the size of the fibroid.

Dietary Changes

There have actually been some studies that indicate that women who eat large amounts of beef, ham, or other red meats are associated with an increased risk of fibroids. Questions are frequently raised regarding the impact of hormones found in beef on fibroid development. Unfortunately, no studies indicate that changes in diet influence the numbers of fibroids or the symptoms they produce.

Chinese Herbs and Others

It would be nice if herbs worked, it really would. But they don't, otherwise gynecologists would recommend them and no one would need surgery. There are often anecdotal stories, but there is not one evidence-based study to prove the safety or efficacy of these preparations. The only people who benefit from these alternative treatments are the people who sell them. They are just as profit-motivated as the pharmaceutical companies and they're making out like bandits.

Chapter 6

Removing Fibroids

Myomectomy is, quite simply, removing the fibroids and leaving the uterus behind. This can only be done surgically. The location and size of the fibroids determine which of three routes—traditional, hysteroscopic, or laparoscopic—makes the most sense. No matter how the fibroid is removed, certain caveats apply.

Recurrence of fibroids after myomectomy is a certainty in 50 percent of women. Just because a fibroid comes back, however, doesn't mean that subsequent therapy will be necessary. Most studies show that 10 to 25 percent of women who undergo myomectomy will require another surgery. Most experts agree, therefore, that women who desire children are the most appropriate candidates for myomectomy. It makes perfect sense to take a 25 percent risk that you may need further surgery ten years later if during that time interval you are able to have successful pregnancies.

Myomectomy, rather than hysterectomy, is also reasonable for women who are within five years of menopause. It's unlikely that there will be a recurrence in that short time that will require treatment, and, if the myomectomy can be done laparoscopically or hysteroscopically, it makes sense to do so. Recurrence rates are also much lower in women who have a solitary fibroid as opposed to multiple fibroids.

The woman who has multiple, large, symptomatic fibroids, who is not interested in pregnancy, and is younger than forty-five years old, should realize that myomectomy is not definitive therapy. Hysterectomy is very often her best option and results in a far superior resolution of both short- and long-term problems. Some women, however, strongly desire uterine preservation. As long as they know the negatives, the choice is obviously theirs to make.

PREOPERATIVE CONSIDERATIONS

It doesn't matter what type of myomectomy is planned; preoperative preparation is absolutely the key to a good outcome. Ultrasound is generally used to determine the number and location of fibroids. The quality of the scan is important and should be done by someone who can count, measure, and locate every fibroid that is big enough to see. Generally, transabdominal and transvaginal ultrasound are both necessary to get an accurate picture. It is also important that the ovaries are visualized and appear normal. A disastrous possibility is that a presumed fibroid is actually an ovarian tumor, which is then ignored. Magnetic resonance imaging (MRI), saline-infused sonography (SIS), or hysterosalpingograms (discussed in chapter 4) are also useful to determine exact locations and types of fibroids and should be considered if the ultrasound is not definitive.

Since blood loss during myomectomy is inevitable and can be significant, it is important to correct anemia prior to surgery. This is most easily accomplished by iron supplementation, which should ideally be started months prior to surgery. If a woman is having the surgery because of heavy bleeding (a common scenario), pretreatment with GnRH (described in detail in chapter 5) shuts off bleeding and allows the anemia to correct itself. Once the anemia is corrected, if there is time, autologous blood donation is also a consideration (see chapter 15).

Often a woman undergoes myomectomy because she has fibroids and is unable to conceive. Sometimes, however, the fibroids aren't even the problem. Every woman having a myomectomy to enhance her fertility should have a full evaluation, including documentation of ovulation, hysterosalpingogram, and analysis of her partner's semen, to ensure that there isn't a totally unrelated factor responsible for infertility. Too many women undergo surgery only to learn that they are still unable to become pregnant.

Likewise, if a woman has a myomectomy after a pregnancy loss, it's important to be sure that the fibroid was the reason for the loss. A sonohysterogram, hysteroscopy, or hysterosalpingogram is useful to evaluate the relationship of the fibroids to the cavity of the uterus in order to determine if the fibroids might have been responsible. Fibroids that do not infringe on the uterine cavity rarely cause miscarriage.

GnRH is useful prior to myomectomy for a variety of reasons. It not only corrects an anemia, but also shrinks the fibroids. Smaller fibroids mean the surgery is quicker, easier, less bloody, and more likely to be accomplished laparoscopically or hysteroscopically. There is, however, a downside to pretreatment with GnRH beyond the expense and side effects. It undoubtedly will make the big fibroids smaller and more manageable, but it also makes small fibroids invisible so that sometimes they can't be found or removed at the time of myomectomy. These tiny fibroids remain behind and continue to grow for years after surgery, increasing the chance of recurrent symptoms and need for repeat surgery down the road. This is especially common when multiple fibroids are present and menopause is not imminent.

TRADITIONAL MYOMECTOMY

In a traditional myomectomy, an abdominal incision is made. Usually this is in the bikini line, but in some situations a vertical (pubic to belly button) incision is needed. The decision is made using the same principles as in an abdominal hysterectomy (see chapter 10). Once the surgeon is in the pelvis, an incision is made in the uterus. The fibroids are then removed by separating and cutting them away from normal uterine tissue. An attempt is made to remove as many fibroids as possible through a single incision in order to minimize blood loss and scarring, but sometimes multiple uterine incisions are necessary. Once the fibroids are removed, the uterus is reconstructed by sewing the uterine wall closed in multiple layers.

The surgeon always prefers not to enter the cavity of the uterus during the course of the procedure but it is sometimes unavoidable if the fibroid is large, intracavitary, or submucosal. If the cavity is entered, a cesarean section is recommended in the event of a subsequent pregnancy since there is concern that the repaired uterine wall will not have the strength to withstand labor. Uterine rupture is a possible complication of pregnancy after myomectomy, and usually, but not always, occurs in labor.

COMPLICATIONS OF ABDOMINAL MYOMECTOMY

Most women are surprised to learn that complications and recovery time after abdominal myomectomy are usually much greater than hysterectomy. Intuitively, it seems it would be better and easier to remove just the fibroids rather than the whole uterus, but in fact, the opposite is true. This is particularly the case if there are multiple fibroids that involve the deeper layers of the uterus.

Virtually every complication described in abdominal hysterectomy can occur during abdominal myomectomy. The three general categories of complications still hold: bleeding, infection, and injury to surrounding structures.

Blood loss during abdominal myomectomy is considerably greater than hysterectomy. During hysterectomy, the vessels are identified and controlled before they are cut so that a hysterectomy usually results in negligible blood loss. During a traditional myomectomy, the fibroid is removed through a uterine incision (or incisions, in the case of multiple fibroids), which bleed until all the fibroids are out. Only then can the incisions be sewn, but blood loss is inevitable.

Certainly, many things are done to minimize bleeding, but the fact still remains that most women are anemic to some degree after surgery, even if they start with a normal blood count. It's not unusual for there to be further blood loss from the uterine incision site in the days after surgery, even if everything was "dry" when the surgeon finished. Twenty percent of women require transfusion after abdominal myomectomy, which is why it is so crucial to start with a normal blood count and have blood on hand, either autologous or donor-designated. In contrast, transfusion after hysterectomy is rare.

Infection after myomectomy is rarely a problem, but does occur. Fever, however, is very common and occurs in approximately fifty percent of women in the days after surgery. The fever isn't harmful; it just makes the recovery unpleasant. In general, people just feel lousy for days after myomectomy due to pain, fever, abdominal distention, and slow return of bowel function. Many women who have a hysterectomy had a myomectomy first and invariably report that the recovery after the myomectomy was by far the more difficult one.

Any abdominal surgery can promote the formation of adhesions (scar tissue), but abdominal myomectomy is one of the worst. No matter how meticulous the surgeon, and no matter how many precautions are taken to prevent scar tissue from forming, it is almost impossible to go back after a myomectomy and not find some adhesions. The incision line on the uterus is like Velcro to anything that touches it during the healing process, which is why re-operation can be complicated by bowel, omentum, or bladder sticking to the uterus. Adhesions are less likely to occur if the incision is placed on the back wall of the uterus, and most surgeons try to do this whenever possible.

Fortunately, most women are not aware of, or troubled by, adhesion formation. In other women, adhesions are responsible for life-long problems like bowel obstruction or pain. The real problem occurs when a woman who has adhesions from myomectomy needs further surgery. Adhesions can make the surgery far more difficult, the complication rate higher, and may eliminate the possibility of a laparoscopic procedure. Since up to 25 percent of women who have a myomectomy require another operation within ten years, this can be a significant problem.

The most serious complication of abdominal myomectomy is the possibility that during the course of the procedure, a hysterectomy will be needed as a life-saving procedure. It is extremely rare, but there are times when removal of a fibroid creates bleeding that cannot be stopped unless the uterus is removed. It usually occurs if a fibroid is extremely large, or is located on the side of the uterus as opposed to the front or the back. A repeat myomectomy is the most likely to result in hysterectomy. Sometimes all goes well at the time of myomectomy, but delayed bleeding two or three days after the surgery requires a return trip to the operating room, at which time there may be no choice but to do a hysterectomy.

The potential need for hysterectomy is impossible to predict before surgery, and every woman needs to know that there is a possibility that she will leave the operating room without her uterus. Most surgeons have their patients agree to a "possible hysterectomy" when they sign the consent form for myomectomy. It is also appropriate to tell your surgeon that you prefer a fibroid to be left behind rather than risk hysterectomy. Fortunately, this is a rare occurrence.

In spite of all this, most women do very well after abdominal myomectomy and are pleased that they had the procedure. Unlike in other methods of myomectomy, the fibroids can almost always be entirely removed. Postoperatively, many women are able to conceive a baby, carry the pregnancy to term, and deliver vaginally. Fifty percent of women are never troubled by fibroids again; 75 to 90 percent never need another operation.

There is another advantage to abdominal myomectomy that should not be minimized. Unlike the many new, minimally invasive procedures, this is a procedure virtually every gynecologist is comfortable and experienced performing. Abdominal myomectomy has been routinely done during the last fifty years and most women can be confident that if their gynecologist offers the procedure, she can do the procedure (see chapter 13).

HYSTEROSCOPIC MYOMECTOMY

One of the most underutilized uterus-sparing techniques available is hysteroscopic myomectomy. It's already been established that most fibroids are asymptomatic and require no treatment, but, as any good real estate agent knows, it's all about location, location, location. If a fibroid does cause problems, it's most likely because of where it is, rather than its size. There's no worse location than submucosal and intracavitary fibroids. These are the fibroids that push into, or are actually *in,* the cavity of the uterus. These are the fibroids that create problems with infertility, early miscarriage, and preterm delivery. These are the fibroids that cause extremely heavy periods and profound anemia, even if the fibroid is not particularly big. These are the fibroids that can be removed hysteroscopically.

A hysteroscope is a scope with a camera and light attached to it that is inserted through the cervix in order to visualize the uterine cavity. In operative hysteroscopy, instruments can be passed through the scope that cut, burn, and grasp whatever is in the cavity that shouldn't be, including polyps, tumors, and . . . you guessed it, fibroids. Thanks to technology that urologists have been using on prostates for years, an instrument called a resectoscope actually slices through fibroids in order to shave off chunks that can then be removed, a process known as resection (Fig. 6-1).

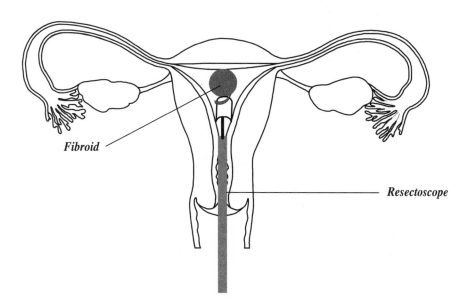

Fibroid

Resectoscope

Figure 6-1. Hysteroscopic resection.

The surgery itself is generally done as an outpatient procedure, with general anesthesia, since any movement can be dangerous. After the hysteroscope has been inserted through the cervix, sterile fluid then continuously flows through the hysteroscope into the uterus to distend the cavity of the uterus so the surgeon can see. The resectoscope is used to cut the fibroid into small pieces, which are then removed through the hysteroscope. It sounds simple and straightforward. Sometimes it is. Sometimes it is technically very difficult.

Before the Procedure

Once it is determined that the fibroid is amenable to removal, most gynecologists pretreat with Lupron (GnRH agonist), the hormone that turns off estrogen production. Pre-treatment accomplishes multiple goals. It makes the fibroid smaller so there is less tissue to remove and the surgery is technically easier. It also makes the fibroid and uterine wall less vascular so there is less bleeding and better visualization at the time of surgery. In women pretreated with Lupron, less fluid is absorbed during the myomectomy, which increases safety if longer surgery is required. Finally, pretreatment allows a woman who has been bleeding heavily to stop and catch up so that she's not anemic at the time of the procedure. Most gynecologists give one or two monthly injections of Lupron; some treat longer, particularly if the fibroid is large.

Candidates for Hysteroscopic Myomectomy

Like any alternative to hysterectomy, the key to success is appropriate pre-operative evaluation so inappropriate patients never get to the operating room. The first step is to determine if a fibroid is even amenable to hysteroscopic resection. This can be done by an SIS, a hysterosalpingogram, or hysteroscopy.

All three of the above techniques are appropriate and give similar information; the choice usually depends on what is available and the personal preference of the gynecologist. If the fibroid is not protruding into the uterine cavity, or is predominately in the wall of the cavity, hysteroscopic resection is the wrong choice.

The Downside of Hysteroscopic Myomectomy

Hysteroscopic myomectomy is one of those procedures in which experience is key. Even with experience, sometimes it is very difficult to get to the fibroid due to its location in the uterus and the limitations of a rigid hysteroscope. Sometimes visualization is difficult, especially once there are chunks of fibroid floating around and obscuring the view. There is also a limitation to how much fluid is safe to put in the uterus. Some fluid always gets absorbed, and if the fibroid is very large and surgery time long, an excessive amount of fluid can be absorbed, resulting in complications such as pulmonary edema (fluid in the lungs) or a life-threatening fluid imbalance. Sometimes a large fibroid needs to be resected in more than one session. If your surgeon says she couldn't resect the whole fibroid in one session, your surgeon is not a bad surgeon; she is a safe surgeon.

Another potential problem is uterine perforation. Since the fibroid is essentially being shaved off and carved out of the uterine wall, sometimes a hole can inadvertently be poked in the wall during the process. For that reason, many gynecologists always do a laparoscopy at the time of hysteroscopic resection so that they can simultaneously watch the inside and the outside of the uterus. Sometimes it's not automatic, but you may be told that a laparoscopy is possible depending on how things are going.

Right now, the biggest hurdle to this procedure is finding a surgeon to do it. In 2003, fewer than one third of gynecologists reported that they offer hysteroscopic myomectomy to their patients, or are comfortable performing it. As with many of the newer techniques, if a doctor completed her training more than ten years ago (which would include the majority of practicing gynecologists), it's possible she wasn't trained in the procedure. Even if someone is motivated to learn, training is not always accessible and it takes experience (and someone experienced around) until someone gets really good. So even if you are a good candidate, it may be hard to find someone do it, particularly if you don't live in a big city (see chapter 13).

Like most uterus-sparing, alternative procedures, hysteroscopic myomectomy is not one-stop shopping. First the cavity must be evaluated (with a procedure), and then one has to go through at least a month of hormonal suppression, followed by the procedure itself, which may need to be repeated. More than once.

That's right. The fibroids often come back. It's rare to get the whole fibroid since you're shaving the part that protrudes into the cavity rather than removing the entire thing. So, yes, it's possible for the patient to be right back where she started a few years later. If someone is interested in achieving a pregnancy, or buying a few years if she is close to menopause, that may be enough. If someone is forty years old, done with babies, and has twelve years until menopause, she may not gain a whole lot. Certainly, many women never have a recurrence, but a significant number do. In general, after any kind of myomectomy there is an approximate 50 percent recurrence rate, less if a solitary fibroid was removed, as opposed to multiple fibroids. Roughly 18 to 20 percent of women end up with a second procedure within ten years of the original hysteroscopic myomectomy.

Wouldn't It Be Simpler to Just Do a D&C?

It would be nice if the fibroids could be scraped away and, in fact, that question is frequently asked. A D&C (discussed in detail in chapter 8) is commonly done to evaluate bleeding in which the cervix is dilated (the "D") and then the uterine lining is scraped using an instrument called a curette (the "C"). Unfortunately, doing a D&C to scrape away fibroids is like raking the leaves and expecting to remove the boulder stuck in the ground.

Why Do a Hysteroscopic Resection?

In experienced hands, the complication rate is very low. The recovery is minimal and usually only involves a day or two of mild cramping and bleeding. For many women, particularly if they have one fibroid sitting in the cavity, the procedure is definitive. Even if fibroids do recur, it may be after someone has had a successful pregnancy, or they may be less symptomatic and not require treatment. Some women would rather have two or three hysteroscopic resections over the years than a hysterectomy.

It's a reasonable option in many situations. It's probably the best option for women who desire pregnancy and have a problematic submucosal fibroid.

LAPAROSCOPIC MYOMECTOMY

Laparoscopic myomectomy, used to remove subserosal or pedunculated fibroids (the ones on the outside of the uterus), can either be a terrific quick fix or a challenging surgical nightmare. Again, it all depends on the correct person, doing the correct procedure, on the correct patient. Unlike women with submucosal or intracavitary fibroids, women with subserosal and pedunculated fibroids rarely suffer from excessive bleeding. If they do, the diagnosis needs to be seriously questioned.

A subserosal fibroid is located under the outermost layer of the uterus. While a subserosal fibroid originates in the myometrium, it grows away from the uterine cavity. The pedunculated version has pushed completely outside the uterus and is attached only by a stalk.

Before the Procedure

As always, preoperative evaluation is key. Ultrasound is the standard way to evaluate fibroids; however, there is ultrasound, and there is ultrasound. An ultrasound report that reads, "There are multiple uterine fibroids, some very large," is inadequate, to say the least. An ultrasound report that reads, "There is a 5 × 7 cm subserosal fibroid on the anterior (front) wall of the uterus without infringement on the uterine cavity," is the sort of report a surgeon needs. If it is difficult to tell the exact location, or if a stalk is present, a three-dimensional ultrasound, sonohysterogram, or MRI may give additional information. There's no substitute for actually looking inside, but you want as much information as possible before proceeding.

What's Involved

As with all laparoscopy, general anesthesia is required (see chapter 14). Once the laparoscope is placed, the surgeon first takes a look to evaluate the situation. On occasion, the surgeon immediately realizes that laparoscopic myomectomy is not technically feasible because the actual situation is different than what the preoperative ultrasound suggested. The laparoscope is then removed, and depending on the preoperative agreement with the patient, either the patient goes home or the procedure is converted to a traditional myomectomy with an abdominal incision or a hysterectomy.

If it seems appropriate to proceed, additional ports are placed in the lower abdomen, as described in the setup for laparoscopic hysterectomy (see chapter 12). If the fibroid is on a stalk, the procedure is easy. The stalk is simply cauterized, then cut, to free the fibroid from the uterine wall. The trick, of course, is getting the fibroid out, which may be the size of a cantaloupe or bigger. There are three methods. *Morcellation*, or cutting the fibroid up, is the easiest and makes the most sense if your surgeon is trained in that technique. This is the same technique used to remove the whole uterus when a laparoscopic hysterectomy is done. Another option is to remove the fibroid through the vagina by making an incision in the back of the vagina and pushing the fibroid out of the pelvis and into the vagina, where it is "delivered" by the gynecologist. The incision is sewn up with dissolvable stitches and the patient isn't even aware of the incision. This plan can actually work pretty well, but is limited by the size of the fibroid, and, quite frankly, by the size of the vagina. It's fairly easy to remove an orange-size fibroid through the vagina of a woman who once delivered an eight-pound baby. The same size fibroid is simply not going to fit through a virgin's vagina without major difficulty. The third option is to make a small incision in the bikini line to remove the fibroid, but this defeats the whole purpose of using the laparoscope, since an incision is still made.

Laparoscopic myomectomy gets considerably more complicated if the fibroid is not pedunculated, but incorporated into the muscle of the uterus. It's not terribly difficult to remove the fibroid from the uterus laparoscopically. That's done by making an incision in the uterus over the fibroid and dissecting the fibroid away from normal uterine tissue. The fibroid can then be removed using morcellation.

The challenge is in dealing with the defect left in the uterine wall where the fibroid used to be. That defect needs to be repaired in order to reconstruct the uterine wall and stop the bleeding. In a traditional open myomectomy, the surgeon simply sews the wall in multiple layers to reconstruct normal anatomy. This is pretty standard surgery that any gynecologist can comfortably do. Laparoscopically, it's not so easy. The uterine wall can be sewn laparoscopically, but few surgeons have the laparoscopic skills to do it well and quickly. Keep in mind that until the uterine wall is repaired, it is bleeding. Sometimes it's bleeding a lot and the surgeon needs to move fast to prevent significant blood loss. Probably fewer than 5 percent of practicing gynecologists have the advanced laparoscopic skills required to do a laparoscopic myomectomy that requires reconstruction of the uterine wall, particularly if a large fibroid is involved.

The other concern is the strength of a laparoscopically repaired uterus. In an open, standard myomectomy, the wall is repaired in multiple layers. In a laparoscopic repair, one layer closure is typical. Doctors have questioned if the single layer is strong enough to hold a full-term pregnancy. There have been cases reported of uterine rupture during the eighth month of pregnancy in women who had laparoscopic myomectomies. Until more data are available, women who desire pregnancy and require myomectomy should go with the multilayer standard closure used in abdominal myomectomy.

Any time a laparoscopic myomectomy is done, the woman needs to consent to a possible abdominal incision as situations may present themselves where the procedure cannot be completed laparoscopically due to uncontrollable bleeding. This occurs about 8 percent of the time. There are also women who go back to the operating room for delayed bleeding (hours or days after the procedure). And yes, a small number of women do end up with a hysterectomy due to bleeding that can't be controlled any other way. Most prudent physicians inform women of this possibility and have them sign consent forms to that effect. Fortunately, that is a rare occurrence.

As with all myomectomy techniques, there is the issue of fibroid recurrence. For some reason, the recurrence rate seems to be higher after laparoscopic myomectomy than open myomectomy. Not enough data are available to know if this is always the case.

The bottom line is that while laparoscopic myomectomy is a viable option, most gynecologists are only capable of doing the easy ones, when the fibroids are small or pedunculated. The real question is, do most of those fibroids even *need* to be removed?

LAPAROSCOPIC MYOLYSIS

This is the latest technique and refers to laparoscopic destruction of fibroid tissue with a laser. The advantage is the technique is easier than resection and no suturing is needed. The disadvantage? It's very new, the numbers are very small, and at this time it is not recommended for women who desire pregnancy since little data about pregnancy after myolysis are available and there have been reports of a higher rate of complications. There also seems to be a greater tendency for adhesion formation after myolysis than after other laparoscopic procedures.

AREN'T THESE PROCEDURES LESS EXPENSIVE THAN HYSTERECTOMY?

The cost? Myomectomy can be expensive, both in time and money. If someone has one successful, minimally invasive procedure, the cost is lower than hysterectomy. An open myomectomy actually costs more than a hysterectomy since it often takes longer and generally involves a longer hospital stay and recovery. If someone is a frequent flier and you add the cost of multiple diagnostic hysteroscopies, pretreatments with Lupron, possibly more than one hysteroscopic resection, a laparoscopic myomectomy, and multiple intervening ultrasounds and doctor visits, it is *far* more expensive than one laparoscopic hysterectomy. So once again, don't assume your physician has recommended a hysterectomy to make more money.

In the long run, the woman who has recurrent fibroids is more likely to be the high roller in patient revenue. Your insurance company, on the other hand, does better with multiple procedures over time. First of all, they are hoping you will need only one procedure. If you do need repeat procedures, you pay for a big chunk of each one since you pay a new deductible each year. If they get really lucky, you may switch insurance carriers over the years (a common occurrence) so they only pick up one procedure. Those who accuse doctors of recommending hysterectomy over alternative procedures for financial gain are wrong. If your doctor doesn't recommend an alternative procedure it is usually because you are not a good candidate, or your gynecologist is not trained in the procedure.

After completing this whirlwind tour through the land of fibroids, you may decide that an alternative or uterus-sparing therapy is the way you want to go. But, if you would prefer to avoid multiple procedures, continued surveillance, and frequent visits to your gynecologist, you may want to consider definitive therapy. Once you've decided that hysterectomy is your best choice, or your only choice, the goal is to make it as positive an experience as possible. For most women, it usually is.

Chapter 7

Uterine Prolapse

While the majority of hysterectomies in this country are performed due to problems from fibroids, there are many other non–life-threatening yet indicated reasons for hysterectomy. Uterine prolapse is one of the most distressing gynecologic conditions and spares no age group. For many women, hysterectomy is truly the best option, but there are also appropriate reasonable alternatives for the woman who would like to avoid hysterectomy.

Uterine prolapse is just what it sounds like: the uterus drops down into the vagina, and in severe cases, *outside* the vagina (Fig. 7-1). It occurs from injury to the fascia, the tissue that supports and holds up the uterus. Weakened ligaments that support the uterus and loss of pelvic floor musculature also contribute to the loss of the normal uterine position.

Women who have uterine prolapse frequently have other displaced organs due to weak pelvic tissues. A *cystocele* (Fig. 7-2) results when a prolapsed bladder bulges through the vaginal roof; a *rectocele* (Fig. 7-3) occurs when the rectum bulges through the vaginal floor.

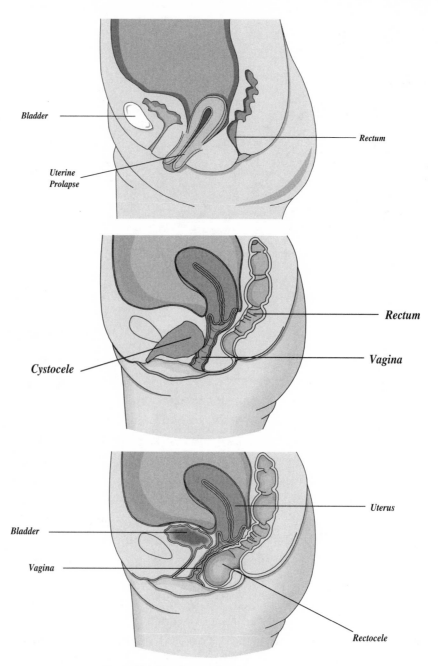

Figure 7-1. Uterine prolapse.
Figure 7-2. Cystocele.
Figure 7-3. Rectocele.

WHO GETS A PROLAPSED UTERUS?

Vaginal deliveries, particularly if the labor is long and the baby large, are the greatest risk factor for pelvic relaxation. It's not the only risk factor since most women who deliver vaginally don't end up with uterine prolapse. Family history seems to be a major factor. Tissue prone to damage is an inherited tendency and it's not unusual for a woman with uterine prolapse to mention that her mother and grandmother had the same problem. Take a genetic predisposition, add a nine-pound baby and three hours of pushing . . . something is going to give. Once the tissue is damaged, it never completely regains its strength and elasticity; the effects of gravity and age then compound the problem.

Smoking is also a major risk factor. Smokers have poor tissue in general and chronic coughing weakens tissue even further. Long-distance runners may also have a greater propensity for prolapse. The running probably doesn't cause the weakened tissue; it just makes an already tenuous situation worse from the constant pounding.

Incidence is directly related to age, and since women are living longer, increasing numbers of women are destined to suffer from uterine prolapse. It's not unusual for women with only a slight prolapse to not be aware of the problem until they go through menopause. Vaginal and pelvic tissues depend on estrogen to maintain their strength and elasticity. The decline of estrogen, which occurs at menopause, can result in a sudden worsening of symptoms, particularly if a woman chooses not to take hormone therapy. Many women who stop postmenopausal estrogen replacement find that pelvic organ prolapse is far more bothersome than the hot flashes.

HOW DO YOU KNOW IF YOU HAVE A PROLAPSE?

Symptoms are generally related to the degree of the prolapse—in other words, how far the uterus has dropped. In a *first-degree prolapse*, the uterus is only slightly lower than its normal position and most women are totally unaware that something has shifted unless their gynecologist points it out. A further drop creates a *second-degree prolapse*, which is the point when some women become aware that something is not quite right. Still, many women with a second-degree prolapse have no symptoms. By the time the uterus drops low enough for the vagina to be completely filled and the cervix reaches the opening of the vagina (*third-degree prolapse*), most women are definitely aware there is a problem. Even the most oblivious woman notices when her uterus drops outside her vagina (a *fourth-degree prolapse*), prompting an emergency visit. One woman actually called from her bathtub, appropriately upset, crying, "Something is *floating* out of my vagina . . . and I think it's my uterus!"

The most common symptom is the feeling that "something is falling down," which is not surprising since that is exactly what has happened. Nine times out of ten, a woman correctly diagnoses her own prolapse before any doctor lays eyes on her. Many women, in addition to constant pressure, actually feel a mass or bulge at the vaginal opening. A quick look in the mirror (a hand mirror with a long handle works well) and you can see something pink bulging out. Low back pain and discomfort during intercourse are common. If the cervix is outside the vaginal opening, there may also be bleeding, discharge, and pain. In severe cases, there may be an inability to have a bowel movement or urinate.

DOES ANYTHING PREVENT IT FROM HAPPENING?

Avoiding vaginal delivery is not necessarily the most practical way to prevent prolapse, but it is the best way to avoid it. Women who have never been pregnant almost never have a significant prolapse. Women who labor, but ultimately end up with a cesarean section, are at less risk than if they had delivered vaginally, but still at some risk.

There are actually a growing number of women who are requesting elective cesarean sections to prevent prolapse and associated incontinence problems. It's been estimated that 20 percent of the hysterectomies done each year because of prolapse could be avoided by giving women at risk (family history, big baby) the option of elective cesarean section without laboring. As radical as this sounds, it's not a ridiculous notion given the fact that today a cesarean section is as safe (or even safer, in some instances) than a vaginal delivery. If one accepts the premise that women should have autonomy in decisions regarding their route of delivery, once they understand the risks and benefits of each, the birth plan of the future may look very different.

SURGERY

Once the damage is done, what options are available to treat uterine prolapse? Surgery is the ultimate treatment, almost always a vaginal hysterectomy. The first hysterectomy, as a matter of fact, in 200 A.D., was a vaginal hysterectomy for a completely prolapsed uterus. During the 1860s, doctors at the Women's Hospital in New York City routinely sliced off the cervix if it was hanging outside the vagina. Since the technique of hysterectomy was not yet known, it was the only available cure for women suffering from prolapse. The 50 percent of the women who survived the operation were evidently pleased with the result, but it fell out of favor when it became evident that the cervixless women were unable to carry a pregnancy. The good doctors decided that there was no point in a procedure that rendered a woman infertile, regardless of how it might improve her life. The high mortality rate was not a factor in discontinuing the procedure since all surgery at that time had similar risks.

Today, vaginal or laparoscopically assisted vaginal hysterectomy is the standard treatment for symptomatic uterine prolapse. The details of vaginal hysterectomy for prolapse are discussed in chapter 11, along with associated surgical procedures for cystocele and rectocele. Sometimes, depending on other needed procedures, an abdominal approach is also appropriate.

NONSURGICAL TREATMENT OF UTERINE PROLAPSE

Nonsurgical options are available and useful in the treatment of uterine prolapse. They are most appropriate if the condition is not severe, or if a woman is a poor surgical candidate. Some women simply want to avoid surgery or need to delay surgery until a more convenient time.

Estrogen

There is no question that estrogen can improve pelvic relaxation. It's well established that vaginal tissues and supporting structures depend on estrogen for their strength and elasticity. Women in low-estrogen states (menopause, breast-feeding moms) often are the most symptomatic. The use of estrogen in the form of pills, vaginal rings, patches, or vaginal creams will often improve a mild prolapse so that no other treatment is needed. Severe prolapse (third or fourth degree) will rarely respond to estrogen therapy alone, but can be useful as an adjunct to other therapy.

Menopausal women who are scheduled for surgery will have a better result if they are pretreated with estrogen for at least a few weeks before surgery. The tissue is much easier to work with and will be more supportive. Gynecologists will often recommend continuing the use of vaginal estrogen creams after surgery to maintain surgical results, particularly if the vaginal tissues are dry and thin.

Exercises

Every woman who has ever had a problem with incontinence or prolapse has been instructed in the fine art of Kegel and other pelvic muscle exercises. If the Olympics had a Kegel event, the United States team would have millions of potential contenders skilled in the art of squeezing their vaginal muscles and stopping their urine midstream. Unfortunately, most would be disqualified since their prolapsed uteruses would preclude them from participating. With all due respect to Dr. Arnold Kegel, the exercises he developed strengthen the muscle but do little for the weakened fascia, which is what really holds the uterus in position.

Picture a hammock that's been used too long. If someone lies in an old hammock, his or her bottom sinks through the middle. Even if the fabric on the sides of the hammock is strong and supportive, the middle is still loose. Now picture a *cystocele*, which is the bladder bulging through the roof (the hammock) of the vagina. Kegel exercises can strengthen the sides but not the middle. The only way to strengthen the middle is by surgically repairing the loose area using stronger tissue. Kegels help in mild cases of incontinence, but are not particularly worthwhile in severe cases or to improve prolapse.

Does It Make Sense to Wait It Out?

Surgical treatment should never be considered in a woman with prolapse who recently had a baby. Tissues damaged during childbirth, once given the chance to heal, often improve. Many women panic when they discover that in addition to all the other new surprises that come with motherhood, they are also unable to make it to the bathroom without losing urine. Before running out and buying diapers in two sizes (newborn *and* adult), it's important to not overreact. A symptomatic prolapse in the first few weeks after delivery, especially in breast-feeding moms who have lower than normal estrogen levels, is not an indication of a long-term problem. There is always improvement after nursing is concluded and hormones return to prepregnancy levels. Often the problem completely resolves.

If a woman already has normal estrogen levels and has eliminated smoking and high-impact exercise from her routine, further spontaneous improvement is unlikely. What nobody can predict is, will it get worse? Therein lies the difficulty. Many women can endure the situation as it is, but are worried that as the years go on, their prolapse will progress to an intolerable point. They will then be in the position of needing surgery when they are much older and potentially too sick to safely undergo an operation. The vision of lying in a nursing home with diapers and a pessary is one scenario most people would like to avoid, but it is difficult to predict which women with moderate prolapse will ultimately end up with a severe prolapse. Another reason some women opt for surgery before they absolutely need it is that pelvic reconstructive surgery (like a face-lift) holds up better if it is done with younger, more elastic tissue.

Having said that, expectant management is appropriate if symptoms are tolerable and as long as the uterus is not actually hanging outside the vagina. Once that happens, treatment is no longer elective. Cervical and uterine tissue, when exposed to air, dries out, breaks down, bleeds, and over time becomes macerated and potentially infected. That situation is potentially life-threatening and requires immediate surgery.

Women who choose to wait it out in hopes that things won't get worse should be seen at regular intervals to ensure that the situation is not deteriorating. Most women, though, know when something has changed.

Pessaries

Pessaries are not new. In fact, devices placed temporarily in the vagina to lift up the uterus have been around long before modern medicine. There is documentation of a Roman medicated pessary as early as 30 A.D. Modern pessaries can be left in place for up to three months at a time with interval physician visits for cleaning and replacement. Younger women are usually able to clean and replace their pessaries themselves, allowing for less frequent visits.

In the past, pessaries were often recommended for women who were felt to be poor surgical risks due to age or chronic illness. Pessary use is far less common in recent years since improved surgical and anesthetic techniques have made surgery a safer, more reasonable option for older and sicker patients, but there are still some situations in which a pessary is useful and appropriate.

Some women simply don't want to go through surgery and are willing to live with the inconvenience—and limited relief—of a pessary. Some women are so elderly or sick, surgical intervention would be dangerous or inappropriate. If young women with symptomatic prolapse desire more children, a pessary is a good option to alleviate symptoms until her family is complete and she is ready for definitive surgery. Some women with slight prolapse are only symptomatic at certain times, such as when they are playing golf or tennis, and find a pessary useful to use on an as-needed basis.

Short-term pessary use is appropriate for women to make them more comfortable if a planned surgery needs to be delayed. Women with postpartum prolapse are good candidates for a pessary. Given time (and return of normal estrogen levels), the situation will likely improve. Some women are even advised to wear pessaries during pregnancy to elevate an uncomfortable, prolapsed enlarged uterus.

There are multiple types of pessaries and finding the right pessary, in the right size, is the key to success. Many women have a miserable pessary experience and feel that they were not good candidates, when it fact, the pessary was the wrong type or did not fit properly.

There are rings, rings with a rubber support (much like a diaphragm), cubes, doughnut shapes, and inflatable balls. The type of pessary is dependent on the degree of prolapse and presence of other pelvic defects, such as a cystocele or rectocele. Each type of device comes in multiple sizes. If the wrong size is used, problems such as pain, vaginal ulceration, infection, or inability to urinate or have a bowel movement can result. The pessary also won't stay where it's supposed to, or hold up the uterus, if the fit is wrong. If the pessary fits properly, complications are rare.

Fitting takes time, and before a woman leaves her doctor's office with a new pessary, it is imperative that she walk around, urinate, bear down, and then have the placement rechecked to make sure that slippage has not occurred. It's not unusual to require multiple fittings to get it right. Within one week of placement, a return visit is required in order to make sure that the pessary is not rubbing or pressing on the vaginal wall, which can cause bleeding, ulceration, and infection down the road. Sometimes, a good fit—which supports the uterus, stays in, and is comfortable—is impossible, despite multiple attempts with different shapes and sizes.

Once the correct pessary is in place, most women can be taught to take out and replace it for cleaning. Some women are unable or unwilling to do this, in which case they must return at least every three months for cleaning and examination.

Most women who are motivated to use a pessary do well and are generally satisfied with the device, at least in the short term. One study showed that approximately 50 percent of women fitted for a pessary were still using it and were satisfied sixteen months later.

Why would someone be dissatisfied? The discharge, for one. Women who are unable to clean and replace their pessary themselves frequently have a malodorous, watery discharge. Even women who are fastidious about cleaning and replacing their pessary report a chronic odor and discharge. Pessaries also interfere with intercourse for women who are sexually active. Sometimes a pessary makes incontinence *worse* due to displacement of the urethra. Most women simply find the pessary to be inconvenient and inadequate.

Fitting a pessary is often better done by an experienced (translation: older) gynecologist. A newly trained gynecologist may be great for innovative, high-tech laparoscopic or hysteroscopic procedures, but may have not had a lot of experience with good old-fashioned pessaries. If your gynecologist has only one type of pessary in his or her office, that's probably an indication that pessaries are not his or her forte.

Suspension Procedures

If pushing up from below doesn't work, there's always hoisting up from above. If something is falling down, it seems reasonable to tie it up. This is more complicated than it sounds. Through the years, multiple attempts have been made to come up with a way to surgically suspend the uterus to keep it from falling down, and ultimately out.

Today, suspension procedures (also called *uteropexies*) are rarely done, and are generally major abdominal operations in which a woman's own tissue is used to reposition the uterus. One procedure involves actually sewing the uterus to the abdominal wall. Several techniques have been described, but little long-term follow-up is available.

While uterine prolapse is not currently the most common indication for hysterectomy, it is likely to continue to contribute to a significant percentage of hysterectomies in the future due to longer life spans, active lifestyles, and an increased reluctance to take estrogen replacement.

Chapter 8

Pain and Abnormal Bleeding

Many women have bleeding and pelvic pain that result in a significant number of hysterectomies each year, unrelated to fibroids. While there are many problems that can potentially cause pelvic discomfort, there is no question that endometriosis is the culprit for the vast majority of women who suffer from chronic pelvic pain.

ENDOMETRIOSIS

Basically, endometriosis is a condition in which the endometrial tissue that normally lines the uterine cavity appears other places, such as the lining of the pelvis, fallopian tubes, ovaries, bowel, bladder, and even unusual places like the lung. Each month during menstruation, this tissue responds to hormonal changes, just like the tissue that lines the uterine cavity. Since it is not where it's supposed to be, various problems can ensue, such as scar tissue, inflammation, ovarian cysts, painful intercourse, infertility, and excruciatingly painful periods that get worse with time. The degree of pain is not necessarily related to the severity of endometriosis. Women with minimal endometriosis sometimes suffer the most.

Who Gets Endometriosis?

Any menstruating woman can have endometriosis, but it is most commonly found in women who have no children and who are between the ages of twenty-five and forty. It is estimated that approximately 7 percent of premenopausal women have endometriosis. Historically, teenage girls just weren't supposed to have endometriosis. The monthly pain that would make an otherwise healthy sixteen-year-old eat ibuprofen like candy, miss school, and crawl into bed on a Saturday, was just "bad cramps." It is now known that menstruating females of any age can have endometriosis. In fact, one study showed that 52 percent of teenage girls with severe chronic pelvic pain had surgically proven endometriosis.

There can also be a genetic predisposition for endometriosis. Women with an affected first-degree relative such as a mother or sister are at higher risk than women with no family history. Women with shorter intervals between periods and women who bleed eight days or longer are also at increased risk. Pregnancy is protective, since no menstruation, and hence no shedding of glands, occurs for months at a time.

How Do You Get Endometriosis?

There are lots of theories for how the endometrial glands get outside the uterus, but no single one explains the disease in everyone. *Retrograde menstruation*, in which some menstrual blood flows backward into the tubes and out into the pelvis instead of flowing out the vagina, is one of many possible explanations most experts accept. Most researchers in the field feel that many mechanisms are responsible rather than one explanation. Everyone agrees that it is not infectious or sexually transmitted.

How Do You Know If You Have It?

Unfortunately, the only way to know unequivocally if someone has endometriosis is to look inside and see. This is most commonly done laparoscopically. Frequently, however, endometriosis is serendipitously discovered when a woman has surgery for another reason.

Often, endometriosis is suspected on the basis of symptoms and pelvic examination, but one can never be absolutely certain without surgery, since endometriosis cannot be diagnosed on an ultrasound or X ray. Obviously, it's not appropriate for every woman with severe cramps to have surgery to determine if endometriosis is the cause. Women who probably do need a laparoscopy are women who continue to have pain despite treatment, women with persistent ovarian cysts, or women who are infertile. Women who desire surgical treatment, either conservative or definitive, should have the diagnosis confirmed before proceeding.

TREATMENT OPTIONS FOR ENDOMETRIOSIS

Most conservative treatments for endometriosis do not require definitive diagnosis. If a woman has horrible periods and painful intercourse, and endometriosis is suspected, it is perfectly reasonable to try different medical treatments for improvement. If things are no better despite treatment, a laparoscopy is appropriate.

Treatment is divided into two categories: medical and surgical. Sometimes medical and surgical treatments are combined. Choice of treatment depends on the age of the patient, the desire for pregnancy, and the severity of the symptoms.

Expectant Management

It is reasonable to do nothing in a known case of endometriosis if a woman has minimal or no symptoms and is not interested in conceiving. Typically, the patient who requires no treatment is the woman who is found to have endometriosis at the time of surgery for some other reason. However, if a young woman is found to have endometriosis and has no pain but would like to maintain fertility for pregnancy later on, expectant management is not a great idea. If her endometriosis is not suppressed, she may find that ten years later the disease has progressed to the point where not only does she have symptoms, but she is also infertile as a result of scarring and inflammation.

Another group in which expectant management is reasonable is the woman who is on the cusp of menopause. After the ovaries shut down, endometriosis almost invariably becomes quiescent.

Nonsteroidal Anti-Inflammatory Drugs (NSAIDs)

Drugs such as ibuprofen have always been useful to treat the pain associated with endometriosis, but they are usually not adequate for women with severe problems. It helps if the medication is started as soon as there is any pain, or even better, *before* there is pain. Women who have predictable periods usually start medication before bleeding starts, and get much better relief than if the pain is well established. Some women can't take NSAIDs due to gastrointestinal intolerance or kidney problems.

Oral Contraceptives

It would be nice if combination estrogen/progesterone pills were known by a name other than "birth control pills." Women who require oral contraceptives, of course, have the side benefit of preventing pregnancy, but that may not be the main issue. For many women, the contraceptive benefits are totally irrelevant.

Oral contraceptives are traditionally taken for three weeks of the month, followed by one pill-free week in which a withdrawal bleed, or period, occurs. The reason for the week off is controversial. Some say the pill was designed that way so women would feel like things were still "natural" and would be more comfortable taking it. There is also documentation that the early developers of the pill naively thought that the Catholic church would accept the pill as "natural birth control" and permit its use since it maintained normal cycles. Some say that misguided (male) scientists thought that women taking the pill would still want to get their period—to make them feel young and womanly!

However, there is no medical reason for a woman to take a week off and get her period if she is taking oral contraceptives. For many women, such as those with endometriosis, there is a significant medical benefit in *not* having a period. Some women are uncomfortable with the idea of suppressing menstruation and worry that there will be a build-up of tissue or that it is in some other way unhealthy. In reality, women on the pill have thin uterine linings that do not require monthly shedding, and it is in no way detrimental to long-term health or fertility to not get a period.

The real problem is that most insurance companies only cover twelve packs of pills a year, no matter how many polite letters explaining things (using small words) they are sent. Either they don't get it, or more likely, it is beneficial to them *not* to get it. The best way to suppress mild to moderate endometriosis is to suppress menstruation, and the best way to do it over the long term is by taking continuous oral contraceptives. One brand of pill has recently become available that is packaged, and FDA approved, to be taken continuously for three months. It is likely that other companies will follow their lead.

There are some women for whom this method is not an option. While most women feel well on the pill, some women simply don't tolerate oral contraceptives and despite multiple attempts with multiple pills continue to have problems with break-through bleeding, headaches, depression, etc. With more pills continually being developed, this is an infrequent occurrence, particularly in the motivated patient. Some women can't take oral contraceptives, such as those with a history of blood clots, smokers older than thirty-five, or women with breast cancer.

The rare woman with endometriosis who does want to get her period (a few do exist) can take oral contraceptives cyclically and get some relief, but in general, pills work better if taken continuously. The development of birth-control patches and rings expands options for the woman who finds it difficult to take a pill every day. While those newer devices have not been studied, there is no reason to think that they will not be as beneficial as pills, as long as menstruation is suppressed or minimized.

GnRH Analogues

Gonadotropin-releasing hormones (GnRH) are discussed in full in chapter 5 under treatment of fibroids. GnRH analogues were actually originally intended to be used for the treatment of endometriosis, not fibroids. Since GnRH shuts off estrogen production and suppresses menses, it causes endometrial implants, inflammation, and cysts to become inactive and regress. GnRH is not recommended for more than six months since low estrogen levels over a long period of time may result in osteoporosis. Once GnRH is stopped, endometriosis recurs.

An important role for GnRH is to suppress endometriosis before conservative surgery so that the implants are smaller and more amenable to surgical ablation. In addition, the use of GnRH is a great way to test a woman to determine the source of pain. In some women, it's not clear if chronic pelvic pain is from endometriosis or some other cause, such as interstitial cystitis or gastrointestinal disease. If a woman has complete relief of her symptoms after a few months of GnRH, that is a good indication that her problem is endometriosis and she may chose to have definitive surgery. If her pain continues with suppression of estrogen, a hysterectomy is not going to help.

Progestins

Continuous progesterones in the form of pills or injections have long been used as another way to stop menstruation and suppress endometriosis. The advantage of progestins is that they can be continued indefinitely since estrogen is not turned off, and women are not at risk for bone loss. It is also an inexpensive therapy compared to GnRH and/or surgery. The downside is that most women don't tolerate the side effects, which include unpredictable breakthrough bleeding, nausea, breast tenderness, fluid retention, and depression. If a woman doesn't have those side effects (and not every woman does), progesterone therapy is a reasonable option for symptom relief.

Danazol

Danazol (discussed in chapter 5) works great in endometriosis. Eighty percent of patients who use Danazol find relief of symptoms within two months of use. However, almost 100 percent of patients who find relief refuse to continue the medication due to the weight gain, acne, hot flashes, and mood changes. Side effects from GnRH are a walk in the park compared to how women on Danazol feel. This is not a drug to buy stock in.

Surgery

In conservative surgery, the effects of endometriosis are removed but the uterus is preserved. Definitive surgery is hysterectomy, with or without removal of the ovaries. The decision is made based on severity of symptoms, age, desire for pregnancy, and personal preference.

Conservative surgery is almost always laparoscopic and involves various methods of removing visible endometriosis and scar tissue. Burning, laser, and cutting are all used to restore pelvic anatomy, remove implants of endometriotic tissue, and resect ovarian cysts. Surgery is generally more successful if menstrual cycles have been eliminated with GnRH for a few months prior to surgery.

One of the limitations to conservative surgery is that you can only zap what you see. Endometriotic glands are always present microscopically within tissue, invisible to the naked eye, and therefore go untreated. If pregnancy does not follow surgery, suppression with continuous oral contraceptives is recommended to delay or prevent recurrence. Unfortunately, recurrence in most women is inevitable and it's not unusual for women with severe endometriosis to have three or more surgeries during their reproductive years.

Presacral Neurectomy

Presacral neurectomy is a procedure in which pain fibers that run in the pelvis are surgically cut in order to relieve pain from endometriosis. Years ago, it was a popular adjunct to conservative surgery in hopes of increasing pain relief. While pain decreased in some women, the results were not as beneficial as hoped. In addition, many women developed complications such as constipation and urinary urgency. It is rarely done now and only in extreme cases.

Laparoscopic Uterosacral Nerve Ablation (LUNA)

LUNA, like presacral neurectomy, destroys nerve fibers, but it is done laparoscopically. Less of the nerve is destroyed and the complication rate is lower. There are no well designed studies with large numbers of patients that have accurately determined how efficacious it really is; however, there are anecdotal cases of women who report significant improvement.

The role of conservative surgery is primarily for the young woman who desires preservation of fertility, the perimenopausal women who only has a few years to go, or the woman who declines hysterectomy.

Hysterectomy

Hysterectomy is appropriate if pregnancy is not desired and if debilitating symptoms persist despite medical and conservative surgical treatment. Removal of the ovaries in young women is controversial. Since endometriotic implants occur outside the uterus, removal of the uterus alone will not prevent endometriosis from persisting in the ovaries, pelvic lining, bladder, and other organs if the ovaries remain and continue to cycle. Traditionally, the recommendation for women with endometriosis is to remove the ovaries in order to assure that no residual endometriotic implants are stimulated. Estrogen replacement in the young woman is appropriate and recommended and has not been shown to cause recurrence of symptoms.

Many women are reluctant to undergo a surgical menopause, and in spite of severe endometriosis, choose to preserve their ovaries. While there will definitely be improvement of symptoms, issues related to endometriosis may still occur until natural menopause occurs. If a woman is made aware of that, preservation of ovaries is an option.

When hysterectomy is done for endometriosis, preservation of the cervix is probably not a good idea. Endometriotic glands and scarring are often present in the cervix and structures that attach the cervix to the pelvis. Painful intercourse may continue to be a problem if the cervix is preserved.

ADENOMYOSIS

Adenomyosis refers to a condition in which the uterine glands that usually line the cavity of the uterus reside in the muscle (the myometrium) of the uterine wall. This results in an enlarged uterus, softer than usual and quite tender. Painful periods and abnormal bleeding are common in women with adenomyosis, but many cases have no symptoms at all and are only discovered when the uterus is removed for another reason. The diagnosis of adenomyosis is rarely made with certainty, since the only way to be certain is to look microscopically at a uterus that has already been removed.

Adenomyosis doesn't show up on ultrasounds, X rays, or pelvic examination. You can't see it during laparoscopy or hysteroscopy since the glands are microscopic and buried in the wall of the uterus. MRI can sometimes be useful in the diagnosis, but is rarely done due to its expense.

Most physicians suspect adenomyosis in a patient who suffers from painful periods and abnormal bleeding, and has a large, soft uterus with no evidence of endometriosis or fibroids. Since the only way to diagnose it with certainty is to do a hysterectomy, it's reasonable to try less radical options first.

Treatment options for adenomyosis are essentially the same as for endometriosis. Prior to surgery, a trial of continuous oral contraceptives, or GnRH, may be beneficial. If hormonal therapy or NSAIDs don't result in adequate relief, the definitive therapy continues to be hysterectomy. Symptoms resolve with the onset of menopause, so waiting it out is always an option.

ADHESIONS

Adhesions, or scar tissue, are responsible for a myriad of problems including bowel obstruction, infertility, and in some cases, chronic pain. Most women with adhesions have no symptoms and are unaware of their presence. The only way to prevent adhesions is to avoid surgery.

Most surgeons do a number of things to prevent adhesions from forming, but it is impossible to totally prevent them. Some types of surgery are more likely to result in adhesion formation than others. One of the many advantages of laparoscopic surgery is that subsequent adhesions rarely form.

Interestingly, the way a skin incision heals is not a reflection of the way things heal on the inside. Many women with invisible abdominal scars have terrible intra-abdominal adhesions, yet someone with a poorly healed keloid scar may be perfect inside.

Once someone has adhesions, short of more surgery, very little can be done. More surgery, of course, can cause more adhesions. Sometimes it is possible to do a laparoscopic procedure to cut away painful scar tissue. Exploratory surgery can be done in women with pelvic pain from adhesions and sometimes resolves the pain, but of course, more adhesions might result. On occasion, hysterectomy may eliminate pain from adhesions, particularly if bowel is stuck to and pulling on the uterus and/or ovaries. Pelvic physical therapy, discussed as follows for women with chronic pelvic pain, can be useful in the woman with known adhesions.

CHRONIC PELVIC PAIN

Ten percent of women who go to gynecologists complain of pain that is not associated specifically with menstruation and has been present for at least six months. Twenty percent of laparoscopies are done for evaluation of chronic pelvic pain, and 12 percent of hysterectomies are done as a direct result of that diagnosis.

Most chronic pelvic pain can be attributed to endometriosis; however, a significant number of women who have pelvic pain are not suffering from a gynecologic problem, but have gastrointestinal, bladder, or other issues. Pelvic infections, irritable bowel syndrome, and interstitial cystitis all cause lower abdominal pain and can be mistaken for a gynecologic problem.

It's important to pin down the right diagnosis, since many women have hysterectomies only to find that the pain persists after surgery since the problem was not gynecologic in the first place. In addition to urologic and gastrointestinal sources, fibromyalgia and other musculoskeletal and myofascial disorders have been identified as important sources of chronic pelvic pain. The percentage of women with each diagnosis who present to doctors vary widely in different groups of women, but endometriosis fairly uniformly ends up being the most common problem. There are actually more than fifty conditions that may be responsible for chronic pain other than endometriosis, including:

- ▼ Adhesions
- ▼ Constipation
- ▼ Irritable bowel syndrome
- ▼ Ovarian cysts
- ▼ Uterine infection
- ▼ Tuberculosis of the tube
- ▼ Adenomyosis
- ▼ Fibroids
- ▼ Interstitial cystitis
- ▼ Bladder cancer
- ▼ Diverticular disease
- ▼ Fibromyositis

Frequently, no cause for the pain is identified. These are often the women who are told, "It's all in your head." While some psychiatric conditions or a history of sexual abuse are known to create pain syndromes, it is certainly not a common etiology.

Once a cause of the pain has been determined, treatment can be instituted. If no diagnosis can be found, a laparoscopy, if not already done, should be considered. The majority of women with chronic pelvic pain who undergo diagnostic laparoscopy are found to have endometriosis even if it was not originally suspected. A significant percentage of women without endometriosis have their symptoms resolve after the reassurance gotten from a normal laparoscopy.

Treatment Options

All treatments discussed for endometriosis can be considered for treatment of chronic pelvic pain that is known to be gynecologic, or suspected to be gynecologic. If pain persists despite treatment, it is important to make sure the issue is not from a urologic or gastrointestinal source. Sometimes the best way to know is to suppress things hormonally with GnRH to see if pain improves. If pain persists, a urologist or gastroenterologist should be consulted.

If the pain is clearly gynecologic and/or myofascial (a not uncommon scenario), pelvic physical therapy can be an appropriate intervention. Pelvic physical therapy is an underutilized treatment that has dramatically improved the lives of many women who suffer from chronic pelvic pain. Pelvic physical therapists are physical therapists who have done additional training in the treatment of pelvic disorders, including gynecologic, urologic, muscular, and neurologic problems. Many women are skeptical when advised to seek the help of a physical therapist for pelvic pain. Those same women usually become the greatest advocates of the treatment.

The experienced pelvic physical therapist not only treats the source of the problem, but also is integral to determining the source of the problem. She can usually differentiate myofascial pain syndromes from fibromyalgia or other issues. In performing a thorough musculoskeletal evaluation of the pelvis, spine, and hips, she will often find pelvic asymmetry and muscle imbalances in the individual with pelvic pain. For example, tight hip flexor muscles tilt the pelvis and cause tension in the pelvic floor muscles which, in turn, contribute to pelvic pain and dysfunction. Often the location of the pain is not where the pain originates. Once the source of the pain is identified, the therapist uses a number of modalities for treatment.

The information gleaned from the initial evaluation is critical in designing a comprehensive treatment plan that may include "hands-on" techniques such as myofascial release, joint mobilization, and trigger-point release. It may also include biofeedback training, electrical stimulation, therapeutic exercise, education, posture education, and body mechanics. Soft tissue work of the larger, more external pelvic muscles and tissues is helpful by itself, but it is especially useful prior to any joint mobilization techniques that may restore symmetry in the pelvis.

Manual soft tissue work and trigger-point release can be done directly on the pelvic floor muscles through the vagina. (This is definitely a "hands-on" technique!) These techniques really work to eliminate muscle spasm, improve tissue integrity via increased circulation and tissue oxygenation, and restore normal resting muscle tone and length.

Biofeedback, or neuromuscular re-education, is an excellent way to "see" what the muscles are doing. Women with chronic pain have muscles that remain tense and contracted at all times, as opposed to muscles that are able to relax completely when they are not needed. When a contraction is attempted, it should be strong and coordinated.

Biofeedback involves placing electrodes either externally or internally to register the electrical activity of the muscles so that it is clear what is going on. In this way, a woman can learn how to control pelvic floor muscle tension and recruit the muscles effectively when needed. The end result is a lot less pain.

In some women, electrical stimulation of the pelvic floor muscles and nerves, directly or indirectly, greatly reduces certain kinds of pelvic pain. While this sounds like a variation of a medieval torture, it is not in the least bit painful. Most women actually find it to be quite soothing. Occasionally, it is appropriate to inject trigger points to alleviate painful spasms. Usually a physician or anesthesiologist does this.

Unfortunately, experienced pelvic physical therapists can be difficult to find. Some major medical centers might have a pelvic therapist within the physical therapy department, particularly if there is a chronic pelvic pain center or urogynecology department. Many good gynecologists are not familiar with this area of physical therapy and thus are unable to make a referral. If your gynecologist doesn't have access to a pelvic physical therapist, contact the Section on Women's Health of the American Physical Therapy Association (www.sowh@apta.org) to find a therapist in your area.

Abnormal Bleeding

Like everything else in life, "normal" encompasses a great many variations. Normal also does not necessarily mean average. Having said that,
normal bleeding is bleeding that occurs at intervals no closer than
twenty-one days, and no further apart than thirty-five to forty days.
Normal bleeding should not result in anemia and should last between
two and seven days, requiring a pad or tampon to be changed no more
than every three to four hours. Most importantly, normal is what has
always been normal for you. If there is a deviation from your normal
bleeding pattern, particularly if persistent, there may be a problem that
is worthy of evaluation.

Anovulatory Dysfunctional Uterine Bleeding

The most common cause of abnormal bleeding in pre- or perimenopausal women is anovulation. Anovulation is just what it sounds
like—the absence of ovulation. In a normal cycle, women make estrogen, release an egg from an ovarian follicle, make progesterone, and
then get their period. Women who don't ovulate do make estrogen; they
just don't release an egg. The lining of the uterus gets stimulated with
estrogen alone and essentially bleeds at random times. Sometimes the
bleeding can be quite heavy or prolonged. It is usually totally unpredictable and women rarely have the premenstrual prodrome of breast
tenderness, premenstrual syndrome (PMS), and cramping that typically
occurs in ovulatory cycles.

Anovulatory cycles are more common in women who are under
stress, dieting, traveling, or have medical problems such as thyroid dysfunction. It is also more common in women who are in their forties,
which is one reason why fertility is diminished in that age group even if
menopause is years away. The other end of the spectrum is the adoles-
cent who is making estrogen, but hasn't yet started ovulating.

The diagnosis is often suspected in young women with irregular
cycles, and since other problems (such as uterine cancer) are rarely seen

in the under-thirty crowd, it is reasonable to treat presumptively; that is, without doing a biopsy to confirm.

Perimenopausal Dysfunctional Uterine Bleeding

Perimenopausal bleeding is generally caused by anovulatory cycles that occur during the years in which the ovaries are winding down. Again, the ovaries are secreting estrogen, but no egg is released and no progesterone is produced.

Many other conditions can potentially cause abnormal bleeding in the perimenopausal years. Therefore, it is essential to make a definitive diagnosis rather than assume that irregular or abnormal bleeding is from anovulation. Endometrial biopsy is required to assure that no pre-cancerous cells are present. Ultrasound and SIS (described in chapter 4) are useful to determine if fibroids or polyps are present since they are potentially responsible for abnormal bleeding.

Postmenopausal Bleeding

Postmenopausal bleeding is always abnormal and must be investigated. Ninety percent of postmenopausal bleeding is *not* cancer, but must be checked out nevertheless. Benign polyps, atrophic (very thin tissue) endometrial lining, fibroids, and cancer are all conditions that can cause postmenopausal bleeding.

Growths (Polyps, Fibroids)

Benign growths in the uterus are commonly responsible for abnormal bleeding. Fibroids generally cause heavy bleeding during menstruation, while bleeding from a polyp is noncyclic and unpredictable.

Polyps are benign growths that project from the surface of the uterine lining. It's not unusual for someone to have multiple polyps, or have recurrence of polyps once removed. Ten to twenty percent of women will have polyps at some point in their lives, but most do not bleed. The most common time to have polyps is in your fifties, but they can occur any time after age twenty.

While polyps originate from the uterine surface, it is not unusual for one to be on a stalk and actually emerge through the cervical opening. It's common for women who have such a polyp to have spotting after intercourse.

Postmenopausal hormone replacement and birth control pills don't seem to influence the formation of polyps and should not be discontinued just because a woman has them.

EVALUATION OF ABNORMAL BLEEDING

The most important thing, of course, is to be assured that no precancerous or cancerous cells are responsible for the bleeding. Once that is determined, the goal is to discover what *is* causing the bleeding and then decide how to best eliminate the problem. In the 1950s to 1980s, abnormal bleeding almost always resulted in dilation and curettage (D&C), which was not only done to find the cause of the bleeding, but to make it go away. Today, D&C is rarely the first step.

Pelvic Examination

This may seem obvious, but the first step in evaluation of abnormal bleeding *is* a pelvic examination by a gynecologist. Bleeding is not always from the uterus, and the site of bleeding needs to be determined before further testing is done. It's not uncommon for diagnosis to be made with no further testing needed. Cervical polyps, pregnancy, infection, or fibroids are often discovered on an initial exam and no further diagnostic tests may be needed.

Ultrasound

Imaging the uterus and ovaries is frequently the first step after pelvic examination in the evaluation of abnormal bleeding. Ultrasound identifies fibroids, large polyps, and ovarian growths. An ultrasound is also useful to measure the thickness of the uterine lining.

In a menstruating woman, the lining should be thin in the first half of the cycle (between 4 and 8 mm), and thicker in the second half (between 8 and 14 mm). Excessively thick linings may indicate hyperplasia or other abnormalities, which should then be evaluated by endometrial biopsy, particularly if the woman is over thirty-five.

Postmenopausal women, whether they take estrogen or not, should have very thin, inactive linings. Any thickness greater than 5 mm warrants furthers evaluation.

Saline-Infused Sonography (Sonohysterography)

SIS, described in detail in chapter 4, is the best way to find polyps without doing a D&C/hysteroscopy. In one study, SIS was 93 percent accurate in finding uterine polyps, as opposed to ultrasound, which only detected polyps accurately 65 percent of the time.

Normally, the uterine cavity is not well seen on ultrasound since the cavity is only a potential space. Like a balloon that is not blown up, the walls are collapsed together. In SIS, sterile saline is instilled into the uterine cavity in order to see what protrudes into the cavity. Fibroids and polyps pop into view, allowing much more accurate diagnosis than ultrasound alone. This is currently one of the most valuable, but underutilized means available to evaluate abnormal bleeding.

Endometrial Biopsy

An endometrial biopsy sounds a lot worse than it is. Although the word biopsy is used, no cutting is involved; therefore, most gynecologists prefer to refer to the procedure as endometrial sampling, or aspiration. Pipelle is the brand name for a type of catheter that is commonly used to obtain the sample, so it's not uncommon for the procedure to be referred to as a Pipelle aspiration. After a speculum is inserted in the vagina, the cervix is cleansed with antiseptic. A very thin, flexible catheter is then threaded through the cervix into the uterine cavity. Once the catheter is in the right place, a suction device is used to aspirate loose tissue from the surface of the uterine cavity while rotating the catheter.

During the procedure, most women feel mild to moderate cramping, which lasts about thirty seconds. Some women aren't even aware that a sample is being taken. Occasionally someone experiences severe pain, but that's *really* unusual. Usually the amount of discomfort is directly related to how tight the cervical canal is. Someone who has had multiple vaginal deliveries usually has a wider canal, making the procedure quick and easy. Someone who has never delivered vaginally may have a tight cervical opening, which results in a lot more cramping. Sometimes the procedure is made more difficult due to a cervix that isn't straight, or a uterus that is tilted sharply forward or backward. While anesthesia is never used, 400 to 600 mg of ibuprofen an hour before the procedure is a good idea. Most women truly have minimal discomfort, and if there is pain, it is short-lived. Most women who have had the procedure agree that it is much preferable than going through a D&C.

Tissue from the uterine sample is then sent to the lab, where a pathologist analyzes it. Basically, the goal is to make sure there are no cancerous or precancerous cells. The pathologist then describes the tissue in terms of hormonal stimulation (estrogen effect, progesterone effect, anovulatory pattern), or any benign growths, such as polyps that might appear.

One of the limitations to endometrial biopsy is that it won't detect most polyps or fibroids that will be detected on SIS or hysteroscopy. In addition, even in an appropriately done aspiration, the entire uterus is never sampled, making it possible to miss something. There are also women who can't tolerate the discomfort of an office sampling, or in whom the opening to the uterus is too narrow to admit the catheter. In other words, if the answer is not definitive, or the problem persists, a D&C is an appropriate next step.

D&C/Hysteroscopy

The ultimate way to know what's going on in the uterine cavity is to look inside and see. Hysteroscopy was designed for just that reason. Before the advent of ultrasound and office endometrial sampling, virtually every woman underwent D&C for treatment of abnormal bleeding. Up until the 1980s, a D&C was done as an inpatient procedure using general anesthesia and was intended to be treatment more than a method of diagnosis. Even at that time, there was an awareness that a D&C, while able to sample representative tissue, often missed things, including fibroids and polyps. It was the invention of fiber-optic technology that permitted visualization of the uterine cavity with a hysteroscope that enabled evaluation of the entire uterine cavity.

Currently, D&C with hysteroscopy is usually not the first line for diagnosis but may be used if ultrasound and/or endometrial biopsy is not definitive. Operative hysteroscopy, in which instruments are passed through the hysteroscope, is used for removal of fibroids and polyps. On occasion, hysteroscopy is done without a D&C, particularly when it is an office procedure for the purpose of making a diagnosis.

Dilatation is a procedure in which the cervical opening is widened using a series of graduated pencil-like dilators. The surface of the uterus is then scraped (curettage) with a rake-like metal instrument in order to obtain tissue. Today, a D&C is almost always done in conjunction with a hysteroscopy. The procedure takes place using local anesthesia, sedation, or general anesthesia, depending on personal preference and how difficult the procedure is expected to be. Situations in which D&C/hysteroscopy would be appropriate include the following:

▼ Known uterine polyp that requires removal
▼ Unsuccessful uterine biopsy (no tissue or inability to pass catheter through cervix)
▼ Patient declines office endometrial biopsy or is unable to tolerate procedure
▼ Known hyperplasia with atypia, requiring additional tissue for evaluation
▼ Mass on ultrasound or SIS that requires further evaluation.

TREATMENT OPTIONS FOR ABNORMAL BLEEDING

Treatment, of course, is dependent on the cause of the bleeding, which is why it is essential to make an accurate diagnosis. The process of evaluating the bleeding will sometimes also treat the problem, particularly if a diagnostic D&C/hysteroscopy is needed.

Hormonal Therapy

If bleeding is found to be secondary to the perimenopausal hormonal roller coaster, treatment with hormones will almost always straighten things out. In a nonsmoking woman, oral contraceptives work well. Sometimes progesterone given orally for two weeks each month will correct the problem. It's not unusual for treatment to be necessary for only a few months since things will sometimes revert to normal spontaneously. A progesterone intrauterine device (IUD) is also a useful way to supply progesterone.

When young women have anovulatory cycles, treatment depends on if she is trying to avoid or achieve pregnancy. If she is sexually active and does not want to become pregnant, oral contraceptives will generally solve the problem. If she is trying to conceive, ovulation can be induced using various fertility treatments. The sexually inactive women can be treated with birth control pills, progesterone, or if the bleeding is not severe, nothing, since normal cycles will often eventually kick in. Any women who goes three months or longer without a period (unless she is taking hormones or birth control pills) is at risk for developing hyperplasia (see chapter 9) and should talk to her gynecologist about regulating cycles.

Polypectomy

The way in which a polypectomy is done depends on the location of the polyp. If the polyp is visualized emerging through the cervical opening, it can be removed very easily in the office. There is essentially no pain other than a tugging sensation and possibly some mild cramping. If the polyp was detected on ultrasound or SIS, it can only be removed by direct visualization during a hysteroscopy. Sometimes the procedure can be done in the office but most operative hysteroscopy is done in an outpatient surgical setting with sedation and local anesthesia. Either way, the whole procedure takes about thirty minutes followed by a day or two of light bleeding. Most women return to normal activities the next day.

Endometrial Ablation

Since abnormal bleeding accounts for 30 percent of hysterectomies in the United States, and since the lining of the uterus is the source of the problem, why not just eliminate the lining, instead of getting rid of the whole uterus? That's the idea behind endometrial ablation, another alternative therapy that was first introduced in the 1980s. The endometrium lines the cavity of the uterus and is the tissue that sloughs off during normal menstruation and in abnormal bleeding. The original patients who underwent endometrial ablation were women who had failed medical treatments for heavy bleeding and required hysterectomy but were too ill to undergo surgery. The laser was the trendy surgical accessory in the 1980s, and everyone was trying to find uses for this new surgical toy. In 1981, a laser was successfully used to destroy the uterine lining, resulting in a significant decrease in bleeding. Since then, multiple methods have been developed that are much easier, safer, and less expensive than laser, but accomplish the same thing.

While there are many different ways to destroy the endometrial lining, available methods can be divided into two groups. Standard endometrial ablation techniques all use a hysterocope, the instrument inserted through the cervix to visualize the cavity of the uterus. The surgeon then uses one of a variety of devices attached to the end of the hysteroscope to cut and/or burn the lining of the uterus. The entire procedure is done under direct visualization with a camera attached to the hysteroscope so that the surgeon can watch what she's doing on a monitor.

The disadvantage of most standard techniques is that they must be done in an operating room by a gynecologist experienced and skilled at operative hysteroscopy, along with the various tools used to destroy the endometrium. Training is not widely available and many gynecologists don't have the opportunity to become adept at the procedure. Complication rates are low, but there is a small risk of uterine perforation or bleeding from the procedure.

Global techniques are newer technologies in which the entire lining of the uterus is destroyed by a device that will then burn or freeze the tissue away. Hysteroscopy is generally not used for global techniques and there is no visualization of the uterine cavity. As the procedure is simple and takes a minimal amount of training, many gynecologists are able to safely offer this option to their patients.

One of the most popular methods available is Thermachoice, a hot water balloon that is inserted into the uterine cavity through the cervix, filled with saline, then heated such that the lining of the uterus is destroyed (Fig. 8-1). The balloon must be in close contact with the uterine lining to work, so if a woman has an irregularly shaped uterus or fibroids, the treatment is ineffective (Fig. 8-2). Pain fibers are stimulated during the procedure, so anesthesia is required. The results? Recent data show that 13 percent of women who underwent the procedure never bled again, 67 percent had light periods, and 20 percent continued to have heavy bleeding.

In an attempt to correct the problem of the irregularly shaped uterus, other methods are awaiting, or have recently been granted, Food and Drug Administration (FDA) approval. Hydrothermal ablation has recently been developed in which no balloon is used, but hot water is put directly into the uterus using a hysteroscope. With cryoablation, a probe is inserted through the cervix and liquid nitrogen used to "ice" the uterus. A three-dimensional mesh has been developed that generates heat, and microwave ablation has been used in Europe. Another laser technique is on the horizon, the Elitte system, in addition to a new balloon, which uses radio-frequency waves.

What all these systems have in common is destruction of the uterine lining in an attempt to stop bleeding and avoid hysterectomy. The

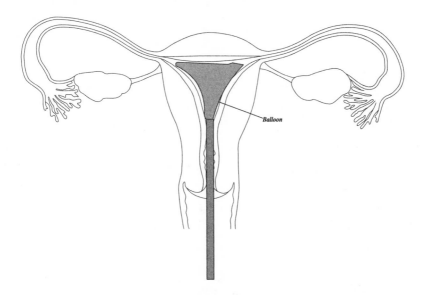

Figure 8-1. Balloon ablation system.
Figure 8-2. Unsuccessful balloon ablation due to fibroid.

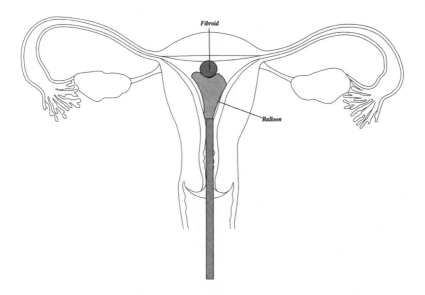

bottom line? For some women, it's a great option. However, approximately 15 percent of women who have the procedure end up with a hysterectomy anyway and there are many women who simply are not candidates for the procedures in the first place.

Who's Not a Good Candidate?

Women who desire pregnancy obviously should not destroy the lining of their uterus. The procedure is ineffective for women who are bleeding from fibroids or uterine polyps; therefore, it's advisable to have a hysteroscopy prior to an ablation to evaluate the cavity and make sure there is no other reason for bleeding. If there is *any question* as to the cause of the bleeding, the treatment should not be done. All women should have an endometrial biopsy prior to the ablation to assure there are no precancerous or cancerous cells present. If a woman desires a single definitive therapy and is not willing to have a preprocedure hysteroscopy and possible future procedures, thermal ablation is the wrong choice.

Since the procedure is easy to do and quite lucrative, many women are offered the procedure inappropriately. A typical scenario is the woman with fibroids who requests that her gynecologist try something other than a hysterectomy. She may even specifically request ablation. Her doctor complies, possibly to please the patient, hopefully not for the financial benefit of what is sure to be a failed procedure.

Who Is a Good Candidate?

A woman who bleeds heavily, has not responded to medical therapy, doesn't want to become pregnant, doesn't have fibroids or polyps, wants to keep her uterus, and is at low risk for uterine cancer is a good candidate for this procedure. Patient satisfaction in appropriate women is high and complications are low. There is virtually no recovery needed and many women feel they have nothing to lose. So what is the down side?

Why More Women Don't Have This Procedure

Many gynecologists are reluctant to advise endometrial ablation in spite of its low complication rate and easy recovery. The biggest concern on the part of gynecologists is the lack of long-term follow-up of women who have undergone ablation. Uterine cancer strikes approximately 32,000 women each year, but is frequently diagnosed at an early stage due to the presence of abnormal uterine bleeding, which prompts a uterine biopsy. Early detection ensures that the cancer is diagnosed before it has spread, when it is almost always curable.

Gynecologists are concerned that women who have had uterine ablation who then go on to develop uterine cancer later in life will not have an early warning sign since their uterus will be incapable of bleeding. Endometrial ablation doesn't increase the risk of uterine cancer, but if women do develop cancer years after the procedure, it might not be detected until a late stage, leading to a worse prognosis. Women need to be informed of that possibility, and until more information is available, decide if they want to take that risk. Many gynecologists aren't willing to take that risk and choose not to do the procedure unless there is no alternative.

Hysterectomy

Some women do end up with hysterectomies for abnormal uterine bleeding, but they almost always have other issues requiring hysterectomy, such as fibroids or prolapse. Many are unable or unwilling to use hormonal therapy. Some women have such high recurrent rates of endometrial polyps that they require yearly D&Cs and simply want definitive therapy. There are many women who prefer to avoid frequent visits, ultrasounds, and endometrial biopsies necessary for evaluation of ongoing abnormal bleeding. Other women are anxious about potential malignancy despite reassurance and elect to proceed with removal of the uterus. For the woman who requires frequent ultrasounds, endometrial sampling, hysteroscopy, and D&Cs, there is no question that the cost, both in time and money, is much higher than in the woman who has one definitive procedure.

Chapter 9

Precancerous Conditions and Cancer

F ear of cancer is a powerful motivator. Many women end up with unnecessary hysterectomies because someone has planted the idea, "Well, it *could* turn into cancer." In many of the following conditions, progression to cancer is actually extremely unlikely and treatments less radical than hysterectomy are far more appropriate.

CERVICAL DYSPLASIA

Every year, 3.5 million women get that stomach-dropping phone call or letter, "Your Pap smear is abnormal, you need to come back for further testing." Out of that 3.5 million, only 13,000 are likely to have a true cancer. The rest either will be found to have nothing wrong with their cervix, or they will have an easily treatable, precancerous condition called dysplasia.

First of all, what is a Pap smear? In 1928, Dr. George Papanicolaou (who really wanted to be a musician, but went to medical school to make his family happy) was trying to make a living in medicine. (Some things never change.) For a variety of reasons, he decided to look at his wife's cervical cells under a microscope every month to see what changes occurred. Unbelievably, she put up with this for *twenty years* and stayed married to him in a show of true love. He then reported his observations about the normal changes that take place in cervical cells. The Pap smear was born, and the rest is history. Mrs. Papanicolaou died at the age of ninety, proving that regular Pap smears prolong life.

The impact of the Pap smear on the early detection and prevention of cervical cancer is one of the most dramatic success stories in public health. In developing countries, where Pap smears are not done, cervical cancer is still the leading cause of death among women aged thirty-five to forty-five. In the United States, the rate is has been extremely low since the 1960s, when routine Pap smears were introduced.

A Pap smear is a sample of the cells from the surface and canal of the cervix, which normally grow and then slough off every few months. During a routine gynecological exam, a speculum is placed in the vagina and a sample of cells is taken with a brush or swab and placed on a slide or in a solution. The cells are then evaluated for the presence of normal growth patterns. If the cells appear abnormal, it is referred to as *dysplasia*, also known as cervical intraepithelial neoplasia, or CIN. A Pap smear only screens for cervical abnormalities and is *not* intended to be a screen for uterine or ovarian cancer.

If a Pap smear is abnormal, the next step is usually colposcopy, which is nothing more than a microscopic examination of the cervix done in the office. While a Pap smear samples random cells, colposcopy allows the gynecologist to inspect the surface of the cervix under magnification so that the abnormal area can be targeted and biopsied. This is done using a local anesthetic gel; most women are aware of a momentary pinch or cramp. The small sample of tissue removed is then sent to a pathologist, who will report one of the following:

▼ **Normal tissue.** Frequently, the cervical cells are normal, indicating that the cells have reverted back to a normal growth pattern. Occasionally, abnormal cells are present high up in the canal, beyond the view of the colposcope, which is why a follow-up, short-interval Pap smear is always done.

▼ **HPV changes.** Human papilloma virus is responsible for almost all dysplasia and cervical cancers. Sometimes cellular changes indicate the presence of the virus, but there are no actual precancerous cells. More on this below.

▼ **CIN I.** Mild dysplasia or low-grade squamous intraepithelial lesions.

▼ **CIN II.** Moderate dysplasia or high-grade squamous intraepithelial lesions.

▼ **CIN III.** Severe dysplasia or high-grade squamous intraepithelial lesions, also known as carcinoma *in situ*.

▼ **Invasive cancer.** True cancer that has infiltrated surrounding tissue and has the ability to spread.

How Do You Get Dysplasia?

Dysplasia is almost always the result of HPV infection. HPV is a sexually transmitted virus, which is why cervical cancer is considered to be a sexually transmitted disease. Before you plot your boyfriend or husband's murder, keep in mind that less common types of cervical cancers do occur that have nothing to do with HPV. Also, an HPV exposure could have occurred *years* before dysplasia shows up and may not be related to a current partner. It is also the reason why lesbians and nuns have a very low incidence of cervical cancer.

Almost all women with cancer have HPV, but most women with HPV *never* get dysplasia or cancer. HPV is extremely common; some studies show that it is present in the cervixes of almost 50 percent of sexually active women. There are over 70 subtypes of HPV; some types are more likely to progress to cancer than other subtypes. It is increasingly common to check the HPV subtype of women with abnormal Pap smears to determine their risk of progression to a more serious condition. Since the vast majority of women with HPV don't get significant dysplasia or cancer, what factors increase the risk?

High-risk HPV subtypes are more likely to progress than low-risk groups. Cigarette smoking significantly increases the risk that women will have dysplasia in the presence of HPV. Breakdown products of cigarette smoke, such as nicotine, have been found in cervical mucous and are considered to be carcinogens. A woman who is immunodeficient, such as a human immunodeficiency virus (HIV)-positive woman, is also at increased risk. There is also new data that suggests a genetic predisposition to cervical cancer.

Treatment Options

Treatment is never based on a Pap smear alone. A colposcopy is required to determine the appropriate course of action. Treatment recommendations are then determined by the extent and severity of the dysplasia.

Expectant Management

Low-grade abnormalities (CIN I) have minimal potential for progression to cancer and will almost always go away on their own. There is no need to treat a colposcopically proven CIN I lesion unless it has persisted for years or progressed to CIN II or III. In the event that a CIN I is destined to progress to cancer, it is a progression that generally takes years, not months. If someone is being watched closely, a CIN II or III generally is detected and can therefore be treated long before actual cancer occurs. The appropriate treatment of a CIN I, therefore, is repeat Pap smears at close intervals. If a Pap is persistently abnormal, repeat colposcopy is also required. Some women choose to treat a CIN I to relieve anxiety, or if follow-up is unlikely or inconvenient.

Cryotherapy

Cryotherapy is a technique in which the cervix is frozen using nitrous oxide or carbon dioxide. The frozen tissue (including the abnormal tissue) then dies and sloughs off. Cryotherapy is easy to do, costs little, and has a low complication rate. It was commonly done through the 1980s, but is now rarely done since the loop electrosurgical excision procedure (LEEP) is far superior. The downside to cryotherapy is that since tissue was not removed, it was impossible to know if all abnormal cells were treated. Patients also complained about the smelly, copious, watery discharge that lasted for up to two weeks. Recurrence rates from cryotherapy are higher than the rates seen in other treatments. Some physicians still recommend cryotherapy for low-grade dysplasia, which frankly, probably don't even need treatment.

Laser Ablation

Laser ablation had a short, popular run in the late 1980s when physicians were trying to find an alternative to cryotherapy and new uses for laser. The advantage to laser ablation done under colposcopic guidance is that it is very precise in its ability to vaporize the abnormal area while not harming healthy tissue. The disadvantage is that it is very expensive, no tissue is obtained for analysis, the procedure is potentially dangerous, and it requires significant training. It is rarely done.

Cone Biopsy

Prior to the development of LEEP, cone biopsy (or cold-knife conization) was the treatment of choice for women with dysplasia. A cone biopsy is a surgical procedure requiring general anesthesia in which a cone-shaped segment of cervix is removed using a scalpel (hence, "cold knife"). The major disadvantage to cone biopsy is the need for general anesthesia and the risk of complications such as bleeding, infection, and damage to the cervix, which might complicate future pregnancies.

Loop Electrosurgical Excision Procedure

LEEP (also known as large loop excision of the transformation zone, or LLETZ) is the treatment of choice for women with persistent mild dysplasia or moderate or severe dysplasia. LEEP procedures are almost always done in the office using local anesthesia. After inserting a speculum, the gynecologist injects anesthesia in the cervix, totally numbing the area. A wire loop that cuts and cauterizes tissue is then used to scoop out the area of the cervix that contains the abnormal cells. (Figure 9.1) No stitches are needed and the tissue heals beautifully within a few weeks. The specimen is sent to a pathologist for evaluation to determine if all the abnormal tissue has been removed.

Complications such as infection, bleeding, and damage to the cervix are possible, but occur at a much lower rate than the rate seen in cone biopsy. It is an ideal treatment since the success rate is high, yet the cost and complication rates are low. Cure rates are generally in the range of 85 to 90 percent, depending on the size of the abnormal area and the type of HPV present. In addition to treating dysplasia, LEEP is used for diagnostic purposes if the problem area can't be seen on colposcopy.

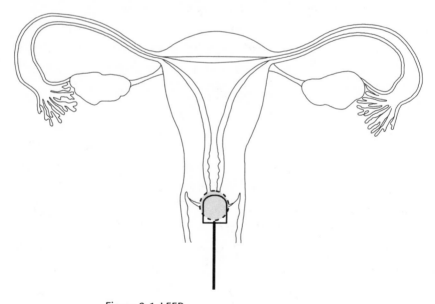

Figure 9-1. LEEP.

Vaccination

There is currently a great deal of research to implement an HPV vaccine that could theoretically wipe out the majority of future cervical cancer cases. Unfortunately, if you already have HPV, it's too late. The purpose of the vaccine is to inoculate young women before they become sexually active to prevent them from acquiring the virus.

Hysterectomy

Removal of the uterus is almost never considered as appropriate first-line treatment for cervical dysplasia. There are a few exceptions:

▼ If a woman is having a hysterectomy for another reason and also has dysplasia, then it makes sense to remove the cervix along with the rest of the uterus. A woman who has a history of moderate or severe dysplasia, even if it has been successfully treated, is not an appropriate candidate for a subtotal hysterectomy.

▼ A woman who has completed childbearing and is unwilling or unlikely to follow up after treatment of dysplasia may be better off with a hysterectomy.

▼ If a woman with CIN II or CIN III has a recurrence after LEEP and desires definitive therapy, hysterectomy is an alternative to a repeat LEEP procedure.

▼ If a woman has had two LEEPS, followed by a recurrence, and has completed her family, it's time to seriously consider hysterectomy.

▼ Very rarely, there are persistent high-grade abnormalities on the Pap smear, yet no abnormal tissue can be seen on colposcopy or in a LEEP specimen. The probability is that abnormal tissue is very high in the canal and the only way to get to it is by removing the whole uterus and cervix.

▼ Despite the fact that their dysplasia is unlikely to progress to invasive cancer, some women are terrified to the point of dysfunction due to cancer phobia. For these women, frequent surveillance is simply unacceptable. Peace of mind is worth a lot; as long as they clearly understand that hysterectomy is not their only option, it may be the right choice for them.

▼ Some women would simply prefer to have one definitive procedure rather than return to their gynecologist every three months for Pap smears, possible colposcopies, and interval treatments. As long as they understand that less radical options are safe and available, that choice is theirs to make.

▼ Hysterectomy is required if invasive cancer is detected; it is a life-saving procedure in that situation.

ENDOMETRIAL HYPERPLASIA

Endometrial hyperplasia is a condition in which the uterine lining gets excessively thick due to unopposed estrogen stimulation. This condition is most likely to occur in women who produce estrogen but don't ovulate, and therefore have no progesterone to counteract the effects of estrogen on the uterine lining. Women with hyperplasia generally have heavy bleeding, postmenopausal bleeding, or irregular bleeding, sometimes proceeded by months of no bleeding. Any women who has unopposed estrogen is at risk for hyperplasia. This includes not only women who don't ovulate, but women with polycystic ovarian syndrome, obese women, perimenopausal women, and postmenopausal women who take estrogen but no progesterone. Women who take tamoxifen for treatment or prevention of breast cancer are also at increased risk. Some women develop hyperplasia without having any risk factors.

Making the Diagnosis

An ultrasound may show an unusually thick lining, but the only way to know for sure that a women has hyperplasia is to sample the lining of the uterus by doing an endometrial biopsy, or a dilation and curettage (D&C).

There are different types of hyperplasia, and the type of hyperplasia determines the potential for uterine cancer down the road. In other words, not all hyperplasias are precancerous conditions. Hyperplasia *without* atypia means that no precancerous cells exist and the progression to uterine cancer is extremely unlikely. Hyperplasia *with* atypical cells is more serious and considered to be potentially precancerous. While treatment with medication is usually successful, 28 percent of women with atypical hyperplasia ultimately develop uterine cancer.

Treatment

Treatment options for hyperplasia are usually determined by the likelihood that cancer will develop, and personal preference.

Hyperplasia Without Atypia

Progesterones are used to treat hyperplasia by counteracting the effect of unopposed estrogen. Usually progesterone pills are given daily for three to six months. An endometrial biopsy is then repeated to make sure that the hyperplasia is gone. It's important to figure out why the hyperplasia occurred in the first place so that recurrence can be prevented. Women who don't ovulate can often be successfully treated with birth control pills or monthly progesterone. Postmenopausal women are a little trickier since theoretically, they should have very low estrogen levels. On occasion an estrogen-secreting tumor is the problem. Obese women, who make extra estrogen in fat cells, are also at risk for postmenopausal hyperplasia and are usually successfully treated with progesterone supplementation.

Hyperplasia With Atypia

Treatment of hyperplasia with atypia is a whole other matter. All women with hyperplasia with atypia should have a D&C in addition to an endometrial biopsy to assure that no cancer cells are already present. Many women, because of the significant progression rate to uterine cancer, opt for hysterectomy. If someone would like to avoid surgery, medical treatment is an option. The decision is made based on personal preference and the ability and willingness to have close surveillance. In that case, treatment consists of high-dose oral progesterone followed by a biopsy three months into treatment. Most women tolerate progesterone pretty well, but many women complain of bloating, depression, and continued irregular bleeding. Progesterone also has a negative effect on cholesterol and lipids.

While medical treatment with vigilant follow-up is an option in selected women, most gynecologists would agree that *recurrent* hyperplasia with atypia is best treated by hysterectomy. If atypia is no longer present, cyclic progesterone therapy should be continued with follow-up biopsies every six to twelve months. A postmenopausal woman who has had atypia is at high risk for recurrence of hyperplasia, and potentially, cancer.

Inability To Sample the Uterine Lining

One problem that occasionally arises is the woman with bleeding who cannot be properly evaluated and assured that her bleeding is not a manifestation of cancerous or precancerous cells. It is usually simple to do an office uterine lining sample for women who are having abnormal bleeding. If an office sample can't be done because it is too painful or technically not possible, a D&C can be performed. Very rarely, it is technically impossible to sample the lining of the uterus, even by doing a D&C. If that is the case, the only way to assure that no cancer exists is to actually remove the uterus.

GYNECOLOGIC CANCERS REQUIRING HYSTERECTOMY

While the majority of precancerous conditions do not require hysterectomy, the same cannot be said when an invasive cancer is present. Many women are reluctant to undergo a hysterectomy since they feel that treatment of their cancer may be futile and just prolong the inevitable. Nothing could be further from the truth. Early detection and improved treatment of many gynecologic cancers has resulted in dramatically reduced mortality rates. While options occasionally exist, treatment for the following gynecologic cancers is fairly standard. Almost all of these cancers are best treated with the involvement of a gynecologic oncologist, even though your general gynecologist usually makes the diagnosis.

Uterine Cancer

Uterine cancer, also known as endometrial cancer, is the most common gynecologic malignancy and the fourth most common cancer to occur in women. Most invasive uterine cancer is diagnosed in its early stages when a woman first experiences abnormal bleeding. Since it is usually diagnosed early, relatively few women die from it. Five-year survival for women diagnosed when their cancer is stage I is 96 percent.

Risk factors for uterine cancer are identical to risk factors for endometrial hyperplasia. It also occurs more commonly in women with a history of breast and/or ovarian cancer. While most cases of uterine cancer occur after menopause (the average age is sixty-one), 25 percent of cases are diagnosed in women who are premenopausal. Interestingly, women who use oral contraceptives have a significantly lower chance of developing uterine cancer (and ovarian cancer) than women who have never taken oral contraceptive pills.

Women with uterine cancer almost always have abnormal bleeding. In a premenopausal or perimenopausal woman, abnormal bleeding is anything that varies from a normal monthly flow. Heavy bleeding, constant spotting, or irregular cycles may all indicate a problem. *Any* bleeding in a postmenopausal woman should be evaluated. Keep in mind that the overwhelming majority of abnormal bleeding is not an indication of uterine cancer, but does need to be checked out.

Similar to hyperplasia, the diagnosis of uterine cancer is determined by taking a sample of tissue from the cavity of the uterus by an office endometrial biopsy or a D&C. A Pap smear may occasionally show abnormal uterine cells, but is inadequate for diagnosis. Ultrasound is also useful. Normally, the uterine lining of a postmenopausal woman is thin and inactive. If the lining on ultrasound measures thicker than 5 millimeters, a sample should be done to assure that no abnormal cells are present.

Treatment for uterine cancer is a total abdominal hysterectomy, bilateral salpingo-oophorectomy, and pelvic and para-aortic lymph node sampling. During surgery, the entire abdomen is evaluated to see if cancer is present in locations outside of the uterus. This procedure is known as *staging* and requires a midline incision that extends from the pubic bone to a few inches above the belly button in order that the liver, spleen, kidneys, and bowel can be evaluated. Ultimately, staging determines the need for further treatment. Women with early cancers usually require no further treatment beyond the hysterectomy and removal of tubes and ovaries. In more advanced cancers, postoperative radiation and/or chemotherapy is recommended. Postoperative estrogen replacement is an option for the woman with uterine cancer and most experts feel it will not influence recurrence of uterine cancer.

Ovarian Cancer

One in seventy women will develop ovarian cancer during their lifetime. This is a gynecologic cancer in which early detection is limited. While most ovarian cancers are diagnosed and treated when they have already advanced, hysterectomy can save lives.

Risk factors and detection of ovarian cancer are discussed in detail in chapter 9. Treatment of ovarian cancer is almost always total abdominal hysterectomy, with removal of both tubes and ovaries and a lymph node sampling. Like uterine cancer, staging is an essential part of the procedure and requires a midline incision to evaluate the entire abdomen. Postoperative chemotherapy is also essential to treatment.

Cervical Cancer

The plummet in invasive cervical cancer rates is one of the cancer success stories of the twentieth century. Due to detection of treatable precancerous lesions on Pap smears, the rate of cervical cancer has dropped by 75 percent so that cervical cancer currently accounts for only 1.7 percent of cancer deaths in women. Cervical cancer can occur in any sexually active age group, but is most common in women forty-five to forty-nine years of age with a rate of 16.5 per 100,000 women per year. Cervical cancer generally is asymptomatic, which is why regular Pap smears are recommended.

Treatment of invasive cervical cancer is usually a radical total abdominal hysterectomy with pelvic and para-aortic lymph node dissection. Depending on circumstances and extent of the disease, sometimes the upper part of the vagina is removed as well. Combined radiation and chemotherapy are used in some situations. Removal of the ovaries is not mandatory in young women.

Fallopian Tube Cancer

Fallopian tube cancer is extremely rare, representing only 0.2 percent of gynecologic malignancies. Since it only occurs in 3.6 out of a million women per year, most gynecologists never see a case during their entire careers.

Fallopian tube cancer acts like ovarian cancer in many ways. Most women are asymptomatic until it has progressed to a late stage, accounting for a poor overall prognosis. The treatment is the same as for ovarian cancer: total abdominal hysterectomy, bilateral salpingo-oophorectomy, and pelvic and para-aortic lymph node dissection followed by chemotherapy.

OTHER GYNECOLOGIC CANCERS

Vulvar Cancer

Vulvar cancer is the fourth most common gynecologic malignancy, comprising 4 percent of gynecologic malignancies. The mean age of the woman with vulvar cancer is sixty-five years old. It accounts for 800 deaths per year. Most vulvar cancer manifests itself as a vulvar lesion that doesn't go away. Frequently the skin involved is very itchy. Any suspicious sore or patch of skin should be biopsied.

Treatment of vulvar cancer does not involve hysterectomy. Surgical resection of the vulva and radiation are the standard treatments.

Vaginal Cancer

Vaginal cancer comprises 2 percent of gynecologic malignancies and occurs in 1/100,000 women per year, with a mean age of sixty. Most women experience vaginal bleeding. Vaginal cancer is also diagnosed when an abnormality is seen by the gynecologist or detected on a Pap smear. Vaginal cancer is one of the reasons why you should continue annual visits with your gynecologist even after you have had a hysterectomy.

The location in the vagina, age of the patient, and other factors determine optimal treatment, which involves either radiation or radical total abdominal hysterectomy, lymph node dissection, and removal of at least the upper part of the vagina. Removal of the ovaries is not necessarily required if vaginal cancer occurs in a young woman.

Part III

Surgery and Recovery

Chapter 10

Abdominal Hysterectomy

Abdominal hysterectomy results in the longest recovery time and has the most potential for postoperative complications. It is also the most common route of hysterectomy in the United States, accounting for 70 percent of hysterectomies performed. The fact that a hysterectomy is done through an abdominal incision does not tell you exactly *what* is being removed, just *how* it was removed. A scar on the abdomen has the same appearance whether the hysterectomy is total, subtotal, or includes the tubes and ovaries.

The decision to proceed with an abdominal route, rather than vaginal or laparoscopic, depends on two basic questions: what exactly needs to be accomplished, and is an abdominal incision the safest way to do it?

ADVANTAGES OF AN ABDOMINAL INCISION

An abdominal incision gives the surgeon the most flexibility and the best "hands on" ability of any other approach. While an expert laparoscopic surgeon can generally see the entire contents of the pelvis and upper abdomen, sometimes visibility is greatly limited by scar tissue or a very large uterus. Often scar tissue can be safely dealt with laparoscopically, but sometimes there is no substitute for using your hands to facilitate surgery. It is only through an abdominal incision that the surgeon has this option.

There is another advantage to an abdominal hysterectomy that should never be underestimated. Because abdominal hysterectomy is the most common type of hysterectomy done, it is also the hysterectomy with which gynecologists have the most experience. It is a procedure in which virtually every gynecologist is trained and is expert at performing. While there are many gynecologists who may have had limited experience with newer, minimally invasive techniques, such as laparoscopic subtotal or laparoscopic assisted vaginal hysterectomy, you can be certain that *every* board-certified gynecologist is more than capable of doing an abdominal hysterectomy. There is a lot to be said for having an operation that your surgeon is really good at.

DISADVANTAGES OF AN ABDOMINAL INCISION

The main disadvantage to an abdominal incision, compared with a laparoscopic or vaginal approach, is the increase in recovery time and pain. It usually takes about two weeks until the discomfort of the incision is minimal, and a full four to six weeks until there is no awareness that something was done.

Some potential complications of hysterectomy, such as wound infection, can only occur if an abdominal incision is made. Other problems, such as postoperative adhesion formation, can occur with any type of hysterectomy but are more common with an abdominal approach.

TYPES OF ABDOMINAL INCISIONS

There are three types of skin incisions that are used for abdominal hysterectomy. Multiple factors affect the surgeon's decision to use a midline, Pfannenstiel, or Maylard approach. Ultimately, the choice depends on which incision allows the surgeon to accomplish the procedure most easily, yet optimize safety, recovery time, and a good cosmetic result.

Midline Incisions

A midline incision is a vertical cut that begins just above the pubic bone and continues until just below the belly button (Fig. 10-1). In some situations, it may even go around and continue above the belly button. Contrary to popular belief, the muscle is not cut; it is simply separated where it naturally splits. At the completion of the surgery, normal muscular anatomy is restored.

The major advantage to a midline incision is that the surgeon has maximal ability to see everything in both the upper and lower parts of the abdomen and pelvis. This is particularly important if surgery is for treatment of cancer, but can sometimes be necessary in benign situations as well. It's also the fastest incision to make; this becomes crucial if the surgery occurs in an emergency situation where there is rapid blood loss and minutes count. The most common emergency scenario is during a postpartum hemorrhage requiring an emergent hysterectomy. The cosmetic result becomes secondary when there is a life-threatening situation.

If a woman is known to have a very large uterus and severe adhesions from endometriosis or prior surgery, a midline approach is the best way to reduce her risk of complication. A generous vertical midline incision can significantly decrease injury to surrounding structures. There will be less blood loss, a shorter operating time, and in short, a difficult surgery will go a whole lot better.

The major disadvantage to a midline incision is the cosmetic

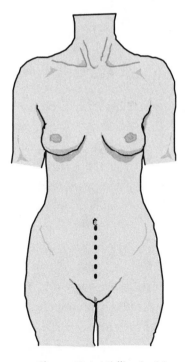

Figure 10-1. Midline incision.

result. The scar does not bother some women, but many women are upset at the daily reminder of their operation and also feel that it gives nosy locker room acquaintances a reason to ask questions. The appearance is variable. Some women end up with a raised, wide, clearly visible scar running the length of their belly; others have a thin, barely discernable line. The outcome has less to do with the technique your surgeon uses than your skin type, weight, and luck.

There is also no question that a midline scar takes a little longer to heal and hurts more than a horizontal incision. In addition, there is a higher risk of wound separation and hernia formation down the road. The placement also makes it difficult to breathe deeply and cough after surgery, resulting in a greater propensity for postoperative pneumonia and respiratory problems.

Few surgeons make a midline incision without a reason for doing so. If your surgeon recommends a midline rather than a bikini incision, it is usually in your best interest. In most cases, the added exposure decreases your risk of serious problems, a far more important factor than any cosmetic or healing problems that are created.

Pfannenstiel Incisions

Pfannenstiel (pronounced fan-in-steel) is the most frequent incision used for hysterectomy and is commonly known as a transverse, or bikini incision (Fig. 10-2). A Pfannenstiel incision is made in a horizontal, semi-elliptical manner approximately one inch above the pubic bone and can be anywhere from five to eight inches in length. Once through the skin, the muscle is separated, not cut, and the pelvic contents are then visible.

The major advantage to a Pfannenstiel incision is the great cosmetic result. It is not unusual for a healed Pfannenstiel scar to be virtually invisible, particularly if it is placed in a natural skin fold. Of all the abdominal incisions, the Pfannenstiel results in the least amount of postoperative pain and heals incredibly quickly since there is minimal tension or pulling on the edges. Most reports also show a lower rate of postoperative adhesion formation than with other types of incisions.

The major disadvantage is the surgeon's limited exposure. Since the incision is low, there is virtually no access to the upper abdomen. That means that the surgeon is unable to see the liver, gallbladder, majority of the bowel, or lymph nodes. If someone is known, or suspected, to have cancer, a Pfannenstiel incision is usually inadequate to explore the entire abdomen and do appropriate staging and lymph node dissection. It also may be inade-

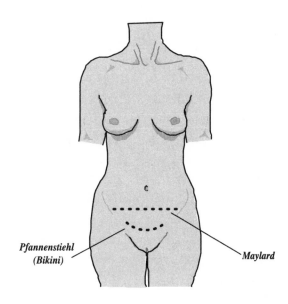

Figure 10-2. Pfannenstiel incision.

quate if someone is known to have adhesions from prior surgery or has a very large uterus. The surgeon must be able not only to see the uterus and ovaries, but other structures as well, such as the ureters and blood supply to the uterus. Sometimes a Pfannenstiel incision just isn't adequate to give the necessary exposure.

The majority of hysterectomies done for benign disease in a woman who does not have adhesions can be done safely through a Pfannenstiel. If your surgeon is planning a vertical incision, it is perfectly appropriate to ask why. The only response that is not acceptable is, "That's the way I always do it."

Maylard Incisions

Maylard incisions are infrequently done, yet in many ways offer the best features of both the vertical midline and Pfannenstiel. A Maylard is a horizontal incision, done anywhere from two to four inches above the pubic bone. The abdominal (rectus) muscle is then cut prior to entering the abdomen. The cosmetic result is similar to the Pfannenstiel incision, but the exposure is significantly greater. While the surgeon isn't able to see the upper abdomen as well as with a midline incision, the view is vastly greater than with a small, low bikini scar. Some oncologists will even use a Maylard incision for cancer surgeries, particularly if the woman is thin.

The disadvantage? It takes a little longer to do, but the time is well spent if it makes the rest of the operation quicker and easier. While cutting the muscle sounds bad, the cut edges heal together beautifully and abdominal muscle strength is not compromised. Healing time is a little longer than with a Pfannenstiel, but shorter than with a large midline incision.

Frequently, a Pfannenstiel is converted to a Maylard. In that case, a low, elliptical skin incision is made. If exposure is inadequate, the surgeon may decide to cut the muscle to see well. Strictly speaking, it is not a true Maylard since the initial incision is low, but it is a way to improve exposure.

Two Incisions?

Very rarely, a surgeon starts with a Pfannenstiel incision for what is presumed to be a simple benign case. If unsuspected cancer is encountered, it is then necessary to make a second vertical incision in order to do appropriate lymph node sampling and a more extensive cancer surgery. While a T incision takes longer to heal, there are times when it can't be avoided.

Situations in Which an Abdominal Incision Is Always Necessary

Known Invasive Cancer

Most cancer surgeons require an incision in order to remove the cancerous tissue and evaluate the pelvic and abdominal contents for the possible spread of cancer. In general, lymph node sampling, a required part of evaluating cancer, can only be done through a generous vertical incision. In addition, the surgeon must feel the bowel, liver, and other structures in order to detect the presence of cancer that might have spread to other organs, making a laparoscopic approach inadequate. A few oncologists are starting to do some early-stage cancers laparoscopically, but that is certainly not the standard of care.

Fortunately, cancer is usually not a surprise. Uterine cancer is almost always diagnosed prior to a hysterectomy, based on endometrial biopsy. Invasive cervical cancer is usually diagnosed after an abnormal Pap smear, which leads to a cervical biopsy. Ovarian biopsies are generally not performed prior to hysterectomy, but the diagnosis is almost a certainty based on an elevated CA125 level (see chapter 21) and ultrasound findings. In cases of known or suspected cancer, an abdominal hysterectomy is virtually always required.

Aborted Laparoscopic or Vaginal Procedure

Any procedure that starts out laparoscopically or vaginally has the potential to be converted to an open abdominal case if it is not safe to continue the surgery by the planned route. Sometimes this is determined at the onset of a procedure after looking through the scope and realizing that a laparoscopic approach just isn't going to work. Sometimes the surgeon will start to operate laparoscopically or vaginally and at some point realize that the exposure is limited, there is bleeding that can't be controlled, or the adhesions are too thick. Your surgeon knows that you prefer the less invasive approach and does not make the decision to switch to an abdominal incision casually. Any time a surgeon chooses to convert to an abdominal procedure it will be in your best interest, and with your safety in mind. All operating rooms are prepared for that possibility, have appropriate instruments available, and can convert to an open abdominal set-up in a matter of minutes.

Emergency Surgery

A true emergency hysterectomy (see chapter 3) must be done through an abdominal incision. When someone is rapidly losing blood, the quickest way is the best way and that is almost never laparoscopically or vaginally.

Bleeding from an Unknown Source

The most common situation in which the source of bleeding is unknown is when a woman arrives in the emergency room in shock with a belly full of blood. It could be a ruptured ectopic pregnancy, ruptured uterus, vascular injury . . . the list goes on and on. In that scenario, the quickest way to find out where the bleeding is from and, more important, to stop the bleeding, is to make a quick vertical midline abdominal incision. To do otherwise is inappropriate and potentially dangerous.

Abdominoplasty

If someone desires an abdominoplasty (see chapter 22), it makes no sense to avoid an abdominal incision since the plastic surgeon will be making one anyway. The typical incision for hysterectomy is low and no more than eight inches long. The scar from an abdominoplasty (tummy tuck) is higher and much longer, extending from hipbone to hipbone.

SITUATIONS IN WHICH AN ABDOMINAL INCISION IS OFTEN NECESSARY

Large Uterus

A uterus that is up to or higher than a belly button is usually a uterus that needs to come out through an abdominal incision. Even if you could get the laparoscope in without skewering the uterus, there needs to be some working space inside the abdomen around the end of the laparoscope. It's simply not technically feasible to do a laparoscopic hysterectomy with a uterus that fills the entire pelvis. (See chapter 12.)

Why not a vaginal hysterectomy? After all, if a nine-pound baby can squeeze through a vagina, why not a large uterus? The difference is that the surgeon needs to be able to see, identify, and tie off uterine arteries before pulling a uterus out of a vagina. The process and mechanics are different, and it simply cannot be done.

Adhesions from Prior Infection, Endometriosis, or Surgery

Many adhesions can be cut through a laparoscope. Sometimes adhesions are so thick that it is impossible to visualize what is being cut along with the adhesion. Rather than chance inadvertently cutting bowel, bladder, ureter, or other structures, an abdominal approach is sometimes the safer way to go. Sometimes that can be anticipated prior to surgery, particularly if someone has had surgery before. Sometimes a low-risk patient is unexpectedly found to have a massive amount of scar tissue from unknown endometriosis or a prior infection at the beginning of a laparoscopic procedure and the operation must be converted to a traditional abdominal incision.

SITUATIONS IN WHICH AN ABDOMINAL INCISION IS RARELY NECESSARY

Chapters 11 and 12 discuss vaginal, laparoscopic, and laparoscopically assisted vaginal hysterectomy and illustrate scenarios in which those approaches are appropriate alternatives to abdominal hysterectomy. In general, assuming a surgeon is skilled in laparoscopic and/or vaginal surgery, an abdominal approach is usually not necessary if hysterectomy is being done for a noncancerous condition, with a small uterus and minimal adhesions.

RECOVERING FROM UNCOMPLICATED ABDOMINAL SURGERY

When Do We Eat?

Most people are aware that no one gets to eat right after abdominal surgery. The real question is, why not? The inability to tolerate food after surgery (otherwise known as throwing everything up that hits your stomach) is due to your bowel function having come to a complete standstill. This occurs as a result of general anesthesia and bowel manipulation, causing your intestines to become inactive and unable to process food.

During the course of normal abdominal surgery the bowel is sometimes pushed, prodded, squeezed, and packed away. If bowel is stuck to your uterus or other pelvic structures, additional manipulation is needed to safely separate it from where the surgery is occurring. All this handling of the bowel results in its shutting down for a few hours, or sometimes a few days. Once your bowel kicks in, it is usually safe to eat without getting nauseated and vomiting.

You'll know your bowel is functioning because you will start passing flatus, your stomach will make gurgling noises, and most important, you'll feel really hungry, as opposed to thirsty. There's a reason why every medical person who walks in your room listens to your abdomen with a stethoscope as if they expect to hear something really interesting and seems obsessed with your ability to pass flatus. While it's tempting to eat before your gastrointestinal system is ready, it might be a big mistake. Most people would agree that it's really unpleasant to throw up. Vomiting with a fresh abdominal incision is even more unpleasant.

There is now data that suggest that *early* introduction of liquids actually helps the bowel kick into action and that delaying feeding actually prolongs the whole process. Pretty much everyone agrees that solids should be held until liquids are tolerated.

Factors that slow down the return of bowel function include longer anesthesia time, increased bowel manipulation, and difficult surgery. Women who have epidural anesthesia usually have quicker restoration of bowel function.

Most patients who have a laparoscopic or vaginal procedure are able to eat within twenty-four hours. An abdominal hysterectomy, particularly if it was lengthy, complicated, or for treatment of cancer, usually results in the longest delay in return of bowel function and typically lasts anywhere from twenty-four to seventy-two hours. Usually liquids are tried first, since they go down (and come up) easier. Considering the quality of hospital food, it's surprising that patients are so anxious to eat, but if someone is hungry enough, even Jell-O and broth for breakfast seem gourmet.

Postoperative Pain

There is no question that the pain after abdominal hysterectomy is greater than the pain after vaginal or laparoscopic hysterectomy. That doesn't mean that the pain is terrible, it just means that there is more of it and it lasts a little longer. Typically, women have pain during the first twenty-four hours, which requires (and responds to) a narcotic. By the second day, it's not unusual to only need an occasional pain pill or even a non-narcotic NSAID such as ibuprofen. Most women describe the pain as minimal by the second day after surgery, with a significant number of patients taking no pain medication at all.

Factors that result in more severe pain would include a bigger incision, a midline incision, smoking (because of the coughing), and slow return of bowel function, resulting in abdominal distention.

Most women are surprised at how little pain they actually have and how manageable it is. Pain control has come a long way in the last ten years.

Staples Versus Stitches

Years ago, all incisions were closed using multiple black threads made out of silk. Those stitches were then removed prior to going home from the hospital or at a return visit. While that is still the case in some circumstances, usually the skin edges are closed using either staples or a subcuticular closure.

A subcuticular closure is a method in which one continuous very thin thread is placed just under the skin layer. The suture used for this closure absorbs over time and is not removed. The stitches are all below the skin and can't be seen except for a thread (which eventually falls off) coming out of the end of the scar.

In the 1980s, stainless steel surgical staples became popular and are now the most common skin closure used. The advantage to staples is that they can be placed very quickly, reducing surgery time and anesthesia time by ten to fifteen minutes.

One slight disadvantage to staples is that they need to be removed. In actuality, it is a disadvantage that only affects the surgeon since it is the surgeon who needs to take the time to remove the staples. Generally, there is no pain involved in staple removal since they literally lift up and out with a staple remover. The prongs are not turned under like paper staples and removal takes about five minutes. Don't panic if they send the brand new medical student to remove your staples. It really is simple, and is something the greenest of students can easily handle.

The big debate is if the scar from staples is as nice as the scar from a subcuticular closure. While some might disagree, most surgeons feel that the ultimate result is exactly the same. There is generally agreement, however, that a subcuticular closure might have a slightly higher risk of infection. This occurs because a subcuticular closure seals the incision much more tightly than staples, sealing any drainage (and bacteria) below the skin. In addition, the tightly sealed skin might obscure early signs of infection or seroma, resulting in later treatment and a longer recovery time.

In thin women at low risk for wound complications, a subcuticular closure is a reasonable choice, but the true advantage is probably minimal other than that many patients seem to prefer it. The fact that staples are stronger than suture is irrelevant. The skin closure provides no strength to the incision; it is simply a way of bringing the skin edges together so it will look nice down the road. The stitches in the fascia (the layer beneath the skin and fat) are what hold you together, and that is always done with a thick, strong suture material.

Whether you have staples or stitches, you will likely have multiple short pieces of tape, commonly known as Steri-Strips, placed across your incision. You can usually remove them yourself five to six days after surgery unless you are given other instructions. Residual gummy adhesive can be removed with a cotton ball soaked in nail polish remover.

What Is Normal Incision Healing?

The bandages are usually removed from the incision the morning after surgery. Don't be surprised if there's a little blood on the dressing. There is no tape over the incision itself, just around the sides, so it will not pull or be painful when the bandages come off. Don't be afraid to look . . . it really won't be scary. You will see either a row of little staples, or a row of little pieces of tape. Nothing will be open or bloody.

After the dressing is removed, a light bandage or dressing is usually placed over the incision, which does nothing but prevent sheets and clothes from irritating it. A sterile dressing is not necessary. In fact, many women find that placing a sanitary pad over the incision and sticking it on their underwear works really well. Many women prefer to have nothing at all on the incision, and that's fine.

Obviously, there is a wide range of normal healing. Most women are relieved to hear that the skin from the incision completely closes within a couple of days. Puffiness around the incision for a few weeks is not unusual and is considered to be normal unless there are hard, tender red areas. If that is the case, an infection may be brewing and you should notify your physician.

Numbness around the incision can last for months and results from small nerves getting cut. Occasionally, someone will have a numb patch for years, or even permanently, but that's pretty unusual.

A slight drainage of clear or blood-tinged fluid is not unusual for a day or two. Drainage is not normal after the first couple of days and should definitely prompt a phone call. It is not always indicative of a problem, but if a problem exists, it's much better to catch it early.

The ultimate appearance of the scar has less to do with what your surgeon or you do than what you are genetically destined to have. The same technique and wound care can result in an invisible scar in one woman and a thick keloid scar in another. It is also important to realize that the way the skin scar forms is not an indication of the way things heal on the inside. You can have an invisible skin scar with massive internal adhesions, or a cosmetically terrible scar with perfect healing below the skin.

Your New Best Friend

A small pillow should go wherever you go the first few days after surgery, and it's not for your head. Whenever you cough, laugh, sneeze, or move, it really helps to place the pillow firmly over your incision. It decreases pain and the sensation that you are going to fall apart. (You won't, it sometimes just feels that way.)

ODDS AND ENDS

What About That Old Scar?

Often, someone has a scar from a prior abdominal surgery. Since the old scar won't go away, it makes sense to use it again since the cosmetic result will be the same. If the old scar was crooked or wide, this is an opportunity to improve what was there before since an old scar can be removed or revised.

If a prior scar is very thin, it will not be removed. The surgeon will simply use the exact same incision line. On the other hand, just because you have an old scar doesn't mean you *must* have an abdominal procedure, or that the same type of incision must be done. Women with prior abdominal surgeries are often good candidates for laparoscopic or vaginal procedures. Women who have an old midline scar can have a bikini scar if they don't mind having two scars on their belly and they prefer a different incision the second time. Keep in mind that there is usually less pain when someone has an incision through an old scar rather than in a new area since some of the original nerve fibers never regenerated. In other words, a second midline incision won't hurt as much as it did the first time.

Anesthetic Concerns

One of the limitations to laparoscopic surgery is the requirement for general anesthesia. An advantage to an abdominal incision is that regional anesthesia is sometimes an option. For women with a fear of going to sleep, this is a major plus on the side of abdominal hysterectomy over a laparoscopic approach. Chapter 14 goes through the details.

Drains

Drains are flexible, narrow tubes that come out through small openings next to the incision. They are usually attached to a suction bulb, which pulls excess fluid out. The purpose of drains is to prevent fluid collection and decrease infection. Drains are not routinely placed during abdominal hysterectomy, but may be done if someone is obese or has had more extensive surgery due to cancer or bladder procedures. Drains are almost always placed if an abdominoplasty (tummy tuck) is done.

While the idea of a drain is scary, it really is a minor inconvenience. Determining where to put the drain when you put your clothes on may take some creativity and a few safety pins. Sometimes the drain is only in for a couple of days. If a drain needs to remain beyond the hospital stay, it can easily be dealt with at home. Removal is painless and takes about five seconds. The small skin incision where the drain has been placed closes within a few days and is usually invisible within weeks.

Staying in the Bikini Line

Okay, it's vanity time. If you are in the 2 percent of the population that considers a tiny bikini as part of your public wardrobe, and if you are worried that your scar might show, put your worries aside. Visit a tanning booth prior to your surgery, wearing your bikini. Arrive at the hospital with a great tan and then request that your surgeon stay within those tan lines. This is a relatively rare request, but it's nice to know it's an option for those so inclined.

Complications of Abdominal Surgery

Complications of hysterectomy are discussed in detail in chapter 18. Complications that are unique or much more likely to occur after an abdominal hysterectomy than after other types of hysterectomy would include wound infection, seromas, hematomas, adhesion formation, ileus, and wound dehiscence.

A Word to the Wise

Ultimately, the decision to do an abdominal procedure rather than a less invasive procedure will lie with your surgeon, not you. If your surgeon tells you that he or she never offers vaginal or laparoscopic surgery in any situation, it most likely means that your surgeon does not do a high volume of gynecologic surgery. If it is not an emergency and you are able to get a second opinion, this is a good idea. If there is no time or no choice, don't try and talk him into doing a procedure that he doesn't want to do, or you'll really have a long recovery.

If your surgeon is experienced and routinely performs laparoscopic, vaginal, and abdominal hysterectomies, but feels that an abdominal hysterectomy is in your best interest, it probably is. If you get enough opinions, you will eventually find someone who agrees to do it another way, frequently resulting in a complication, or a procedure that starts laparoscopically and ends abdominally.

Chapter 11

Vaginal Hysterectomy and Treatment of Urinary Incontinence

Y ou don't hear much about vaginal hysterectomy anymore, which is interesting because it was the first, and for a long time the only, way a hysterectomy could be done. The first reputed vaginal hysterectomy was thought to have occurred in the second century A.D. when Soranus of Ephesus solved the problem of a uterus that had prolapsed out of a vagina by simply cutting it off. A few brave surgeons tried the operation during the early 1800s and a few hardy women even survived. It wasn't until the late 1800s that advances in surgical techniques resulted in decreased mortality so that the procedure could be refined. By the 1900s, vaginal hysterectomy was a standard operation for women who suffered from prolapse and other gynecological problems.

Today, vaginal hysterectomy is rapidly becoming a lost art. This route of hysterectomy is performed relatively infrequently and accounts for less than 30 percent of total hysterectomies. Part of the reason for the decline is the replacement of some vaginal hysterectomies by laparoscopic or laparoscopically assisted hysterectomies. While these newer techniques certainly offer a number of advantages, the pure vaginal hysterectomy is still a procedure that has its place in modern gynecology. For many women, a vaginal hysterectomy should be considered as not only a viable, but perhaps, the best option.

How It's Done

The simple explanation is that the uterus is removed through the vagina. Of course, there's more to it than that. Vaginal hysterectomy is one of the hardest operations to describe and medical students are frequently told, "You just have to see it." Through a series of steps, the uterus is dissected away from adjacent structures and each connection is severed until the uterus is completely outside the vagina. The back of the vagina is then sewn shut. The entire procedure is done through the vagina and there are no abdominal incisions.

It seems that in the case of prolapse, it would be a simple operation, and usually it is. Sometimes, however, in cases of severe prolapse, the dropped uterus has also pulled down the bladder and/or ureters and distorted the normal anatomy so that there is an increased risk of injury to surrounding structures. In experienced hands, this is rarely a problem, and in fact only occurs in 1 percent of cases.

Advantages of Vaginal Hysterectomy

Look Ma, No Incision!

The obvious major advantage to vaginal hysterectomy is that there is no abdominal incision. No abdominal incision translates into shorter recovery time, less pain, and a better cosmetic result. Women are able to eat sooner and move better. In addition, there is no chance of wound complications, such as infection or separation. This is particularly important in obese women. The risk of postoperative adhesions is also minimal. Overall, complication rates from vaginal hysterectomy are significantly lower than seen in abdominal or laparoscopic hysterectomy.

Combines Well with Other Vaginal Procedures

Vaginal hysterectomy is the ideal time to correct a cystocele, rectocele, or other structural defect from weakened tissue (see chapter 7). In fact, almost half of the vaginal hysterectomies are done to correct pelvic relaxation issues that have resulted in uterine prolapse, a dropped bladder, or a bulging rectum. Women who suffer from prolapse, cystocele, and rectocele also frequently have problems with bladder control. Therefore, vaginal hysterectomy is often combined with procedures to correct urinary incontinence.

Correction of Urinary Incontinence

Urinary incontinence is the inappropriate loss of urine and can be divided into several categories. Careful preoperative evaluation of incontinence is critical to a good surgical result. Not all types of incontinence respond to surgical treatment, which is why many women who were incontinent before their surgery remain incontinent after their surgery. Sometimes surgery can even make it worse. That is why it is so important to determine the type of incontinence before a treatment plan or surgery is initiated. In women, the majority of incontinence is in one of three categories.

Stress incontinence is the loss of urine with coughing, sneezing, laughing, or anything that increases abdominal pressure. This is the incontinence that makes you grab your crotch when you cough. This is the incontinence that prevents you from playing tennis without at least considering wearing Depends. The problem in stress incontinence is that the bladder sphincter doesn't stay closed to prevent urine from exiting the bladder. This is caused by weakness of the tissues that support the bladder and urethra, allowing the urethra to drop into an abnormal position, so that it is unable to function properly. This type of incontinence almost always occurs as a result of pregnancy.

Urge incontinence, or overactive bladder, is a sudden, irresistible urge to void. In urge incontinence, the bladder muscles contract when they should not. The woman with urge incontinence is fine until she puts her key in the door. If she is lucky, the door will open, she won't drop her packages, and she will make it to the toilet and get her pants down within the next four seconds.

Usually, the cause of urge incontinence is not known but is attributed to age-related changes in the urinary tract or bladder irritation from infection, cancer, or inflammation. Urge incontinence can also be caused by neurologic problems, such as stroke or multiple sclerosis.

It is not unusual to have elements of both stress incontinence and urge incontinence, otherwise known as the third category—*mixed incontinence*. Successful treatment depends on treating the major component, and in some cases, both components.

Once the type of incontinence has been established, treatment options can be explored. The first step in the treatment of stress incontinence is an attempt to strengthen and train those muscles that support the urethra and bladder. This can be done using biofeedback or bladder training techniques. Kegel exercises have traditionally been recommended to strengthen muscles and improve the ability to hold urine. They rarely work in the woman with severe incontinence, but there can be some improvement in highly motivated women who do the exercises properly and consistently. Weighted vaginal cones and electrical stimulation devices have been found to be useful in training muscles to contract properly. An experienced pelvic therapist is instrumental in the success of pelvic muscle strengthening techniques. This is discussed further in chapter 7.

Surgery is usually the best option for women with pure stress incontinence, particularly in the woman who is planning a hysterectomy for other reasons. The surgical method depends on what defect is causing the problem, and what other procedures may be necessary at the same time. All incontinence surgeries attempt to correct inadequate urethral support. The basic problem is weakened tissue, which has caused the urethra to drop. The goal of surgery, therefore, is to put the urethra back in its proper position and hold it in place using a sling made from the woman's own tissue or synthetic tissue. There is always the chance that the urethra will "fall" again, but most repairs last a minimum of ten to twelve years, sometimes significantly longer.

A woman scheduled for a vaginal hysterectomy is an ideal candidate for a sling procedure. There are many different options, but all use various methods to create a hammock to lift and support the urethra. One of the most commonly done sling procedures is known as a TVT (tension-free vaginal tape) procedure and can be done with or without a vaginal hysterectomy. The surgery is done vaginally but requires two tiny abdominal incisions near the pubic bone. While long-term studies are pending, the cure rate is over 90 percent, the complication rate very low, and the recovery short. TVT procedures are considered to be the best first surgery to do for the woman with stress incontinence.

In the event that someone is having an abdominal or laparoscopic procedure, other procedures more compatible to those routes can be chosen. A Burch suspension is done by placing stitches in the tissue next to the urethra to lift it into its proper position. It is usually done through an abdominal incision, but can also be done laparoscopically. The cure rate is 80 to 90 percent, but long-term data is lacking for the laparoscopic approach.

The Marshall-Marchetti-Krantz procedure is similar to the Burch, but involves putting stitches through the pubic bone. It is done abdominally, but is now rarely performed since the Burch is felt to be the superior open procedure.

In contrast, the treatment of urge incontinence is *never* surgical, unless there is also a component of stress incontinence. Treatment strategies that are highly successful include behavior modification, biofeedback, and pelvic physical therapy. There are also a wide range of commonly prescribed drugs that are beneficial in many circumstances.

PERINEOPLASTY

In addition to pelvic relaxation issues, the opening of the vagina can become distorted and lax due to trauma from childbirth. Episiotomies are less frequently done, and are generally felt to be unnecessary as a routine procedure. It's not uncommon that after delivering large babies or multiple babies, the vaginal opening can get stretched out or have tears that don't heal properly. A distorted or scarred vaginal opening can result in painful or problematic sexual function. The time of vaginal hysterectomy is ideal to repair the area and restore things in a cosmetically and functionally acceptable way. Repair of the vaginal opening is known as perineoplasty and is essentially reconstructive surgery to tighten and reshape an introitus that may be lax or distorted as a result of a vaginal delivery.

We've come a long way since the days of the "husband stitch" in the delivery room, when the new father smirked, winked at the obstetrician, and said, "Put a stitch in for me, Doc," during episiotomy repair. Of course, on the rare occasion when that still does happen, the *only* appropriate response is to look piercingly at the guy's crotch and say, "Just how small do you need it?" While a return to that approach is not desirable, sometimes a nip and a tuck are beneficial and appropriate.

ANESTHETIC ISSUES

One advantage to vaginal hysterectomy is that it can comfortably be done with regional anesthesia and is therefore a good option for someone in whom general anesthesia is risky or undesirable. This is particularly true of women with chronic pulmonary or heart disease in whom general anesthesia poses an increased risk. Laparoscopic hysterectomy, on the other hand, requires general anesthesia.

This is frequently the case in an elderly patient with chronic medical problems who needs a hysterectomy, but for whom general anesthesia poses a problem. A vaginal hysterectomy with spinal or epidural anesthesia is a safe alternative and is a common solution for an older woman with uterine prolapse. One spry ninety-eight-year-old woman after her hysterectomy was heard to say, "If I had known how easy this was, I would have thrown out the damn pessary and had this done twenty years ago! At least then I would have got my money's worth!"

LIMITATIONS TO VAGINAL HYSTERECTOMY

With all of those advantages, why are not all hysterectomies done vaginally? Unfortunately, there are limitations to the vaginal route that make it unacceptable in many situations.

Large Uterus

The greatest limitation to a vaginal hysterectomy is the size of the uterus. If someone has large fibroids, they simply won't fit through the vagina. The same vagina that will stretch to accommodate a ten-pound baby could not possibly "deliver" a ten-pound fibroid. The reason is that the baby is not attached to anything, and pushes through the vagina, stretching tissues as it goes. A uterus needs to be pulled through the vagina, and needs to meticulously be separated from surrounding structures. In order to do that, the surgeon needs to see, and get to, all the structures that the uterus is attached to. This is simply not possible if the uterus is very large and bulky.

GnRH (Lupron) or uterine artery embolization (UAE) are useful adjuncts to surgery to facilitate shrinkage of fibroids in hopes that a very large uterus will shrink enough to allow a vaginal hysterectomy to be done in lieu of an abdominal hysterectomy. GnRH and UAE are discussed in detail in Chapter 5.

Small Vagina

In addition to the size of the uterus, the caliber and elasticity of the vagina is a factor as well. Women who have delivered babies vaginally usually have a vagina that is a little larger, with stretchier tissue, resulting in greater mobility of tissues and better exposure for the surgeon. A woman who has never had a vaginal delivery, or who has never had sex, is usually a poor candidate for vaginal hysterectomy since the surgeon has extremely limited room to work.

Adhesions

Adhesions pose a special challenge during vaginal surgery. If scar tissue has caused bowel or bladder to be stuck to the uterus, or if it has distorted the normal anatomy, it is often more difficult to resolve during vaginal surgery than abdominal or laparoscopic surgery in which the surgeon has a full view of the pelvis. For that reason, many surgeons are reluctant to offer vaginal hysterectomy to women who have had a prior cesarean section, pelvic operation, or who have known endometriosis or a history of pelvic infections. Adhesions can't always be predicted and it is always possible that a surgery that starts out vaginally will need to be converted to an abdominal hysterectomy in order to safely separate adhesions and avoid injuring tissue.

Since there is no way of knowing in advance if adhesions, a large fibroid, or distorted anatomy will prevent the operation from safely being completed vaginally, you will most likely be asked to sign a consent form that specifies vaginal hysterectomy *and* possible laparotomy. It doesn't mean it is a likely occurrence, it means it is a possible occurrence. Many surgeons routinely add that caveat on to the consent form.

Conversion to an abdominal approach occurs in 1 to 3 percent of vaginal hysterectomies and is almost always due to adhesions or bleeding that can't easily be controlled. If the surgeon does not have adequate exposure for whatever reason, a laparotomy is not a failure. It is the safe, smart thing to do. Realize that your surgeon has your safety in mind when converting a vaginal surgery to an open surgery. The role of laparoscopy has had an impact on the approach to women with adhesions and is discussed in chapter 12.

Absolute Oophorectomy Not Guaranteed

During an abdominal or laparoscopic hysterectomy, the ovaries are visible and therefore removable, except in rare instances where there are dense adhesions. If a patient wants her ovaries out, it generally can be accomplished without additional risk. During vaginal hysterectomy, the surgeon is not always able to easily see the ovaries. If they can't be seen, they can't be removed.

Picture a long tunnel with two boulders on the other end. If the boulders are large and right outside the end of the tunnel, you will be able to see them and grab them without leaving the actual tunnel. If the boulders are a distance from the tunnel and off to the side, you can't see them and you can't grab them. Similarly, if someone's ovaries are far away from the end of the vagina, high in the pelvis, and off to the side, they simply cannot be removed vaginally. In general, a skilled surgeon can remove ovaries 80 percent of the time during vaginal hysterectomy. If someone doesn't want, or doesn't care, if her ovaries are removed, this is clearly not an issue.

Inability To Visualize and Explore the Rest of the Abdomen

The vagina as tunnel concept is not limited to visualization of the ovaries. During a laparoscopic or abdominal case, it is a nice bonus that the surgeon can visualize the abdomen and take a look at the liver, gallbladder, bowel, appendix, and other organs. Sometimes things are serendipitously discovered, which give valuable information. During vaginal hysterectomy, explorations of the rest of the pelvis and abdomen are not done. It's a small disadvantage for the typical low-risk patient who is unlikely to have other problems, but it is a disadvantage, nonetheless.

The Cervix Must Go

One of the most important limitations to vaginal hysterectomy is that removal of the cervix is obligatory. Since the cervix is attached to the upper end of the vagina, it must be removed in order to remove what's above it. In other words, a subtotal hysterectomy is simply not an option.

For many women this is not an issue, particularly if the reason for the hysterectomy is because of a problem with the cervix, such as recurrent dysplasia, and removal is the point of the surgery. Many women feel strongly enough about keeping their cervix that it is worth an abdominal incision to do so (see chapter 19).

Requires an Experienced Surgeon

One of the problems with the increased popularity of laparoscopic surgery is that new surgeons often have limited experience in vaginal surgery. This is one situation in which an older surgeon may be a real advantage, for it is likely that he is far more expert in vaginal hysterectomy than his younger colleagues. Another reason why today's gynecologists do less vaginal surgery is that there are better ways to manage bleeding from small fibroids, cervical dysplasia, etc., and many of the most common indications for vaginal hysterectomy are no longer valid.

In addition, hysterectomy used to be the only legitimate way to end fertility for many Catholic women when further pregnancies were undesired. While not as frequent an occurrence as it used to be, hysterectomy as a means of sterilization under the guise of abnormal bleeding or prolapse certainly continues to quietly be done. All of the above factors contribute to the fact that most surgeons today have less experience with vaginal hysterectomy than the surgeons of twenty years ago.

As in any procedure, you want your surgeon do the procedure that he or she does well. A newer surgeon may be adept at laparoscopic surgery, but less experienced at vaginal surgery. If your doctor is trying to steer you away from vaginal surgery, it may be that it is not the best or the most appropriate choice for you. It may also be that it is not the most comfortable surgery for him. Either way, never try to talk a surgeon into a procedure that he is reluctant to do; it is rarely in your best interest.

IDEAL CANDIDATES FOR VAGINAL HYSTERECTOMY

So who is the ideal candidate? Uterine prolapse is still probably the most common and appropriate indication for vaginal hysterectomy. A fibroid uterus, if not too large, can also be safely treated vaginally. Another good candidate is the woman who has abnormal uterine bleeding in which medical management either doesn't work or is contraindicated. Women who have failed conservative management of recurrent cervical dysplasia, or who desire definitive therapy of a precancerous condition are also appropriate candidates. The woman who has a surgeon expert at vaginal hysterectomy, but not trained in laparoscopic techniques, is much better off with a vaginal hysterectomy than abdominal hysterectomy as long as she is willing to give up her cervix and does not absolutely require oophorectomy.

If your doctor is not trained in laparoscopic surgery but feels you are a candidate for vaginal surgery, you are still in luck. Your recovery time will be virtually the same. Of course, you must resign yourself to the fact that your cervix has to be removed, but that may be desirable or something you are comfortable with. You also need to be aware that even if you desire oophorectomy, there is a 15 to 20 percent chance that it won't be technically possible.

If your doctor is expert in laparoscopic surgery, a laparoscopically assisted vaginal hysterectomy really offers the best of both options.

Chapter 12

Laparoscopic Hysterectomy

If you are not scheduled for a laparoscopic hysterectomy, you need to know if you should be.

Twenty years ago, every person who needed his or her gallbladder removed ended up with a large incision and weeks of painful recuperation. Laparoscopic cholecystectomy first became available in the late 1980s and within ten years virtually all cholecystectomies were being done with the less invasive technique unless there was a specific reason not to. Most general surgeons learned the procedure and routinely offered it to their patients. If they did not, they were out of business, as patients became aware that a laparoscopic procedure was available.

Contrast that to hysterectomy. Although first developed in the early 1900s (by a gynecologist), it wasn't until the 1980s that laparoscopy was used routinely to make diagnoses, treat ectopic pregnancies, and perform tubal ligations. The first laparoscopic hysterectomy was performed in 1989.

In spite of the fact that laparoscopic hysterectomy has been technically feasible for over fifteen years, and in spite of the fact that it offers many advantages over abdominal hysterectomy, it is rarely offered. More than a decade after the first laparoscopic hysterectomy, less than 10 percent of hysterectomies are performed totally laparoscopically; approximately 70 percent of hysterectomies are still performed using an abdominal incision. The small group of surgeons who are laparoscopic experts would argue that many of those could have, and should have, been done laparoscopically.

Laparoscopic surgery, also known as minimally invasive surgery, is done by placing instruments through tiny incisions and visualizing the pelvic contents, using a camera attached to a scope rather than utilizing a large abdominal incision. Because surgery is less invasive, there is significantly less postoperative pain and a more rapid recovery. While it is certainly not appropriate for every patient, or every circumstance, there are many situations in which it is the absolute best option. Why then isn't it routinely offered? Why are only a small number of women the recipient of this new technology? Why haven't all gynecologists learned this technique and offered the benefits to their patients, or, if not able to do it themselves, let their patients know about the option?

In order to do laparoscopic hysterectomy, one must not only develop the skills to do the surgery, but use those skills frequently enough to be expert. While some gynecologists do a large volume of surgery, others rarely operate and focus primarily on obstetrics, fertility, and office gynecology. One busy gynecologic surgeon may do two to four hysterectomies per week, whereas another busy excellent gynecologist may only do two to four per year.

A surgeon who doesn't operate frequently may have only a few patients a year who are candidates for laparoscopic surgery since many women who require hysterectomy are not appropriate possibilities. A few patients a year are simply not enough to be adept at a new technique or to justify taking the time to learn it.

Contrast that to gallbladder surgery: 700,000 cholecystectomies are done each year, the majority of which can safely be accomplished laparoscopically. Unlike gynecologists, general surgeons spend most of their time in the operating room, not conducting an office practice. The end result is that a busy general surgeon has the opportunity to do a far greater volume of cholecystectomies than a busy gynecologist does hysterectomy.

So, while it is appropriate and reasonable for all general surgeons to offer a laparoscopic option, it is also appropriate that many gynecologic surgeons do not. Most gynecologists simply do not have the kind of surgical volume to make it worth their while to learn and perform advanced laparoscopic surgery safely. Furthermore, not everyone agrees that laparoscopic hysterectomy is the best, or most appropriate, way to remove a uterus. The one thing everyone does agree on is that most problems occur when someone *not* skilled in the procedure attempts to do it.

TYPES OF LAPAROSCOPIC HYSTERECTOMIES

There are actually three different operations that someone may be referring to when they talk about laparoscopic hysterectomy:

- ▼ **Laparoscopically assisted vaginal hysterectomy.** LAVH is the most commonly performed laparoscopic hysterectomy. When an LAVH is done, the surgery is done laparoscopically, but the uterus, cervix, and possibly tubes and ovaries are "delivered" through the vagina to complete the operation.
- ▼ **Laparoscopic subtotal hysterectomy.** This is a subtotal hysterectomy done entirely through the laparoscope. The uterus, along with the tubes and ovaries if desired, is removed through the laparoscope. This procedure is most appropriate in someone who desires preservation of the cervix.
- ▼ **Total laparoscopic hysterectomy.** This refers to a hysterectomy performed entirely through the laparoscope. The uterus and cervix are removed entirely laparoscopically and the top of the vagina is sutured laparoscopically. This procedure is only done by a handful of experts at laparoscopic surgery.

How Many Hysterectomies Are Done Laparoscopically?

The Centers for Disease Control (CDC) compiles statistics on hysterectomy every five to seven years and reports their findings three to four years later. They compile data by analyzing the standard insurance codes found on discharge records that document what surgery was done during a given hospitalization.

The problem is that when a new procedure is developed, the insurance code to match it doesn't exist. Hospitals and physicians have no choice but to use alternative codes when reporting a new codeless procedure. A laparoscopic subtotal hysterectomy in 1999 may have been reported under the code for "laparoscopically assisted vaginal hysterectomy" since that was the closest thing. It may have been reported under "laparoscopy–other," or lumped in with other operative laparoscopic procedures that didn't have exact codes. There are many permutations of laparoscopic hysterectomy, and there is currently no accurate way to tally how many "laparoscopic hysterectomies" are totally laparoscopic, subtotal, or laparoscopically assisted vaginal hysterectomies.

It is for that reason that it is difficult to establish accurate statistics. The general sense is that approximately 10 percent of hysterectomies are done laparoscopically, and the majority of those are LAVH.

How Is It Done?

All three types of laparoscopic hysterectomies start the same way (Fig. 12-1). Once you are asleep (regional anesthesia is not an option), you are positioned in such a way that the surgeon has access to your abdomen and vagina. A small incision is made in the fold of your belly button and a laparoscope (telescope) inserted. A light source and camera are attached to the laparoscope. Gas is then used to inflate your abdomen in order to better visualize pelvic and abdominal structures. Once the surgeon has looked around and determined that a laparoscopic hysterectomy is safe and appropriate, two or three other tiny

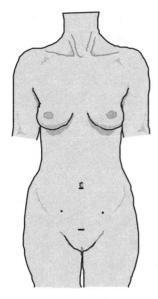

Figure 12-1. Laparoscopic hysterectomy incision sites.

(5-mm) incisions are placed on your belly. Usually one is on the right side just to the inside of your hipbone, with a similarly placed one on the left.

Sleeves (hollow rods) are placed in each incision through which various instruments can be passed during the surgery. The laparoscope has a camera attached to the end with the image displayed on two or three monitors placed at strategic places in the operating room so that the surgeons and the scrub nurse can see the screen at all times.

The same steps done during any hysterectomy are then taken. Structures are identified and cut in order to detach the uterus. Everything is done with long instruments placed through the operating ports while surgeons watch on the monitors. Instruments that can be used to cut, coagulate, tie knots, irrigate, biopsy, and remove tissue have been developed to allow the surgeon to do the same maneuvers that are done in an open incision. The surgeon never directly touches anything with his or her hands. In laparoscopic surgery, the instruments become extensions of the surgeon's hands.

As in all hysterectomies, the blood supply to the uterus has to be severed in order to remove the uterus. During traditional surgery, blood vessels are grasped with instruments, cut, and then stitched with suture. Suturing during laparoscopic surgery is cumbersome. Therefore technology has developed instruments that coagulate (burn) blood vessels before they are cut, resulting in less blood loss than seen in traditional surgeries.

If an LAVH is planned, the surgeon switches to a vaginal approach to complete the operation after key structures have been severed laparoscopically. The uterus, cervix, and possibly the tubes and ovaries are removed intact through the vagina. The back of the vagina is then sewn closed using the same technique as in a standard vaginal hysterectomy.

If a subtotal hysterectomy is planned, the uterus can't be removed through the vagina since the cervix needs to remain in place. Up until a few years ago, there was no way to remove the uterus laparoscopically since even a normal size uterus is far larger than the tiny abdominal incisions used for laparoscopy. The breakthrough in technology that enabled the surgeon to remove a big uterus through a little hole is a device known as a morcellator.

A morcellator does just that. It cuts a large uterus into smaller strips of tissue, which then can be easily removed through a small incision. Most morcellation is done through a 12-mm (half-inch) incision placed in the lower abdomen, just above the pubic bone. Like any other technique, morcellation takes experience and skill, but an accomplished surgeon can morcellate and remove a normal size uterus in ten or fifteen minutes. A large uterus may take an hour or more.

Similarly, in a total laparoscopic procedure, there is no vaginal part of the procedure. The entire uterus, *including the cervix*, is detached and morcellated. Laparoscopic suturing is used to sew closed the top of the vagina. There is a debate among laparoscopic surgeons if there is an advantage to removing the specimen through the laparoscope versus through the vagina. Many surgeons feel that there is rarely an advantage to total laparoscopic over LAVH since it usually takes less time to remove the specimen vaginally then to complete the operation laparoscopically. So few are done that this issue hasn't been studied. Again, personal preference, experience, and the particulars of the patient involved all come into play.

THE ROLE OF DIAGNOSTIC LAPAROSCOPY PRIOR TO HYSTERECTOMY

Often it is advantageous to assess the situation laparoscopically before making a decision as to route of hysterectomy. It makes sense to first do a diagnostic laparoscopy to inspect the pelvis if there is the possibility, but not the certainty, of adhesions, cancer, or poor exposure from huge fibroids. Once the surgeon evaluates the findings, he or she can then proceed with the route of hysterectomy that is most appropriate.

For example, if a vaginal hysterectomy is planned but the surgeon is concerned about possible adhesions from a prior surgery, it is helpful to first take a look and then only proceed with a vaginal hysterectomy if appropriate to do so. Likewise, if there is a mass on the ovary, evaluation by laparoscopy may be appropriate to determine if the mass is benign or malignant. If ovarian cancer is present, an abdominal procedure is done. If the mass is clearly benign, a vaginal or laparoscopic procedure is appropriate. The role of diagnostic laparoscopy at the time of hysterectomy could potentially "save" many women from having to have an abdominal incision.

There are a few downsides to this approach. First of all, you will have no clue until you wake up if your hysterectomy is to be done laparoscopically, vaginally, or abdominally. There will be additional operating time and anesthesia time, adding a minimum of thirty to sixty minutes to the case. The scope may only take twenty minutes, but the operating room staff then has to switch instruments, reposition you, and get things ready for the type of hysterectomy that will be done. While the risk of laparoscopy is low, it is an additional procedure and has its own set of potential complications.

Interestingly, insurance companies generally will not cover a laparoscopic procedure followed by an abdominal or vaginal hysterectomy. Unless there is a good chance that you can avoid an abdominal surgery by starting with a diagnostic laparoscopy, it usually isn't worth the extra time, risk, and expense. Your surgeon will let you know if it's even worth bothering.

ADVANTAGES TO LAPAROSCOPIC HYSTERECTOMY

Recovery/Pain

No one can argue that the major advantage of laparoscopic hysterectomy over abdominal hysterectomy is that recovery, by every criterion, is easier. Pain is minimal and rarely requires a narcotic for more than a day or two. Most women are up and around the day of surgery. Many laparoscopic hysterectomies are outpatient procedures or require only a single night in the hospital. It is typical to tolerate a full diet within twelve hours. The majority of women report that they feel "like nothing happened" by two weeks or fewer from the day of surgery. The most common thing that women report in those two weeks is fatigue, lower abdominal achiness, and slight tenderness around the tiny incision sites. As one women said the day after her laparoscopic hysterectomy, "Surgery? I feel like I should send the flowers back!"

Is the recovery easier than after a vaginal hysterectomy? There have been no good studies that put the two head to head, but if there are differences, they're probably not dramatic. If you are a candidate for a vaginal hysterectomy, a laparoscopic approach probably adds nothing other than expense and possibly a slightly increased risk. The real advantage is in the woman who otherwise would have required an abdominal approach.

Ability to Remove Ovaries

Removal of the ovaries can usually be accomplished vaginally, but there are often times when ovaries are not accessible (see chapter 11). If someone wants to be certain that her ovaries will be removed, a laparoscopic procedure will assure that. An abdominal hysterectomy is the only other alternative in which ovary removal is absolute.

Decreases Need for an Abdominal Approach

For many supporters, the true role of laparoscopic hysterectomy, particularly an LAVH, is to enable the surgeon to do a vaginal surgery in a patient who otherwise would not be an appropriate candidate. That includes the woman with adhesions or a large fibroid uterus or a woman who has never delivered a baby vaginally. The woman who is a candidate for LAVH or vaginal hysterectomy, but who desires preservation of the cervix, is the ideal candidate for a laparoscopic subtotal hysterectomy. Essentially, the primary advantage of these techniques is that they allow many women to avoid an abdominal hysterectomy.

Complete Documentation of the Procedure

Intrinsic to laparoscopic surgery is the ability to make a videotape of the entire procedure. This is beneficial for documentation of surgical findings and is far more accurate than any dictated operative report. (A picture is worth a thousand words.) It is also useful for educational purposes and quality control. In medicolegal claims, there is no question about what happened at the time of surgery. This, of course, can work for, or against, a plaintiff or defendant.

Hospitals do not routinely record or keep videotapes. When they do, they are considered to be part of the medical record. Sometimes patients request a tape. Some surgeons are willing to provide a copy of the tape, others are not. If you are interested, this should be discussed in advance. Keep in mind, there is no sound and you will most likely have no clue what you are looking at. Most surgeons are at least willing to provide Polaroid stills of "highlights," suitable for framing.

Blood Loss, Complications

In experienced hands, blood loss is significantly lower for laparoscopic hysterectomy compared with abdominal hysterectomy. Reports of complication rates are inconsistent. Most studies report them to be similar (in the 2 to 3 percent range) or lower. Other studies have reported significantly higher complication rates.

Accurate complication rates are difficult to determine since the numbers of patients are relatively small and the skill of the surgeons varies widely. One expert laparoscopic surgeon used himself as a control and compared his first seventy cases with his second seventy cases. He found that his complication rate and blood loss were similar to abdominal hysterectomy for the first seventy laparoscopic hysterectomies. In the second seventy, he experienced negligible blood loss and *zero* complications. Experience seems to be the greatest determinant of outcome. There is no question that there is a learning curve that ultimately results in a decreased complication rate.

Another reason that complications should be lower in laparoscopic hysterectomy is that the nature of laparoscopic surgery dictates that certain risks of abdominal hysterectomy can't occur. Since there is no large incision, wound infections, seromas, hematomas, dehiscence, and hernia formation are practically nonexistent. (see chapter 18). Adhesion formation is significantly lower. Pulmonary complications are also decreased since there is no painful incision that inhibits coughing and deep breathing.

Disadvantages to Laparoscopic Surgery

Requires Skilled Surgeon

The biggest roadblock is access to a surgeon who is trained in advanced laparoscopic techniques. If you live in a big city with a major academic medical center, there is usually at least one center that offers the procedure. If you are in a smaller community, you may not have the option (see chapter 13).

Limits Anesthesia Options

Regional anesthesia is not an option. General anesthesia is absolutely required in order to perform operative laparoscopy safely. For the patient who strongly desires an epidural or spinal anesthesia, this may be a drawback.

If LAVH, the Cervix Must Go

If your surgeon is trained to do an LAVH, but *not* a laparoscopic subtotal hysterectomy, you must make a choice of keeping your cervix and having an abdominal procedure, or removing your cervix and having the combined laparoscopic vaginal approach. This is not an uncommon scenario since many surgeons are comfortable with laparoscopic hysterectomy, but are not trained to use a morcellator. If one can't morcellate the uterus, the only other way to take it out is through the vagina.

Complication Rates

Detractors of laparoscopic hysterectomy often cite the fact that complication rates for laparoscopic hysterectomy are higher than those for abdominal and vaginal hysterectomy, particularly relating to inadvertent injury of surrounding tissues such as the bowel, bladder, or ureter. Again, it isn't clear if the occasionally higher complication rates are actually intrinsic to the procedure or if they are related to the inexperience of the surgeons who are doing the procedure. In experienced hands, the complication rates seem to be comparable, or even lower than rates seen in other forms of hysterectomy.

Are You a Candidate for Laparoscopic Surgery?

Assuming you have access to a skilled surgeon (on your insurance plan!) who performs laparoscopic hysterectomies regularly at your neighborhood hospital, are you even a candidate? There are some situations in which a laparoscopic hysterectomy is clearly inappropriate, or simply not in your best interest.

Known or Suspected Cancer

Laparoscopic hysterectomy is rarely appropriate in the face of a known gynecologic cancer. Appropriate cancer surgery requires not only removal of the uterus, tubes, and ovaries, but lymph node sampling and a "hands on" evaluation of the entire abdomen and pelvis. While there are occasional circumstances in which a laparoscopic procedure is possible, most experts agree that currently, abdominal hysterectomy is the standard of care.

If there is uncertainty about the presence of cancer, as in an ovarian mass, it is certainly appropriate to start with a diagnostic laparoscopy to evaluate the situation before proceeding with surgery.

Location of Fibroids

Location of fibroids is a much greater determinant of the ability to do a hysterectomy laparoscopically than size of fibroids. The blood vessels that supply blood to the uterus run along the sides of the uterus. The ureter (the tube that connects the bladder to the kidney) also runs along the side of the uterus. The surgeon must be able to have a good view of those structures in order to do a hysterectomy safely. If fibroids are located on the sides of the uterus, those structures may be difficult to visualize and the anatomy may appear distorted. Technically, a laparoscopic hysterectomy is much easier if the fibroids are located on top of the uterus, even if they are large.

An ultrasound or MRI gives a lot of information about the size and location of the fibroids and frequently it is possible to know prior to surgery if visualization will be adequate. You can't really tell if you will have adequate exposure to safely do the procedure until you actually look at the time of the surgery. Sometimes you don't know until the procedure has started, and it becomes prudent to convert to an abdominal approach.

Uterine Size

Size does matter and each surgeon has a different cut-off for what they are comfortable doing laparoscopically. Some surgeons will only consider uteri that are minimally enlarged. Other surgeons are skilled and confident enough to remove a huge uterus laparoscopically. The majority of laparoscopic surgeons who operate on a regular basis will remove up to a sixteen-week-size uterus, which is a uterus that comes halfway between the pubic bone and the umbilicus. There are some surgeons who will remove a uterus that reaches to the umbilicus, but most experts feel that it is difficult to really visualize the structures and manipulate the instruments when the uterus is that big. The length of surgery is also extremely long. Shrinkage of fibroids prior to surgery with a GnRH agonist, or by uterine artery embolization, may increase the probability of success (see chapter 5).

Known Dense Adhesions

Many women who require hysterectomy have adhesions from a prior myomectomy, endometriosis, or pelvic infection. Most adhesions can be removed laparoscopically, but sometimes adhesions are so dense, the anatomy so distorted, or visualization so obscured, that an abdominal incision is the only safe option. There is rarely a way to predict this before surgery so the women with adhesions need to be aware that conversion to an abdominal hysterectomy may be required. While many women with scar tissue are still candidates for laparoscopic hysterectomy, some adhesions are too severe to be safely dealt with through a laparoscope.

Length of Surgery

Is it better to have a ninety-minute abdominal hysterectomy or a four-hour laparoscopic hysterectomy? This is another area of debate that is difficult to answer. There is no question that it is quicker and easier for a surgeon to remove a uterus that is the size of a basketball though a large abdominal incision. Many experts feel that you are not doing a woman any favors by subjecting her to a four- or five-hour marathon laparoscopic event. The skilled laparoscopic surgeon would argue that the extra operative time is worth it as long as blood loss is not excessive and an abdominal incision is avoided. There is no absolute answer to this debate.

IS YOUR SURGEON QUALIFIED TO PERFORM LAPAROSCOPIC HYSTERECTOMY?

While you can assume that every gynecologist is expert at performing abdominal hysterectomy, the same assumption cannot be made about laparoscopic hysterectomy. The vast majority of gynecologists in this country are not routinely performing laparoscopic hysterectomy, either because they trained before 1990, because they don't have the surgical volume to warrant offering the option, or they were never given the opportunity to learn the technique. Some of the finest gynecologic surgeons in the country have never done a laparoscopic hysterectomy.

How Surgeons Learn New Techniques

Surgeons are not born knowing how to operate. During residency, gynecologists learn to operate by observing, assisting, and ultimately doing a huge volume of surgery, supervised by experienced surgeons all the while. Upon completing residency, new techniques and instrumentation are continually being developed, which a practicing surgeon must then master.

There are a number of ways surgeons can learn new techniques. The best scenario is if someone already expert in the technique is on staff at the hospital where he or she operates. First, like any student, they observe. The experienced surgeon then operates with the surgeon who is learning. This may be once, or it may be many times, depending on the skill level of the surgeon. Once the surgeon is comfortable in the new technique, he or she does it on their own, but the mentor surgeon needs to observe a predetermined number of times in order to certify that the surgeon is capable of doing it on their own.

Some hospitals will bring an expert in to teach a new technique to a number of physicians and be available when cases are scheduled until the surgeons are comfortable. If no one is available to teach a new technique, many surgeons travel to a different institution or take a course where they can learn the instrumentation. The surgeon has the opportunity to observe surgery and practice during labs using animals or models. Remember that these doctors are not new surgeons, but experienced surgeons learning to use new instrumentation or a new approach. Once comfortable with the new technique, they can then incorporate it into their own surgeries, starting with simple cases, and as their skills improve, tackle more challenging cases. When done properly, there is no added risk to a patient.

While these approaches may seem haphazard, they are far from it. Hospitals have strict criteria to ensure that surgeons are not performing dangerous procedures, or surgery they are not ready to do. Operating times, blood loss, and complications are monitored very closely.

Hospital Criteria for Physicians

Physicians, hospital administrators, department chairs, and hospital lawyers are as highly motivated to avoid complications as patients are. Your problems are their problems, and the hospital won't permit an unqualified surgeon to do a procedure he or she shouldn't be doing. Complications create major headaches, not to mention cost major dollars, for hospitals.

By the 1990s, virtually every hospital recognized that guidelines and criteria were necessary to ensure that advanced laparoscopic techniques were done only by qualified surgeons. Quality assurance committees keep track of any untoward events. The fact that your doctor is allowed to do laparoscopic surgery usually means that the hospital has verified his or her competency.

How Many Hysterectomies Constitute Experience?

This, of course, varies from surgeon to surgeon. There is a big difference between the surgeon who has routinely done laparoscopic surgery for ectopic pregnancies, ovarian cysts, and severe endometriosis and then learns how to do an LAVH versus the surgeon who has done virtually no operative laparoscopies other than the occasional tubal ligation. Likewise, a surgeon who is comfortable doing an LAVH does not need a lot of additional training to learn to incorporate the morcellator and do laparoscopic hysterectomies.

How About Your Surgeon?

Go ahead and ask. If you're not sure, it is totally appropriate to ask if your surgeon does advanced laparoscopic surgery, and if so, does he or she perform it on a regular basis? No one is going to say they do it if they don't. No surgeon wants to commit to doing an operation he or she doesn't feel comfortable doing or that their hospital won't let them do.

If your surgeon does laparoscopic hysterectomy, there are also different levels of what they can offer. Many surgeons are comfortable performing LAVH, but not a laparoscopic subtotal or total hysterectomy. Many surgeons are comfortable morcellating a uterus that is not too large, but would not necessarily tackle a bigger uterus. There is a huge range of skills involved for different types of problems, and good surgeons are well aware of the limitations of their own skills.

Surgeons who don't do laparoscopic surgery may try to convince you that you shouldn't have one. You may be told that you are "not a candidate," or that it is "too dangerous." That may be true. Unfortunately, the only one who really can make that kind of judgment is someone who does laparoscopic hysterectomy on a regular basis.

COMPLICATIONS OF LAPAROSCOPIC SURGERY

More than in any type of surgery, the rate of laparoscopic complications is related to the experience of the surgeon. This is why it is critical that you never try to talk your surgeon into doing a laparoscopic hysterectomy if he or she seems reluctant to do so. You are much better off having a surgery that your surgeon is good at, and comfortable doing.

This is not to suggest that experienced surgeons don't get complications. All surgeons have complications even if they are skilled and do everything appropriately. Also keep in mind that any laparoscopic procedure may need to be converted to an open procedure if circumstances arise that would make it unsafe to proceed laparoscopically. It is not a surgical failure to do so; it is surgical safety in your best interest. Any complication that can occur during abdominal laparoscopy can occur during laparoscopic hysterectomy (see chapter 18).

Certain complications are unique to laparoscopic surgery.

Thermal Injury

Since blood vessels can't easily be sutured through the laparoscope, technology has developed instruments that coagulate, or burn, blood vessels so that they can be cut. On occasion, heat generated from one of these instruments can injure a structure adjacent to where the surgeon is working. If bowel or bladder is burned, a thermal injury may occur, which requires repair and possibly laparotomy. This is extremely rare and new instrumentation is designed to protect against this.

Trocar Injury

When placing ports into the pelvis, it is possible to disrupt a small blood vessel and occasionally cause bleeding in the abdominal wall. It is also possible to hit and damage a structure in the abdomen or pelvis as the port is being placed. This rarely occurs since loops of bowel are not fixed and usually move out of the way as instruments are placed in the abdomen. In the event that adhesions have caused bowel to be stuck to the abdominal wall, it doesn't move out of the way as it normally would and could potentially be injured. This is a complication that can occur during any laparoscopic procedure; it is not unique to laparoscopic hysterectomy.

Cost Issues

This is another huge debate. Any analysis of cost must include short-term and long-term costs. In addition, cost to the patient from things such as lost wages and childcare during a prolonged recovery are a different issue than cost for the surgery itself.

There is no question that the instrumentation required for laparoscopic hysterectomy is more expensive than that for standard hysterectomy. High-tech equipment is costly and many of the instruments available are expensive "one-use" disposable instruments. If reusable instruments are used (as is the case in standard abdominal procedures), the cost drops dramatically. In experienced hands, the length of the surgery should be no different, but certainly someone who has not done a lot will take a little longer than the surgeon who has done a large volume. Difficult cases can take a long time even in the best of hands. This all adds up to increased operating room costs.

The money saved is after the surgery. Hospital stays are shorter. Women are back to work quicker, losing less revenue. So while the cost to the insurance company may be higher, the cost to the patient in terms of pain, recovery time, and return to work is substantially less. It all depends on how one calculates cost, and whose cost it is.

A Word About Insurance

It is somewhat surprising that a procedure that has been available for more than ten years is a procedure that many insurance companies have never heard of. It's more understandable when one realizes that there is no specific insurance code for laparoscopic subtotal hysterectomy. When the person in charge of precertification looks at the list on their computer screen, it simply isn't there. It was only in January 2003 that laparoscopic assisted vaginal hysterectomy acquired its very own code. It's difficult enough to get certified for hysterectomy. Try getting certified for a kind of hysterectomy that as far as your insurance company is concerned, is not only more expensive, but doesn't exist.

Many skilled laparoscopic surgeons have spent many years perfecting their laparoscopic skills in order to do laparoscopic hysterectomy, and may decline to be involved in managed care programs that don't recognize or appropriately compensate for a high-tech procedure that few other surgeons offer. If you want one of the experts to do your surgery, you may have to pay for it.

What If My Gynecologist Doesn't Do Laparoscopic Hysterectomy?

This is actually a common scenario. Most women have a long-standing relationship with a doctor whom they trust, like, and want to continue seeing. She has recommended an abdominal hysterectomy, but you are interested in avoiding a long recuperation. When you inquire about the possibility of a laparoscopic procedure, she concedes that you might be a good candidate, but informs you that she does not do them. What options do you have?

You can always find someone else to do the surgery and then return to her for ongoing care. She may not be willing to do that, and you may be uncomfortable doing so. Another possibility may be to see if your doctor can arrange to do the surgery with another surgeon. If there is a skilled laparoscopic surgeon on staff at the same hospital, they may be able to operate together. Your doctor remains involved in your care, and you get access to the less invasive technique.

Also, keep in mind that if you are scheduled for a vaginal hysterectomy, there is no advantage to a laparoscopic approach unless you want to assure removal of the ovaries, or have the option of keeping your cervix. All available data indicate that your recovery and complication rate will essentially be the same. It is only if you are scheduled for an abdominal hysterectomy that the option of a laparoscopic procedure can make a difference.

Many women ultimately choose to have the abdominal hysterectomy with the doctor they know and trust. This is totally reasonable and may be your best bet in the long run. There is a lot of value in a long-standing doctor-patient relationship that should not be minimized. In the big picture, while your recovery will be a little longer, the end result is virtually the same.

The bottom line is that if you are a candidate for laparoscopic hysterectomy and have access to a surgeon who performs it, you are in luck. If laparoscopic hysterectomy is not an option for you either because you are not a good candidate or you don't have access to a surgeon who does the procedure, it is not the end of the world. The reality is that surgical techniques have evolved so that a hysterectomy with an abdominal incision is a much quicker and easier recovery than most women anticipate. What is most important is that your surgery gets done and gets done safely.

Chapter 13

Choosing a Surgeon

Wouldn't it be nice if choosing a surgeon was like choosing a hairdresser? You simply pick the girlfriend whose hair looks fabulous, make an appointment with her stylist, and see what he or she can do for you. If you don't like it? Give it a few months, your hair will grow, and you can try something else. Unfortunately, the stakes are a little higher with surgery, and there's no going back once it's done.

In many ways, your choice of surgeon is the most important decision you make, because the surgeon you choose will affect the options you will be given and the pre- and postoperative interactions you will have. While the main job of the surgeon is done in the operating room, equally important are the preoperative conversations in which options are discussed, alternatives are explored, and potential complications are addressed. In the days and weeks after surgery, postoperative issues often determine what your total surgical outcome will be. For the good surgeon, the operation is not done until the patient has fully recovered.

What About Your Own Gynecologist?

As Dorothy wisely said in *The Wizard of Oz*, "When looking for your heart's desire, (you needn't) look any further than your own back yard. There's no place like home." It may not occur to you that the person who treated your vaginitis and gave you your first birth control pills may also be a skilled surgeon. Even if you think of your gynecologist as someone who "mainly delivers babies," remember that all obstetricians are trained in gynecologic surgery and it may even be their primary interest. Chances are you weren't thinking about a potential hysterectomy when you started to see your mother's gynecologist or picked the first name on the list your Preferred Provider Organization (PPO) gave you. Before you go overboard exploring other possibilities, first consider your own gynecologist with whom you have a relationship and who knows you. If you feel that your own gynecologist doesn't meet your needs, or if your doctor doesn't do surgery, you now need to find a new gynecologist to consult, and potentially to do your hysterectomy.

Insurance Plan Issues

It is a reality of our times that your insurance company has a major say in who your surgeon will be. If your chosen physician happens to participate in your plan, you're in luck. If he or she doesn't, you still have a few options.

Your plan may partially pay if you choose a doctor who is out of the network. Hopefully the hospital is in the network so even if you use your out-of-network doctor, they will still cover hospital costs such as the anesthesiologist, operating room, and room charges. The surgeon's fees only cover the surgery, visits in the hospital, and routine postoperative office visits. It does not include lab work, extra visits if there is a complication, or preoperative consultations.

You may be told that if you go out of the network your insurance will cover up to 60 percent of usual and customary fees. The problem is that the "usual and customary fee," as defined by your insurance plan, is usually what a gynecologist on Mars charges. In other worlds, that 60 percent may only be only 30 or 40 percent of your surgeon's actual fee. You need to get exact numbers to know what your responsibility truly is.

If you have chosen a doctor who is not covered, or only partially covered, by your insurance plan, you will have to pay a significant portion out of your own pocket. Find out in advance what you will owe. Many offices are willing to work out a payment plan, particularly if you have been a patient in the practice for a long time. While some patients ask for discounts, most practices don't offer discounted surgery unless there is a true hardship and a long-standing relationship.

What if you have chosen an out-of-network doctor because he or she is the only one in your town who can do a laparoscopic hysterectomy? If there is no one on your plan who is trained in that procedure, you may be covered for an out-of-network doctor since they offer a procedure you cannot get in the network. It will take a lot of phone calls and letters to explain your circumstances, but it often works eventually.

You can try and enlist the help of the in-network doctor to verify that he is not trained in the particular procedure that is appropriate for you. In general, though, don't expect the physician who is not doing the procedure to spend the time to help you have another doctor do your surgery, unless it was his or her idea in the first place.

Occasionally, patients ask physicians to consider becoming a provider in their insurance plan. Chances are your plan was considered and rejected for a reason, usually poor or slow payment. Even if your physician does take on a new plan, it is usually months from the time of application to participation.

If you live in or near a major metropolitan area, you will have the luxury (or dilemma) of having a lot of physicians to choose from. Again, your own gynecologist is frequently the best choice, particularly if you have a long relationship and feel comfortable with your doctor's recommendations. Don't feel obligated to get a second opinion or look elsewhere unless you are unsure of what has been recommended or want to get another point of view. If you have been receiving care from a family practitioner, internist, midwife, or nonoperating gynecologist, you now need to find a surgeon.

First, Pick a Hospital

If you are looking for a new doctor, it makes sense to pick the hospital first. Certain hospitals are known to be gynecologic centers and have a far greater range of gynecologists to choose from than if you choose a hospital that does not have a large gynecologic department.

Location is certainly a factor, but should rarely be the deciding factor. Choosing a hospital that is a few blocks from home for convenience makes no sense if there is a better hospital ten miles away. Choosing a hospital near home is probably appropriate if a similar hospital is a three-hour drive. If you are picking a hospital that is not conveniently located, keep in mind that there will be trips to the hospital besides the day of surgery and the day home. There may be a preoperative appointment for testing. Your doctor's office may be near the hospital. Most important, postoperative complications may necessitate a trip to the emergency department.

What if you choose an out-of-town hospital? This happens for a number of reasons. Women who live in a rural area often travel to the city to have surgery. Sometimes people travel so that they can be close to family members who may be caring for them after surgery. Sometimes there is a particular doctor who is expert at a procedure that no doctors close to home can do. If that is the case, plan on staying in the vicinity of the hospital for roughly two weeks after surgery. Virtually every serious complication or issue that could potentially occur usually occurs in that time frame. If you don't have a good friend or relative to stay with, the hospital may have an arrangement with a nearby hotel for a special rate.

Don't count on your local gynecologist to provide postoperative care if you have gone to another doctor for surgery. By choosing another surgeon, you have effectively ended the relationship and it is simply inappropriate to return for routine postoperative care or annual exams. The exception is if you travel for procedures your doctor does not offer, or if you go out of town to be near family. If that is the case, the situation should be discussed before surgery so that you can ask if your original gynecologist is comfortable with continuing care. It is equally offensive to go to another surgeon because the insurance coverage is better, but then return to your original physician for Pap smears and vaginitis. If you leave your gynecologist for another, plan on continuing with the new gynecologist. If that is not practical, face the fact that you may need to find a new local doctor.

In general, if the procedure you need is available with your current gynecologist, having your surgery locally is usually in your best interest. An abdominal hysterectomy at the Mayo Clinic is *identical* to the abdominal hysterectomy you will get in Boise, Idaho. The postoperative care you will get at the Mayo Clinic will be nonexistent, as will the relationship with your doctor.

Many women worry about location in terms of the convenience of their visitors. Erase that thought.

Teaching Versus Non-Teaching Hospitals

Contrary to popular opinion, there are a number of advantages to a teaching hospital over a non-teaching hospital. The main advantage is that new techniques and state-of-the-art equipment are more likely to be available at a large academic center than at a small rural hospital. Even if you don't need the latest innovation, there are other advantages.

Teaching hospitals, unlike non-teaching hospitals, have physician coverage when your surgeon is not physically in the hospital. Most gynecologists spend their days in the office and their nights at home. If you are in the hospital after surgery and develop a fever, bleeding, or unexpected pain, your physician will not be physically available to immediately evaluate you. In a teaching hospital, a resident physician who is very familiar with your situation will be available to see and examine you and report to your doctor what is going on. The attendings work with the residents regularly, know them, and find their input to be extremely valuable.

Another major advantage to a large academic hospital is that a higher volume of patients translates to a higher volume of personnel, which translates to more specialization. If a small hospital does only three to five gynecologic procedures per week, you will likely be on a hospital unit with patients who have had an appendectomy or gallbladder surgery. The nurse taking care of the appendectomy patient is the same nurse who will take care of the hysterectomy patient. A large hospital will likely have a gynecological floor, or even a women's hospital where the nurses, doctors, and associated personnel only take care of patients who have had gynecologic procedures. The scrub nurses only scrub on gynecological operations, and the entire staff is geared towards the care of a gynecologic patient.

A large hospital also has access to multiple specialists. In the unlikely event of a complication during surgery that requires a urologist or bowel surgeon, it is nice to know that there is not one, but probably a choice of multiple specialists who are available to come to the operating room to lend a hand. The small hospital might only have one or two urologists on staff, who might or might not be readily available.

Many women worry that if they are at a teaching hospital, "students" will be doing their surgery and taking care of them, resulting in substandard care. They envision a brand-new medical student brandishing a scalpel and saying to a fellow medical student, "So, where should we make the incision today?" while the attending doctor eats a corned beef sandwich in the doctor's lounge. A frightening thought, but nothing could be further from the truth. While a student will likely be present during your surgery, it is your attending physician, assisted by the resident physician, who will actually be doing the surgery and taking care of you (see chapter 16 for details).

The presence of students and residents actually frequently ensure a better quality of care. Every single surgery is discussed during teaching rounds in terms of appropriateness of procedure, complications, and outcome. In other words, unnecessary surgery is virtually never done since someone is always evaluating each procedure. If a physician on staff at a teaching hospital was doing unnecessary operations, or was having a higher-than-acceptable complication rate, the teaching staff and residents would notice it immediately and deal with it appropriately.

So what are the disadvantages to a teaching hospital? Things tend to move more slowly. Teaching hospitals focus on providing care that is state of the art, while educating residents and medical students at the same time. When you arrive for surgery, the student may need to take your history, followed by the gynecologic resident, followed by the anesthesia resident, followed by your attending doctor. Redundancy seems to be the rule, not the exception. Research is also a large aspect of academic institutions and you may be asked to participate in a clinical study. If you prefer not to participate, feel free to decline.

Another disadvantage? Teaching hospitals often aren't as "nice." Community hospitals attract patents because they are usually smaller, more pleasant, and a more comfortable place to spend a few days. A small hospital has the advantage of more personalized attention, fewer patients on a unit, and a quieter feel. It is much more consumer-oriented and focused on "hotel amenities." It is hard to pass up the hospital known for beautiful rooms and great food, which is in the nice part of town. Keep in mind that while it's always nice to be in lovely surroundings, those criteria should be reserved for the vacation you take after your hysterectomy. The best care is not always in the best "hotel."

Is this to suggest that you can't get fine care at a community non-teaching hospital? Of course not. The majority of non-teaching hospitals provide outstanding care and have surgeons that are just as talented and experienced as those at a large teaching institution. Hysterectomy is not an uncommon operation; even small community hospitals view it as a routine procedure that is frequently done. If your gynecologist practices at a small local hospital, you certainly shouldn't feel that you need to travel to a major medical center or find a new gynecologist unless you feel that your needs won't be met or you desire a procedure that isn't offered. In other words, if all else is equal, go for luxury. It shouldn't be the deciding factor in your decision.

FINDING A SURGEON

Once you have picked the hospital, you need to find a surgeon who is on staff at the hospital. You may not be limited to one hospital if there are a number of appropriate options available to you, in which case you can broaden the search.

Referral Services

Most hospitals have a physician referral service. The downside? Obviously you will only be referred to staff doctors at that hospital. However, if you have chosen that hospital because it is well known to be a leader in gynecologic surgery and the place where you want to have your surgery anyway, then the hospital referral service is a great way to find the right doctor. Keep in mind that the people who work at hospital referrals are obligated to refer to all physicians on staff, so if you just call up and say, "Hi, I need a hysterectomy. Who on staff is good?" you'll essentially be given the name of whoever's next on the list. You need to ask specific questions that will lead you to the surgeon who is most appropriate for you. For example, instead of saying, "I'm looking for a good gynecologist to do my hysterectomy," say, "I'm looking for a board-certified gynecologist who has been in practice for at least five years, but less than twenty years. I would prefer someone who trained at a university and who has experience in laparoscopic hysterectomies. I would like someone who also offers alternatives to hysterectomy." You can get a lot of information from physician referral and it is well worth your time to tell them exactly what is important to you. The referral service will also be able to answer questions about office location and accepted insurance. Frequently, they will facilitate your getting an appointment even if you can't get one just by calling yourself.

Hospital referral services are not the same as commercial referral agencies that operate independently of a hospital. Referral agencies that advertise in magazines, the Yellow Pages, or on TV are not a great source. Participating physicians pay to be part of the service and tell them what to say. As with any paid advertisement, healthy skepticism of claims is appropriate.

Professional Societies

Professional societies such as the American Medical Association, American College of Obstetricians and Gynecologists, and the American Association of Laparoscopic Surgeons are all potential sources of referrals, particularly if you are looking for an out-of-town doctor. The lists they have will not be comprehensive, since a physician needs to join one of those organizations to be on their lists, but it is certainly a reasonable starting place.

Doctors Who Advertise

Years ago, it was unheard of for physicians to advertise. It was considered to be unprofessional and simply wasn't done. Most people picked physicians based on the referral of other physicians or family members. The first to break that rule were the plastic surgeons. They recognized that marketing was a powerful tool for a consumer-driven specialty, and advertisements that touted their various successes (complete with before and after pictures) became standard. Other specialties soon followed, particularly if they were trying to attract patients for a "gimmick" or new procedure. Today, most physicians, particularly in academic settings, don't advertise. Referrals are still primarily through other physicians or word of mouth.

Having said that, just because a physician advertises doesn't mean he or she isn't good. It does mean that he or she has paid to say that they are "the best" and offers an "innovative surgery" that is unavailable or not as good elsewhere. The claims may be valid or they may be just that . . . claims. It helps to know what the practice is in your area. If all the gynecologists have paid advertisements in local papers describing the services they offer, that is probably the norm in your area. If only one group advertises, don't take their claims at face value. You may be better off with the surgeon who doesn't need to advertise to stay busy.

It should go without saying that the Yellow Pages is not an appropriate way to pick a doctor, yet this is done surprisingly often.

Other Great Sources for Referrals

Your internist or family doctor is also a good place to get a recommendation. The only downside is that your internist may have standard referrals that he has used for years, particularly if he is older, and his recommendations may not be the most up-to-date. Your child's pediatrician is another helpful source. They work closely with obstetricians and gynecologists and generally know them pretty well. Your pediatrician may be able to ask around and find a good laparoscopic surgeon more easily than your internist.

A commonly overlooked but valuable source are ob/gyn residents. Gynecologists in training are the only ones who operate with *all* the doctors on staff and really know who's good and who's not. They have no vested interest in who you choose and are usually brutally honest. More than one enterprising patient has called a large academic institution and paged the senior gynecologic resident on call to get a referral to the best surgeons on staff. If you happen to know an operating room nurse, he or she also knows who's who.

In general, beware of the friend or acquaintance who insists that her gynecologist is the only one to consider. She may be right, but she also may have no clue about the expertise of her own doctor. Just because she was pleased with her surgery, or has a personable, pleasant doctor, doesn't mean that doctor is the best choice for you.

The exception, of course, is that savvy friend (and everyone has one) who did an exhaustive search of eligible gynecologists in the area, interviewed twelve doctors, and found out who was doing what prior to her hysterectomy. Some friends just *think* they know—the onus is on you to know the difference.

WHAT IF THERE IS NO CHOICE?

You may live in a town where there is only one hospital and one gynecologist. Travel to a distant hospital may not be feasible or desirable. You may have an emergency procedure with little time to interview surgeons. While not an optimal situation, it is still possible to ensure that you have options and get the best care available to you under the circumstances.

Request a preoperative consultation and be prepared. If you are told you need a particular procedure over what you perceive to be the more desirable or appropriate procedure, don't hesitate to ask in a nonconfrontational way why a particular recommendation has been made. There is probably a reason why you have been told that you need an abdominal hysterectomy rather than a vaginal hysterectomy. If an experienced but older gynecologist is planning to remove your cervix and you think you are a good candidate for a subtotal hysterectomy, ask if that is a possibility. Frequently an option your surgeon does not initially offer you may be something he or she is willing to consider, even if it is not initially recommended or the usual procedure.

Sometimes you have to be realistic about the available choices. If you are interested in a laparoscopic hysterectomy but the only gynecologist in town has never done one, you don't want to be the first. You are much better off going with what your surgeon is experienced in and comfortable with, even if it's not exactly what you want. Don't ever try to talk a surgeon into something he or she doesn't want to do.

MAKING THE APPOINTMENT

Once you have decided whom you would like to see, you need to schedule a consultation. When you call the office, mention specifically that you think you may need surgery. A surgical consultation requires more time than a routine annual visit, and you want to be sure the appropriate amount of time is scheduled. Ask what you should bring. It's usually better to bring ultrasound reports, pathology, etc., with you, rather than have them sent to the office. It's unlikely that anyone will look at your records prior to your appointment, and you'll be sure that they are there if you bring them with you. Have an extra copy to keep for your own records in case you choose to get another opinion.

Find out if the physician participates in your insurance plan. If he or she doesn't, it's best to know that before the appointment so you can decide if you want to incur out-of-network costs.

If you would like information about a surgeon's qualifications, ask to speak to someone regarding board certification, years in practice, ability to do laparoscopic hysterectomy, or whatever is important to you.

While it's tempting to ask the receptionist who makes the appointment, she rarely has the time to sit on the phone with you and answer lots of questions. Ask if there is someone (often the practice manager) who can speak to you regarding qualifications.

Sometimes patients want to talk to physicians in advance to get a feel for their recommendations or see what their approach would be. Don't expect and don't ask to have the physician call you. Most physicians are not willing to do a preoperative consultation on a patient they have never met, haven't examined, and know nothing about.

What If You Can't Get an Appointment?

This is actually a fairly common problem. You have your heart set on a particular doctor who you are convinced is the most qualified surgeon to do your hysterectomy. The problem is, this doctor's first opening is three months away. There are a few strategies to get a quicker appointment.

First of all, keep in mind that the receptionist is the gatekeeper. If you are nasty to this person, the first opening may then be four months away. The receptionist is the person you should be really nice to since he or she will keep you in mind if there is a cancellation. Be sure and say that the reason for the appointment is that you need to have surgery, or are thinking of having surgery. You are more likely to get an earlier appointment than if you are just coming in for an annual visit and Pap smear.

Call frequently for cancellations. Every gynecologist's office has cancellations on a regular basis. Women get their periods, obstetric patients deliver ahead of schedule, etc. It helps to find out the scheduler's name and call every day or two to see if anything has opened up. Inevitably, a receptionist who you talk to regularly and to whom you are really nice will find a way to get you in. Chocolates and flowers are probably not necessary.

It doesn't hurt to enlist the help of someone who may have an inside avenue to the office. Your internist may be willing to make a call on your behalf and speak directly to the surgeon, who will then go out of their way to fit you in. Keep in mind that when that happens, the surgeon is probably coming in early, staying late, or skipping something to see you, so there may not be a lot of flexibility in the times offered.

THE CONSULTATION

Arrive on time or a few minutes early. Fifteen minutes late may not sound like a lot to you, but if someone has forty-five minutes to get a history, examine you, and then discuss recommendations, fifteen minutes late means a third of your time is gone. If you made an appointment that you have decided not to keep, a call to cancel is really appreciated rather than simply not showing.

Even if another doctor has just examined you, expect to be examined again. Surgical recommendations can't be based on an ultrasound or someone else's report of your pelvic examination.

Bring someone who is capable of listening and taking notes. It's a real advantage if this person has a medical background or has been through surgery herself, since he or she will be more familiar with a lot of the terminology. This is really important. Chances are, you will be given a lot of information and will retain only a part. It's amazing what is forgotten or not heard.

Bring all pertinent records. The consultant has no interest in and will not look at fifteen years' worth of Pap smears and annual exams. What you will need are any radiology (ultrasound and X ray) reports, surgery reports, pathology (biopsy) reports, recent blood tests, and recent hormone levels. It will save a lot of time if everything is readable and in chronological order, particularly if there are multiple pages. If records were sent directly to the office, make sure they arrived before you arrive for your appointment. Don't assume that just because you requested records to be sent that it actually happened. Your best bet truly is to bring a copy of the records with you to ensure that they are readable, complete, and there.

KEY POINTS TO DISCUSS

Do You Need Surgery?

This is not as obvious as it seems. Many women are told that they need a hysterectomy and search for a surgeon, when surgery is not their best or only option. Central to every consultation is whether a hysterectomy is appropriate and the best option. The possibility of alternatives should always be mentioned, even if the consultant says there are none, confirming what you have already been told.

How Often Does She Do Hysterectomies?

You may not need to ask. If you are seeing someone who is known to be a busy, skilled surgeon, it's silly to ask how often he or she does a certain procedure. The absolute number of hysterectomies that someone has performed is actually unimportant. What is important is that the surgeon operates on a regular basis. There is no question that a surgeon who operates regularly is better than the surgeon who does a handful of cases a year. The real question is, how many procedures does it take to make someone experienced? How often does someone need to operate to keep his or her skills sharp?

Surgeons today do a lot less surgery than gynecologists did twenty years ago, simply because hysterectomy is a less frequently performed operation. The trend over the last ten years has been to avoid hysterectomy unless absolutely necessary, resulting in far fewer operations. A busy gynecologist in 1980 would easily do two to four hysterectomies per week. A busy gynecologist in 2004 may only do two to four hysterectomies per month. There is no absolute number of surgeries that a surgeon needs to do to keep skills sharp, but clearly the surgeon who does only three or four hysterectomies per year is not going to be as skilled as the surgeon who operates on a more regular basis.

It is perfectly reasonable to ask how often he or she does major procedures if you think your gynecologist rarely operates. You don't need an exact number, just the sense that he or she operates frequently. Even if your surgeon has only been in practice a year or so, he or she may actually have a lot of surgical experience. A recent graduate from residency has recently operated a lot, probably every day. In addition, they are also knowledgeable about the latest techniques.

Strategies for Bowel or Bladder Injury

Fortunately, injuries to surrounding structures such as the bowel, bladder, or ureter are rare occurrences (see chapter 18). It does happen, however, and when it happens, it needs to be repaired. Many gynecologists (particularly gynecologic oncologists) are comfortable and capable of fixing injuries to a surrounding structure and need not call in a specialist. If that's not the case, how available is the urologist or bowel surgeon? Are they likely to be in the hospital, or do they need to be called from home?

Strategies for Unexpected Cancer

On occasion, a hysterectomy for a benign problem, such as fibroids, turns out to involve an unsuspected malignancy. Most general gynecologists are not trained to do the required lymph node sampling and cancer staging. In many hospitals, particularly large academic institutions, a gynecologic oncologist (cancer specialist) is readily available to participate in the surgery. In the event that an unsuspected malignancy is discovered and no gynecologic oncologist is available, someone will have to be called in, which may take hours, or may not be an option. If no gynecologic oncologist is available, a second surgery on a later date will need to be scheduled. Either way, it's not optimal and if there is any concern about a possible malignancy, it's prudent to ask who will be available.

Is Laparoscopic Hysterectomy an Option?

This is a major issue that is addressed in detail in Chapter 12. Suffice it to say that unless the surgeon you are consulting with does laparoscopic procedures, any declaration that you are not a candidate needs to be confirmed by someone who does do laparoscopic hysterectomies.

Cervix and Ovary Decisions

You may be planning on keeping your cervix and/or ovaries. Your surgeon may or may not be amenable. Don't assume anything; it needs to be discussed at the time of the visit. You don't need to come to a decision at this point, but there should be a dialogue at that time to explore if there is an option, and the pros and cons of each (see chapters 19 and 20, regarding the cervix and ovary decisions).

Postoperative Issues

Some surgeons are truly interested only in the surgery. They have no interest in dealing with postoperative hormone replacement issues, annual Pap smears, and ongoing gynecologic care. If you have another gynecologist who will be doing follow-up care, this may not be an issue. If you are interested in a surgeon who will be willing to continue to provide routine care, make sure that is a possibility.

How Quickly Can Surgery Be Scheduled?

Don't assume that the surgeon of your choice will be able to do your operation on the day of your choice. Some surgeons schedule cases months in advance, while others are able to get you on the schedule in a matter of days. Keep in mind that even if your surgeon is available, an operating room may not be. The further in advance the whole thing is planned, the better chance you'll get the time you want.

How Important Is It To Like Your Surgeon?

You're not looking for a new friend. If your surgeon is not warm, witty, or charismatic, do you really care? You have plenty of people to invite to parties and have lunch with. You are looking for someone who has the skills you need and whose judgment you trust. Quite frankly, the reason so many women have gynecologists whom they trust to do their Pap smear, but not their hysterectomy, is that they were picking a gynecologist using "the gynecologist as friend" criteria. Your gynecologist need not be your friend.

Age of Surgeon

The right age for your surgeon is an age where they are experienced, still keep up with new innovations, and are likely to still be in practice when it's time for your postoperative visit. For most surgeons, a reasonable age is between thirty and sixty-five. For some surgeons, it's never.

Gender of Surgeon

It really doesn't matter. *Really*. The exception? If you are totally uncomfortable being examined by a man or talking to a man about intimate issues, you will be better off with a woman physician. If you feel somewhat guilty discriminating in that way, consider the number of men who go to women urologists. On the other hand, it would be foolish to go with the less qualified doctor based solely on gender.

Should You Get a Second Opinion?

If you are comfortable and confident about everything your surgeon has told you, a second opinion is probably not necessary. If you think there may be options you're not being presented with, or are not entirely comfortable with what you have been told, you should definitely seek a second opinion.

If you are going to get another opinion, it's really important that you see someone who is truly expert in the area. Start by asking your gynecologist whom she or he would recommend for a second opinion. If he or she is put off and acts insulted that you would like to get a second opinion, that should send off major alarm bells. Any surgeon who is confident in what they have recommended will be totally comfortable with the fact that you would like to seek another opinion. He or she should be happy and willing to give you names of appropriate people. If he or she is unwilling to do so, it's even more reason to get a second opinion.

What If Your Gynecologist Doesn't Do a Procedure You Want?

It's entirely possible that the gynecologist you like and have gone to for years is not trained in laparoscopic hysterectomy. If that's the case, ask if it is possible for your gynecologist to do the surgery with a colleague who can do the newer procedure. That way, your own gynecologist stays involved, but you get the benefit of the new technique. It's not unusual for a surgeon to learn new techniques by doing just that, so it may be a more viable option than you think. If that's not an option, you have to decide if having the minimally invasive procedure is important enough that you find a new doctor who may be a lot less convenient.

BEWARE

There are certain red flags that should make you hesitate before you schedule surgery. In general, question a surgeon who is reluctant for you to get a second opinion, seems very eager to operate, or is insistent that you schedule surgery before you leave the office, unless it is truly an emergency.

Very often those are the same surgeons who suggest that your fibroids "could be cancer," and therefore must come out. A surgeon who doesn't discuss risks to the procedure, or insists that complications never happen, either can't be trusted or operates very little. Finally, if you don't feel confident, even if you can't figure out exactly why, do yourself and the surgeon a favor and find another surgeon.

Chapter 14

Anesthetic Issues

I t's not unusual for the savvy patient to spend extensive amounts of time researching surgical options and surgeons, but give only a passing thought to the person who actually makes sure they survive the surgery. That's right, it's the anesthesiologist, not the surgeon, who keeps you alive. Now that you're in a total panic, be assured that anesthetic complications are astonishingly rare and actual death due to anesthesia even rarer. But the anesthesiologist is important, and there are issues to consider before the day of surgery.

In the dark ages, when people were admitted to the hospital the night before their procedure, patients had an opportunity to meet the anesthesiologist and ask questions in a more leisurely fashion than the current system of meeting the anesthesiologist minutes before you roll into the operating room. More important, quite frankly, was that the anesthesiologist had an opportunity to meet you and go over pertinent details of your medical history.

Every hospital has a different system, but many hospitals have a pre-op day when you meet an anesthesiologist with whom you can discuss anesthetic issues. Notice you don't necessarily meet *your* anesthesiologist,

203

you meet *an* anesthesiologist. Logistically, it is more efficient for one anesthesiologist to meet all the pre-op patients that come in on a given day
since it is impossible to know who will be assigned to your operating
room on the day of your scheduled surgery. In most cases, the anesthesiologist who will be assigned to your care is assigned only the day before.

Many hospitals are moving to a system where an anesthesiologist
only meets with patients who are felt to be particularly high-risk, or
who have significant medical problems. There may be no preoperative
meeting until the actual day of surgery. In some institutions, patients
are screened in preoperative assessment clinics before surgery. Some
anesthesiologist groups screen their patients by telephone. There are
hospitals that provide their patients with computerized screening programs that can be accessed via the Internet. An anesthesiologist then
prepares your anesthesia chart so that on the day of surgery your
assigned anesthesiologist knows everything about you.

While the systems differ, the goal is the same: to get important medical information prior to your surgery in order to plan your upcoming
anesthetic experience. While that might seem to be problematic, it usually
works out fine. The real problem with this system is that some patients are
really anxious about the fact that they won't meet the anesthesiologist until
the day of surgery. If that is a significant issue for you, tell the anesthesiologist at your pre-op visit, and see if something can be arranged.

In most hospitals, particularly large teaching hospitals, your surgeon has no say in the choice of the anesthesiologist. A lot of people
assume that your gynecologist has some hand in choosing who will be
in the operating room. In most hospitals, it doesn't work that way. One
of the reasons it's important to pick a good hospital is that a good
department of anesthesiology goes along with that choice.

THE PRE-OP VISIT

Chapter 15 will go into detail about other aspects of the pre-op visit. In
terms of anesthesia, this is what you need to know. Preparation is key. If
you have a complicated medical history, or have had anesthetic problems in the past, gather as much information as you can before your

pre-anesthetic visit. The following is a list of things to do before you see the anesthesiologist.

▼ **See your internist.** It is important to have your personal internist give what is commonly known as "medical clearance." This means that he or she has examined you and done appropriate testing to ensure that you are in optimal medical condition to go through surgery. This is imperative if you have medical problems such as asthma, high blood pressure, or diabetes. It is not particularly important if you are thirty-five years old with no medical problems.

▼ **Prepare a list of medications.** Write down every medication you take routinely. Include prescription drugs, over-the-counter medications, and alternative or herbal preparations.

▼ **Be prepared to be honest.** This is not the time to hide any less-than-admirable habits. The anesthesiologist is not a new friend you want to think well of you, nor is he or she a disapproving parent. If you smoke, say so and be honest about how much. Recreational drugs? No one will arrest you or be shocked. If you are dependent on alcohol, it's crucial that everyone taking care of you knows. The anesthesiologist doesn't need any surprises after you go to sleep or when you wake up.

▼ **Pre-op laboratory testing.** Electrocardiogram (EKG), blood work, chest X rays, etc., are often done at the pre-op visit, but are ideally done before that appointment so that if there is a problem it can be addressed in time. Sometimes surgery is cancelled due to abnormalities found on pre-op testing that need further evaluation or treatment.

▼ **Get records.** Prior anesthetic records are only necessary if you had a problem or complication from a previous operation. You can obtain records from a prior surgery by sending a release to the medical records department of the hospital or facility where the other procedure was done. Better still, if you had an anesthetic problem, contact your anesthesiologist and get as much information as you can. If the problem is familial, be sure to get your family members evaluated. Your surgeon will *not* have anesthetic records in his or her office.

▼ **See your dentist.** This is not a joke. Sometimes during the induction of anesthesia a loose tooth or other dental work is inadvertently knocked off. This is much less likely to happen if all your dental work is secure. Always let your anesthesiologist know about dental work, special treatments to your teeth, or special appliances.

▼ **Compile a list of questions.** It's not required to have a list of questions. The anesthesiologist will tell you what you need to know without your prompting. However, if you do have specific questions about your anesthetic, this is the time to ask them, as opposed to when you get home and may not have access to your physician.

JUST KNOCK ME OUT!

General anesthesia is the most widely used method of anesthesia for major gynecologic surgery and consists of using drugs to induce a reversible depression of the central nervous system. In other words, you are unconscious and do not have the ability to move or feel pain during your surgery. All functions revert to normal once the drugs are stopped.

Using drugs that are inhaled or injected directly into your bloodstream induces general anesthesia. Most anesthetics today start with medication going through your intravenous line (IV), which quickly puts you to sleep. Drugs administered through the IV and inhaled maintain an unconscious state in the patient. A combination of drugs results in loss of memory for all events immediately preceding your surgery, loss of consciousness, and inability to perceive pain. In some cases, drugs are added that relax your abdominal muscles and affect your ability to breathe on your own.

This concept may be frightening to some people because we all know that the ability to breathe is a good thing. Since you may not be able to breathe for yourself while you are anesthetized, the anesthesiologist will be responsible for taking over this bodily function with the help of a machine called a ventilator. For this purpose, a small tube is put down your throat after you go to sleep, and the tube is inserted into your air passage, or trachea, which leads to your lungs.

During the duration of the surgery, oxygen and anesthetic gasses flow continuously through that tube, keeping you oxygenated and asleep. The tube also prevents material coming up from your stomach from getting into your lungs and causing serious pneumonia.

While you are asleep, an anesthesiologist or nurse anesthetist is sitting by your head every second and making sure that everything is fine. Monitors are hooked up that constantly measure your heart rate, blood pressure, pulse, and oxygenation. In the event that something isn't right, the anesthesiologist knows it immediately and can quickly take measures to correct the problem.

Monitors are also used that measure the depth of unconsciousness. Don't worry about urban legends in which someone went through surgery and felt the whole thing even though they were paralyzed and no one knew they could feel what was going on. Doesn't happen.

REGIONAL ANESTHESIA

Most people are familiar with regional anesthesia because of its widespread use in pregnancy for pain relief in labor. Regional anesthesia renders the patient unable to feel pain, yet she remains totally conscious.

Spinal anesthesia, one form of regional anesthesia, involves placing a needle into the space that contains spinal fluid surrounding the spinal cord in the lower back. A local anesthetic is then injected and provides anesthesia for a set period of time.

Epidural anesthesia is another form of regional anesthesia in which the needle is placed just *outside* the sac of spinal fluid. The local anesthesia may then be continuously infused through a catheter, providing a block as long as it is needed. Spinal anesthesia has a slightly quicker onset, but may not last as long. Epidural anesthesia takes a little longer to put in and a little longer to start working, but has the advantage of lasting much longer since the local anesthesia continues to flow through the catheter.

The advantage? Some people are anxious about going to sleep and are more comfortable with the idea of a regional anesthetic. Some women are concerned about nausea and vomiting from general anesthesia, which can be minimized with a regional anesthetic. There is quicker return of bowel function with regional anesthesia than when a general anesthetic is used since the bowels are not "put to sleep" along with the patient. Epidural anesthesia can be continued after surgery and allows optimal pain relief in the immediate postoperative period, since narcotic and local anesthetic drugs can be put through the catheter to decrease pain.

The disadvantage? Many people have no desire to know what is going on in the operating room and just want to be "out." Remember that even if you are awake, you won't be watching. Drapes are used not only to keep the surgical area clean, but also to keep you from sneaking a peek at your open abdomen. It is common practice to give sedation so you almost always fall asleep during the surgery. Most women who have a regional anesthetic have little or no memory of the operating room and snooze during the majority of the procedure. Often music is played so if someone is awake, they aren't aware of the conversation and noises present in the operating room.

Gynecologic surgery usually occurs below the waist and regional anesthesia is often an appropriate choice. There are, however, some gynecologic surgeries for which regional anesthesia is simply not an option. Laparoscopic surgery cannot be done with regional anesthesia since the gas that enters the abdomen interferes with the patient's ability to breathe adequately on her own; therefore, general anesthesia is the safest choice. Since areas above the waist are not anesthetized, women who are having surgery that may involve manipulation in the upper abdomen are not good candidates. This is commonly the case in women with suspected or known cancer, large fibroids, or known adhesions from severe endometriosis or prior surgery.

Every woman who has a regional anesthetic is made aware that general anesthesia may be needed if the regional anesthesia is not sufficient. This rarely happens. On occasion, particularly if someone has a very curved spine or has had back surgery, it may be technically difficult to get the needle in the appropriate space or impossible to get the local anesthesia to spread sufficiently to provide adequate numbness. The anesthesiologist checks the patient before the surgeon makes her incision to make sure the numbness is adequate for the surgery. If it is not, the anesthesiologist will either fix it or proceed with a general anesthetic if necessary.

COMBINED ANESTHETICS

Combined spinal/epidural techniques are becoming more common. Spinal anesthesia provides quick onset and more reliable numbness. Epidural anesthesia allows longer operating times and pain relief in the immediate hours and days after surgery. Put both together, and the anesthesiologist has the ability to provide all the advantages.

Sometimes an epidural catheter is placed and the patient goes right to sleep. The beauty of this system is that all the advantages of general anesthesia are there and the patient has the advantage of postoperative pain relief through an epidural catheter.

ANESTHETIC COMPLICATIONS

It is truly astonishing how far anesthesia has come in the last fifty years, and how rare anesthetic complications are. In 1950, the risk of dying from anesthesia was one in 1,500. Today, the risk is in the neighborhood of one in 250,000, even though surgeries have become more complicated and are often performed on older and sicker patients.

Virtually every death due to anesthesia is cardiac, and is almost invariably in someone who was high-risk due to heart problems that were present (and known) prior to surgery. The risk of a healthy woman dying during gynecologic surgery from the anesthesia is less than 0.03 percent; in other words, almost zero.

Death, of course, is not the only complication, but is the one that most people worry about. What else can happen? During general anesthesia, it is possible to put the tube in the wrong place (the esophagus rather than the trachea), but this is corrected right after it happens and causes no harm. Sore throats and hoarseness occur occasionally and generally last a day or two. There may be damage to teeth when the tube is being placed, even if dental work is secure. Other less likely complications are related to specific medical problems and would be discussed during the preoperative evaluation.

Complications from regional anesthesia are also rare and most commonly include headache, minor backache, or a high block that creates temporary difficulty breathing during surgery. Transient changes in blood pressure can also occur but are easily corrected with drugs.

Everybody has heard of someone who received a spinal anesthesia and was paralyzed for life. The trouble is, no one ever really *knows* someone. It's always, "My cousin's next-door neighbor had a friend who had a spinal anesthetic and never walked again!" The reason nobody actually knows anyone is because it never actually happens.

Extraordinarily rarely, a hematoma (blood clot) forms in the epidural space, which can cause what is almost always a transient neurological problem. There have been rare cases in which a neurologic deficit does not completely resolve.

Nurse Anesthetists

A nurse anesthetist is a nurse who has received a master's degree in anesthesia and works directly with the anesthesiologist (an M.D. who has done a four-year residency in anesthesia) to place and maintain anesthesia. It's quite common for a nurse anesthetist, under the supervision of an anesthesiologist, to be the one who actually puts you to sleep and stays with you during the surgery. An anesthesiologist is present when you go to sleep, when you wake up, and if there are any problems, but he or she is generally in charge of two or three rooms. The nurse anesthetist is only taking care of one person at a time. It's very similar to the pilot and copilot of an airplane in which both are involved during take-off and landing, but it is the copilot who keeps an eye on things when the plane is at cruise altitude.

A testimony to the skills of the nurse anesthetist is that surgeons often request a particular nurse anesthetist when they themselves have surgery. Keep in mind that the surgeon is ultimately responsible for your well-being; if your surgeon is comfortable with a nurse anesthetist, you should be, too.

WHO'S GOT A VALIUM? STRATEGIES FOR THE TERRIFIED

First and foremost, tell the anesthesiologist how frightened you are. If possible, try and figure out exactly which part of the process worries you the most. Is it fear of feeling the surgery? Fear of going to sleep? Fear of not waking up? Fear of post-op pain? It's easier to help you if someone knows what your fear is. Sometimes a detailed explanation of how something is done is all it takes to relieve anxiety. There are other strategies that can help.

Once your consent form has been signed, the anesthesiologist can give you anxiety relief through the IV before you go into the operating room to quickly get rid of that panicky feeling. If you think you may want drugs, mention it to the anesthesiologist at the pre-op visit. Consent forms can be signed before your surgery date to speed things up and allow you to get drugs sooner. If that is something that interests you, mention it to both your surgeon and anesthesiologist at pre-op visits since they each have their own consent forms.

Some women relieve anxiety by listening to music through headphones while waiting for surgery. Feel free to bring headphones and whatever music relaxes you. If you have general anesthesia, the anesthesiologist will remove the headphones once you're asleep; women with a regional anesthesia can listen to their music throughout the surgery.

There are actually tapes available specifically for use during surgery with "positive thoughts" and music designed to promote healing and decrease anxiety. If this works for you, fine.

What Kind of Anesthesia?

This is one situation where you won't be making the decision. You can certainly voice a preference, but ultimately the anesthesiologist will decide the safest and most appropriate strategy for you.

A lot of factors go into deciding the best method of anesthesia. The type of surgery, length of surgery, expected blood loss, pre-existing medical problems, level of anxiety, and preferences of the surgeon and anesthesiologist all play into the decision. Don't try and talk the anesthesiologists into what you perceive is the best method; it's really not in your best interest.

An anesthesiologist who needed emergency surgery happened to be on vacation in a rural community with a small hospital. The anesthesiologist on call, realizing that his patient was another anesthesiologist, politely asked him, "What kind of anesthesia would you like?" The anesthesiologist replied, "Whatever *you* want, and whatever you do best." There was a lot of wisdom in that statement.

Chapter 15

Preparing for Surgery

Y ou've set the date. Now what? That depends on how much time you have. Many women plan their surgery months in advance; many have less than a week to get everything together. The following timetable is the ideal situation in which there is a minimum of three months to plan. Most things that are really important, however, can be taken care of in a matter of days.

THREE MONTHS BEFORE SURGERY

Stop Smoking

It's not news that smoking is bad for you, yet to be advised to stop smoking when you are about to go through a major life stress may seem ridiculous, if not impossible. It's not uncommon for someone to think, "I just need to get through this surgery and then I'll deal with my smoking problem." Having said that, there are some compelling reasons why this really is the time to quit once and for all.

▼ Any anesthesiologist will tell you that smoking presents an additional risk of lung complications after surgery.

▼ Postoperatively, smokers are at increased risk for pneumonia, bronchitis, and atalectasis. Atalectasis is a condition in which the lungs don't completely expand, resulting in decreased oxygenation and fever. The postoperative use of an incentive spirometer and other lung-expansion techniques helps, but doesn't eliminate the problem (see chapter 18).

▼ Hospitals are no-smoking zones. The first few postoperative days are tough enough without adding the stress of nicotine withdrawal.

▼ Coughing hurts. It is a given that smokers cough more than nonsmokers to get secretions out of their lungs. In fact, after surgery, smokers are encouraged to cough and breathe deeply to help clear secretions. Coughing with a fresh incision on your abdomen is extra pain you don't need, which is why smokers may require more pain medication than nonsmokers.

▼ Smokers have a higher rate of postoperative complications such as poor wound healing, infection, and blood clots.

▼ You need to stop anyway. This is a good time.

Now that you're convinced that this is the time to stop, how do you do it? Every successful smoking cessation program succeeds because the person wants to quit and is ready to quit. Your physician can recommend a program, or you can call the American Cancer Society.

If surgery is less than six weeks away, this is not the time to quit. There will not be enough time for your airways to recover, and in fact they may end up having more inflammation than usual due to reparative changes. Tell your gynecologist and anesthesiologist that you smoke so that lung-expansion techniques such as incentive spirometry, deep breathing, and coughing can be practiced and perfected before surgery. Get an extra pillow to hold over your belly when you cough. Do not sneak a cigarette in your bathroom. Smoke detectors will go off and it will be incredibly embarrassing.

Iron Supplementation

Some blood loss is anticipated during any surgical procedure. Fortunately, blood loss with an uncomplicated hysterectomy is usually minimal and results in no more than a mild transient anemia that corrects itself within a few weeks of surgery. Some women, however, are starting surgery with a low blood count due to prolonged heavy bleeding and are therefore at higher risk of becoming significantly anemic after surgery. The more iron stores your body has, the faster new red blood cells can be made in order to correct anemia. Therefore, it is a good idea to take additional iron as soon as you even contemplate the possibility of having surgery.

You can increase your iron stores by eating iron-rich foods or by taking iron supplements. Iron supplements may cause gastrointestinal upset and turn stool very dark, almost black. Your preoperative blood count will determine how much iron you should take. Even if you have a normal blood count, it's a good idea to take some extra iron . . . money in the bank, if you will.

Autologous Blood

Some women choose to bank their own blood in advance in the event that a transfusion is necessary, otherwise known as autologous transfusion. This became popular in the 1980s and 1990s due to concerns about the risk of contracting acquired immunodeficiency syndrome (AIDS) or hepatitis from a transfusion. In addition, autologous blood also protects against other transfusion complications, such as allergic reactions or transfusion fever.

Autologous donation takes advance planning since only one unit (500 cc) a week can be donated. The last unit must be donated at least

one week prior to surgery so that the anemia that results from the donation can correct itself. If someone is planning on donating her own
blood, she should immediately start taking iron supplementation and
continue it until the time of surgery. Three hundred mg two to three
times a day is recommended if your stomach can take it. Your physician
can arrange for you to donate blood at the hospital or designated facility. Your blood is then frozen and delivered to the hospital on the day of
your surgery. Arranging for autologous donation is not difficult. The real
question is, should you bother?

There are all kinds of reasons why autologous donation for a
routine hysterectomy is unnecessary and perhaps a negative. First of
all, transfusion is extremely unlikely for a routine hysterectomy,
occurring in less than 1 percent of hysterectomies. Most women tolerate a mild to moderate anemia well, particularly if they are young
and healthy. Women who require transfusion usually have uncom-
monly heavy blood loss or were very anemic to begin with. The most
likely people to need a transfusion are anemic to start with and
wouldn't be a suitable candidate to donate their own blood.
Furthermore, if someone truly requires a transfusion, she will
require far more than the one or two units she might have banked
"just in case." If someone gets just one or two units of blood, she
probably didn't need it at all. Donating the blood, aside from being
inconvenient, has the end result of a person going through surgery
iron-depleted and slightly anemic to start with and therefore less
able to recover on her own from whatever normal blood loss she
might experience.

Even autologous blood is not risk-free. Transfusion reactions have
been reported in cases where there is bacterial growth in the banked
blood, or where clerical error has resulted in the wrong blood being
transfused. Studies have shown that a person with autologous blood on
hold is much more likely to receive a transfusion than the person who
did not donate. In other words, the blood may be transfused unnecessarily simply because it is there.

Donor-designated blood is another option. Donor-designated blood
is when someone, usually a friend or relative, donates blood on your

behalf. The advantage is that the person having the surgery does not need to donate her own blood, yet can avoid the "risks" of acquiring a transfusion from the bank. But is the blood from a friend or relative safer than the blood you get randomly from the community blood bank? The answer is, probably not. Multiple studies have shown there is no significant difference in safety, and that donor-designated blood may be slightly riskier. This is not the moment that friends and relatives will choose to announce that they've engaged in unsafe sex or used IV drugs. Studies have shown that donor-designated blood carries a higher risk for hepatitis than banked blood. Your best bet is to take your iron and don't worry about the extremely remote chance that a transfusion, if needed, will be contaminated.

Weight Loss

In the ideal surgical world, everyone would be of normal body weight. There is no question that many surgical complications are directly related to obesity. The problem is, the patient who is significantly, medically overweight will not be able to lose more than about fifteen pounds in three months. While fifteen pounds is a significant weight loss and will probably get you into a smaller pair of pants, it won't make a dramatic difference in complication rates. The patient who really needs to lose weight needs six months to a year to make a significant difference. That's not to say it's not worth losing some weight before surgery, but only if it's done appropriately. Starving is always a bad idea since healing depends on good nutrition.

ONE MONTH BEFORE SURGERY

Precertification

Generally, your surgeon's office will precertify the procedure with your insurance company. Just because a procedure is precertified is not a guarantee of coverage. Read the small print. Talk to a representative from your insurance company yourself if there is any question about coverage. If your insurance says it will pay "usual and customary charges," bear in mind that these probably won't come close to your physician's actual charges. Know what your financial responsibility will be so that a bill won't shock you.

Verify Length of Stay

It is not unusual for your insurance company to precertify you only for a brief stay after your surgery. If they have only given you, say, one night for a hysterectomy, understand that they are willing to give you more if there are medical issues that justify a longer stay. Your doctor's office knows to call your insurance company every day to explain why you are still there, so don't panic if they give you one night and your doctor thinks two or three is more likely. However, be aware that just because your doctor requests an additional day, they will not necessarily cover the cost if they don't agree that it is medically necessary. Your doctor must justify a request with objective data. For example, if your doctor says you would benefit from a longer stay due to a greater than average blood loss, the insurance company will decline coverage unless you are receiving IV fluids or need a transfusion. No one is going to throw you out of the hospital; your insurance just won't pay for it.

See Your Internist

As soon as you know you are scheduled for surgery, it is a good idea to make an appointment with your internist for a general physical. This is the time to determine if you have special needs due to an existing medical condition, such as asthma or high blood pressure. This is extremely important if you have ongoing medical problems. This is less important if you are a healthy thirty-year-old who doesn't even have an internist (see chapter 14).

Schedule Pre-Op Testing

Each hospital has guidelines concerning age and circumstance as to what laboratory tests will be required. Most anesthesiologists do not repeat testing done four to six months prior to surgery unless there is reason to believe that something may have changed.

At a minimum, most women require a blood count prior to surgery. Depending on your age and general medical condition, blood chemistries, EKG, chest X ray, and pulmonary function tests may also be required. Your gynecologist or internist will let you know what you need. Testing is usually done a week or so prior to your hysterectomy, but sometimes it is not done until the morning of surgery if you are healthy or your surgery was scheduled at the last minute.

Ideally, testing should be done far enough in advance so that if anything surprising shows up, it can be addressed without postponing the surgery. You can only imagine how disconcerting an abnormal EKG reading is; it is even more disconcerting if it is found the day before you are scheduled for surgery.

Legal Issues

A will? The last fourteen chapters have assured you that everything is going to be fine, nothing bad will happen to you, and now you're being advised to get a will? The reality is that all adults should have a will, even if they are not about to have major surgery. Most people drive a car every day, and the likelihood of death from a car accident is far more likely than death from a hysterectomy. This is a good time to get things in order. If you don't have a will, get one—not because you are having surgery, but because it is something you need to do anyway.

In addition to a will, it is prudent to think about advance directives in the unlikely event that you are incapacitated or become terminally ill. Again, these are things that all adults should think about, even if they are not about to have surgery. There are two directives that are prudent to have: a health-care proxy, and a living will.

A health-care proxy is also known as a power of attorney for health care. The person designated as your health-care proxy serves as your surrogate in the event that you are incapacitated and cannot make your own health-care decisions. There is no legal requirement that you choose a proxy. If you have not designated a specific person, your next of kin will serve in that role. If that is acceptable to you, you need not appoint some-one else. Many people choose a relative who is medically knowledgeable in the event that complex medical issues need to be considered.

A living will is a document that takes effect if a person is terminally ill, with no chance of recovery, and specifies one's desire to withhold heroic measures. Modifications can be made to detail specific circumstances.

No lawyer is necessary to legally designate a health-care proxy or execute a living will. Simple state-specific forms can be downloaded from www.partnershipforcaring.org/advance, or can be obtained from the hospital. A copy of your health-care directives should be on your hospital chart and in the possession of a close relative.

TWO WEEKS BEFORE

In addition to taking care of all the above matters, this is the time to be aware of any medications that might affect your platelet function and your body's ability to form clots. In other words, it is time to start avoid-ing drugs that might make you bleed more.

Occasional use is not problematic, but regular use of medications that contain aspirin or NSAIDs should be avoided and include: Anacin, Advil, Aleve, Alka-Seltzer, Anaprox, Bufferin, coricidin, Excedrin, empirin, indomethacin, ibuprofen, Midol, Motrin, naproxen, and Ponstel.

Tylenol (acetaminophen) is fine. Keep in mind that many herbal compounds alter clotting and should also be stopped two weeks before surgery. The surgeon and/or anesthesiologist should be informed of any medication you take on a regular basis so he or she can tell you if it is safe to continue taking it.

THE WEEK BEFORE

What To Pack

Don't bring anything that would upset you if it were destroyed or lost. If you are not sure if you will be spending the night, pack a small bag with just the essentials:

▼ Scuff slippers

▼ Socks

▼ Shower cap (You may want to take a shower but not deal with washing and drying your hair.)

▼ Sanitary pads (The hospital will give you some, but you may prefer your own.)

▼ Underwear (Leave your thongs at home.)

▼ Pajamas

▼ Clothes to wear home (think baggy, loose, and comfortable)

▼ Pillow (if you think you'll sleep better with your own)

▼ Sleep mask

▼ Toiletries

▼ Money (for the morning newspaper)

▼ Cheap watch

▼ Pens

▼ Paper

▼ Something to read

▼ Glasses

▼ Phone numbers

▼ Insurance card

▼ Medications, such as daily thyroid medication or your asthma inhaler

Do not bring:

▼ Valuables

▼ Make-up (Visitors should feel sorry for you. You don't want to look too good.)

▼ Work (Come on!)

▼ Anything you would be upset if it was lost, stolen, or broken

Hair Issues (Not the Hair on Your Head)

Most abdominal surgeries require a hair-free belly. A bald vulva and perineum is not required. Studies have shown that shaving the day before
surgery actually increases the rate of wound infection so *don't* shave
your abdomen or vaginal area the day before surgery. If it needs to be
done, it will be done for you in the operating room and will be far less
extensive than what you are probably imagining. Some women prefer to
wax, and this is acceptable as long as it is done days before surgery so
that any inflammation will have subsided. The added advantage of wax-
ing is that you don't have to deal with the uncomfortable itching from
new hair growth. If you are going to wax, the area from your belly button to pubic bone is more than adequate. Again, a hair-free vulva is not
necessary, unless that is something you usually do anyway.

Know How to Get to the Hospital

If you have never been to the hospital where you are to have your surgery,
find out how to get there and where to park. Some hospital complexes are
huge and while you might get to the general area on time, it may take you
another thirty minutes to park, find the right building, and find where
you need to check in. If you arrive even a little late, your surgery may be
cancelled or they may bump you to a different time slot. Operating rooms
make a real effort to run on time, especially if you are the first case of the
day. Figure out in advance where you are going. If they say arrive two
hours before the actual time of surgery, they mean it.

If you are traveling to a hospital far from your home, consider staying in a nearby hotel the night before surgery. There's a lot to be said for
a nice dinner, followed by a massage, an in-room movie, and a good
night's sleep the night before surgery. It's nice to simply wake up, jump
in a cab, and arrive at the hospital in a matter of minutes. Many hospitals have arrangements with nearby hotels and have special rates for
patients. Don't forget the wake-up call, especially if you have taken a
sleeping pill.

Arrangements to go home should also be made in advance. If you are planning on having someone bring you home at the end of the day (when they get off work), keep in mind that most discharges occur in the morning. Your insurance company may charge you for an extra day if you stay until evening. They are not concerned about your convenience or the logistics of finding someone to take you home at 11:00 A.M. The morning of discharge is a bad time to scramble for a ride, so plan in advance.

The Day Before

The most important thing to do the day before is to keep busy so you're not feeling anxious. For some reason, closet-cleaning is a popular activity. After you finish cleaning your closet, it's time to clean your bowel . . . .

Bowel Preps

Bowel prep (cleaning out the gastrointestinal tract) is not required for every hysterectomy. Usually the decision to do a bowel prep is based on the personal preference of the surgeon, or your particular situation. Scenarios in which you should expect to need a bowel prep would include women who are suspected to have ovarian cancer, history of multiple pelvic surgeries, infection or endometriosis, and women who have a gastrointestinal disease such as diverticulitis.

You may be given something to drink that will induce bowel movements; you may be instructed to do an enema, or a combination of both. This may be one of the situations in which it is truly nicer to be in the privacy of your own bathroom instead of in the old days when this was done the night before in the hospital.

Shaving, Shower, Shampoo

Feel free to shave your legs or under your arms, but not your belly. Showering and shampooing the night before is key since you may not be able to for a couple of days.

Pay attention to your belly button. When the nurse in the operating room scrubs your belly, she or he usually uses a Q-Tip to clean it out. You'll want to make sure you're not the rare patient who has a huge amount of black gunk requiring four or five Q-Tips. This is particularly relevant if you are having a laparoscopic procedure since it is a guarantee that your belly button will be scrutinized. Make sure it's clean. Your mother would be mortified.

The Last Meal

Dinner the night before should be whatever you want, as long as it is something that won't give you indigestion. A big heavy meal will make you feel uncomfortable and is probably not a good idea. One glass of wine or beer is fine; more than that will dehydrate you and make you feel lousy in the morning.

Unless otherwise instructed, do not eat or drink *anything* after midnight. Anything. Anything.

Sleeping Pill

In more civilized days when women were admitted to the hospital the night before surgery, it was common to take a sleeping pill to assure a good night's sleep. This is no longer routinely done since women are not in the hospital the night before and need to get up at the crack of dawn to get to the hospital on time. If you think you would like a sleeping pill the night before surgery, your surgeon can prescribe one. Just make sure and take it early enough in the evening that you are able to actually get up and be functional in the morning.

What If You Are Sick?

If you have a bad cold or the flu the morning of surgery, it is likely that surgery will be postponed, unless it is emergent. Let your doctor know right away if you are not feeling well the week before surgery. He or she will most likely want to wait until the day before surgery to decide if you are well enough to proceed. If your surgery was planned well in advance

and you have taken off work, made arrangements, and are psychologically ready to go, this postponement can be devastating to you. Why *not*
go ahead if all you have is a little cold? There are a few studies that suggest that the presence of an upper respiratory infection may increase the
risk of anesthetic or postoperative complications. The numbers are
small, but if surgery is elective, it makes sense to put it off if it might
increase your risk of a problem even slightly. In addition, recovery is
worse if you feel congested and achy. It can also be confusing if you have
a fever after surgery . . . is it from the flu, or is it an indication of a surgical infection? If you show up on the day of surgery and are sick, the
anesthesiologist will ultimately decide if it is prudent to wait.

Most important, maintain a positive attitude. There is no reason to
think that things are not going to go well. You're ready.

Chapter 16

The Day
of Surgery

It's 5:00 A.M. You're feeling anxious, hungry, slightly nauseated, gripping a suitcase, and wishing you were on the way to the airport instead of checking into the hospital to have a hysterectomy. Focus. Remember the bleeding, the pain, and the constant pressure on your bladder. Remember you made this decision because it's the right thing to do and you're going to feel a whole lot better.

Once you arrive at the hospital, check-in may seem excruciatingly slow considering you've preregistered and your insurance has already been cleared. Once you have checked in, depending on the hospital, you will be brought either to the room where you will be staying after surgery, or more likely, to the holding area.

HOLDING

The holding area is where you wait just before going into the operating room. Operating-room time is obscenely expensive, so everything that can be done will be done, prior to actually entering the operating room.

The opening in the attractive gown you are given is not there so everyone can see your butt; it's there so the gown can easily be taken off once you are asleep. You may be given socks or slippers. Don't plan on wearing your own unless you never want to see them again. The matching hat comes later.

The holding area for surgery is very similar to the terminal where airplanes wait to take off. It is where all last-minute safety checks are done in preparation and yes, people in carts are often queued up like planes on a runway. Sometimes there are little cubicles; more often you are separated from your neighbors by a curtain. You usually are allowed to have a visitor stay with you. Make sure it's someone who makes you feel less anxious; perhaps your mother-in-law is not the best choice.

Now that you're in your attractive outfit, with no make-up, no contact lenses, no sleep, and feeling more than a little anxious, you get to meet lots of new people. The *last* thing in the world you're in the mood for is to make a nice impression. Don't worry, no one is making a judgment about how you look and act. Everyone knows you usually look much more attractive. Everyone knows you are wishing you were someplace else. No one expects you to be particularly charming.

THE CIRCULATING NURSE

The circulating nurse is often the first person to greet you in the holding area. He or she is a registered nurse who will get you ready for surgery and then stay in the operating room the entire time. The nurse starts by getting basic information and confirming things that she already has been told, like your name and the specific operation you are scheduled for. She will take your blood pressure, temperature, and pulse.

She usually will ask you to pee in a cup in order to do a urinalysis and pregnancy test. Don't get crazed when the hospital insists on a pregnancy test the morning of surgery. No matter how unlikely pregnancy may be, many hospital policies require pregnancy tests on all menstruating women prior to surgery. The circulating nurse is also the first of many people who seem obsessed with asking you if you have had anything to eat or drink and if you are allergic to anything.

THE GYNECOLOGIC RESIDENT

If you are at a teaching hospital, the next person on the scene is usually the gynecologic resident. The gyneological resident is a licensed doctor, not a medical student. He or she has completed four years of medical school and legally could have gone out and opened an office. Instead, he or she decided to do an extra four years of postgraduate training to specialize in obstetrics and gynecology. As part of their training, they participate in surgery. Many people think that residents only observe other surgeons operate. While certainly there are many instances in which they are observers, they are usually assisting an attending surgeon.

Patients sometimes request that a resident does not participate in their surgery. That's usually not an option since every surgeon needs an assistant and at a teaching hospital, the assistants are always resident doctors. In fact, insurance companies will not even cover the cost of a different assistant if a resident is available.

Residents do a high volume of surgery and are capable surgeons. They are not strangers to your doctor; they operate with him or her every day and know them very well. Your hysterectomy is likely their thirtieth or fortieth; they have been assisting and doing many types of surgeries for years. Residents are assigned to cases that are appropriate for their level of experience and your doctor has a say in who his or her assistant will be. If they are assigned a resident and feel that they need someone more experienced, another resident will be assigned. Your doctor stays scrubbed and in the room for the entire duration of the surgery. At no time is the resident "on their own," with the possible exception of closing the skin although, quite frankly, they are usually totally capable of doing the entire surgery on their own, and will be operating independently within a year or two.

In your case, the doctor you have chosen will be there, will be in charge, will be the primary surgeon, and most importantly, will take responsibility for everything that happens during the course of the operation. Your doctor can't do the surgery herself any more than you can tie your shoe with one hand. Also, keep in mind that your doctor's major concern is that your surgery goes well; the educational process of the resident is secondary.

The gynecological resident will introduce themselves and identify his or herself as the resident who will be assisting your doctor. They will usually know a lot about you, having already spoken to your doctor and read your history. Sometimes they will know nothing about you and will ask you questions that make it obvious that they are not familiar with your case. "What brings you here? Why are you having a hysterectomy?" Sometimes this is annoying. Sometimes it's simply terrifying that this person who knows nothing about you, or the detailed discussions you have had with your doctor about your gynecologic and medical history, is about to assist in your surgery. Why doesn't he or she know? What's going on?

In the days when women were admitted the day before surgery, there was ample opportunity for residents to meet the patient the night before and review all the information. Now, with same-day admissions, that opportunity isn't there. If a resident is assigned to your surgery at the last minute by a change in schedule or request on the part of your doctor, they may not have had a chance to learn about you. Sometimes they simply want to hear your story first-hand. The bottom line: don't worry. Your doctor will be there; your doctor knows everything about you.

THE MEDICAL STUDENT

The medical student is a different story. Medical students are required to rotate through all the specialties during their third year of medical school. They usually spend a week or two on gynecologic surgery as part of their rotation in obstetrics and gynecology. While they often scrub for surgery, they rarely do anything other than hold something the surgeon has asked them to hold; they are essentially observers. They do nothing that will influence your surgery other than provide an extra pair of hands. Very often, your surgeon meets the student the same time you do.

Should you ask that the student not participate? You have that right, but it's usually not in your best interest. Surgeons generally like to have a student scrub and will ask for one if one isn't assigned. They are an extra pair of hands that facilitate the surgery, and most surgeons enjoy pointing out anatomy and asking questions of the medical students. Particularly if you are having a vaginal hysterectomy, a second assistant makes your operation go much faster.

The student has likely been told that they must ask you questions about your gynecologic problems. Again, it can be somewhat irritating that all these people taking care of you seem to know so little about you. On the other hand, talking to students and residents is distracting. They also frequently learn something about you that no one else knew and which ultimately helps in your care. (You have a latex allergy? How interesting!) The medical student will also be seeing you after surgery and, in fact, is sometimes the person you see the most. If you really don't want them around, let someone know.

THE ANESTHESIOLOGIST

The anesthesiologist who will be taking care of you also greets you in the holding area. At the anesthesia appointment (see chapter 14), all issues regarding anesthesia should have been discussed. There are hospitals in which you don't meet with an anesthesiologist until the morning of surgery, particularly if you are young and healthy. If that's the case, many of the issues discussed in Chapter 14 will now be addressed. If a nurse anesthetist is involved in your care, they will also introduce themselves.

THE CONSENT FORM

The next step, if it was not done in advance, is to sign consent forms. Usually there are two forms: one for the anesthesia, another for the surgery. The lawyers, not the doctors, design the consent form. The term "informed consent" is a legal term meaning that the patient has been informed of what the surgery will include, what potential complications might be, what alternatives are available, and what outcome the patient should expect.

The concept of informed consent is an absurd notion. The only patient who can be truly informed of all possibilities that might occur during gynecologic surgery is another gynecologist. There is absolutely no way that a surgeon can tell a patient everything that could potentially happen.

The real reason for a consent form is to satisfy the requirements of the lawyers and hospital administrators. From a surgeon's point of view, informed consent means that their patient goes into a procedure knowing what the plan is, what the outcome is intended to be, and the most common complications that might occur. It is not a contract. Hopefully, this was all discussed in detail before the actual day of surgery.

Consents for surgery are standard forms with areas to fill in the blanks. That means that the consent form for a heart or lung transplant is essentially the same as for a circumcision. All consent forms include waivers, "There are NO Guarantees," and disclaimers. Don't spend a lot of time reading the fine print, crossing things out, and changing things. The reality is that the surgeon can do whatever she deems is appropriate and in the best interest of the patient, despite what the consent form says. Any patient can sue regardless of what she signs, or agrees to. From a doctor's point of view, preoperative discussions, which are documented in the office chart, are far more indicative of what you have been told and what you have agreed to.

There is usually a section that asks for permission to transfuse blood if necessary. Many women cross that section out. Understand that transfusions are only given in life-threatening emergencies. No one is going to give you blood unless you really need it. Most surgeons will not operate without your consent to transfuse. It is extraordinarily rare that a transfusion is needed, but when it happens, your doctor doesn't want to be in the position of having her hands legally tied when trying to save your life. If you are a Jehovah's Witness, or have an issue with this, it should be discussed with your surgeon before the day of surgery.

Another section of the consent form asks for permission to photograph or videotape portions of the surgery. Your surgeon, as part of your medical record, may keep videotapes and photos. If you are interested in having your own videotape as a record of your surgery (or to show at the next family reunion after the videotape of Aunt

Myra's wedding), ask your doctor beforehand.

Now that you're convinced that the consent form is totally worthless, here is what you *should* check for. Make sure your procedure is listed correctly according to your understanding of what is to be done. If you are planning a subtotal hysterectomy with preservation of the ovaries, make sure that is what the consent says. It's not unusual for the form to list your surgery, followed by other potential procedures that you are not planning on. For example, your subtotal hysterectomy with preservation of the ovaries may be listed on the consent form as subtotal hysterectomy, possible oophorectomy, and possible total abdominal hysterectomy. All that means is that your surgeon is planning the subtotal hysterectomy, but has let you know that removal of the cervix or ovaries may be necessary based on what occurs or what is found during surgery. If what was thought to be endometriosis turns out to be ovarian cancer, your surgeon is going to proceed with appropriate cancer staging surgery, even if that wasn't originally discussed.

What's important is that the intended plan has been discussed and you and your surgeon understand it. Obviously, you shouldn't sign anything you're not comfortable with, but keep in mind that "possible" usually means unlikely. All medical words should be explained; don't hesitate to ask if there are things you don't understand.

If you would like to see a consent form when you are not feeling under duress (like when you're rolling into surgery), you can ask to see a consent form before your surgery day. Some surgeons do this anyway so you have the time to carefully read the consent, ask questions, and sign when you are thinking clearly.

Someone usually takes away your glasses after you sign the consent form. You can get drugs now if you want them.

INTRAVENOUS LINE

Everyone must have an intravenous line (IV) in place before surgery since that is the way you get fluids, and ultimately, the drugs that put you to sleep. If you are having a regional anesthetic, you still need an IV since you need to get fluids before your epidural or spinal is placed.

The person who inserts your IV may be the resident, medical student, nurse, anesthesiologist, or in some hospitals, someone from their IV team. You can be sure it will be someone who knows what they are doing since a missed IV means a delay in getting to the operating room. The operating room team is highly motivated to run on time and will not send someone to start your IV who is not experienced.

The IV is usually placed in your arm somewhere on your hand or above your wrist. Blood is generally drawn from the crook of your arm, but IVs are usually not placed there since it will be staying in for at least twelve to twenty-four hours and you want to be able to bend your arm without worrying about dislodging the IV.

Usually, local anesthesia is injected in the skin where the IV is to be inserted. This burns for about five seconds. The IV is a needle with a soft plastic catheter, which is poked through the anesthetized skin and into the vein. Once the catheter is in the vein, the needle is removed and discarded so that only the soft catheter remains. The IV is then hooked up to a bag filled with fluid. When your IV is first started, no drugs are in the bag of fluid; usually it is a saline solution, which may or may not have sugar in it. Any medication that is to go through the IV will be added later.

What if you have bad veins or the person keeps missing your vein? The majority of IVs go in easily on the first try. But everybody, no matter how many thousands of IVs they have started, is going to miss sometimes. Let them try again. If someone misses twice, it is reasonable to ask if someone else is available to try. Some people (particularly drug addicts or people who have spent a lot of time in hospitals), do have tremendous difficulties having an IV inserted. The anesthesiologist is the ultimate IV expert and is usually the end of the line. He or she starts IVs that no one else can, and *will* do it, one way or another.

COMPRESSION BOOTIES

One of the risks of any operation, and gynecologic surgery in particular, is the risk that a blood clot may form in the veins of your legs (deep vein thrombosis). Anytime someone's legs are immobilized for a long period of time, blood can pool and form a clot. The clot in and of it is not dangerous. If that clots travels from your leg and lands in your lung, a pulmonary embolus results, which can have serious consequences. Normally, we move our legs around during sleep, which prevents clots from forming since the leg muscles keep the blood veins moving. During surgery, there is no movement and blood clots may result, particularly if surgery is lengthy. Many different strategies can prevent deep vein thrombosis from occurring (see chapter 22). The most common practice is to use compression booties.

Compression booties are inflatable leg wraps that are placed around your calf and sometimes your thigh as well. Once surgery has begun, the booties inflate and deflate so that your legs are periodically massaged. Essentially, the booties reproduce the effect of moving muscles on the venous system of the lower extremities and prevent blood from pooling. Since the use of compression booties has become standard, deep vein thrombosis is a rare complication.

Sometimes the booties are placed on your legs before you go to sleep in the holding area. Sometimes they are not put on until after you have gone to sleep. They are never hooked up and turned on until surgery is about to begin. If compression booties have not been placed in the holding area, it is certainly appropriate to ask the circulating nurse if you will get them later.

Usually, the booties remain on until you are walking around. For some women, this will be a few hours after surgery; for others, it is the next day. Most people don't mind the booties and even enjoy the leg massage. Some people find them really claustrophobic and want them off as soon as they're awake. As long as you're able to get up and walk, that's usually not a problem.

THE OPERATING ROOM

As you roll out of the holding area on the way to surgery, you'll probably suddenly need to go to the bathroom. It's a combination of nerves and the liter of IV fluid that has gone into your vein and straight to your bladder. Don't bother. You'll be asleep in a matter of minutes and your bladder will be emptied for you.

The Temperature

The first thing you will notice upon entering the operating room is the temperature, which seems to be roughly thirty below zero. The hospital is not trying to save money on the heating bill. The operating room is cold because the huge lights over the operating table generate a lot of heat. Those overhead lights are off when you enter the room, but the room is kept cool in anticipation of when they will be turned on. In addition, the surgeons and scrub nurses wear gowns, gloves, masks, and hats that are really warm. If you are cold, ask for a blanket. They are readily available.

The Table

The operating table is extremely narrow so that the surgeons are right up against you during the surgery. When you scoot on the table from the gurney, they will ask you to put your bottom near an indentation in the table. This is so you won't need to be moved after you are asleep. There is generally no pillow, but there is a small head cushion. Final positioning occurs after you are anesthetized. The table is narrow, but you won't fall off. A safety belt is placed around your hips in the event that you move around. In addition, someone is virtually always by your side.

Frequently, one or both arms are placed on an arm board. A safety strap is often placed on your arms (loosely) to "remind" you not to help during surgery. This is especially important if you have a regional anesthetic, as you will potentially have the ability to move your arms freely. If your arm is not secure, you may inadvertently place it on your abdomen. Since your surgeon does not need an extra hand, your arms will be placed out of the way and loosely secured.

As soon as your arms are strapped down, you will need to scratch your nose. When that happens, and it always does, tell the anesthesiologist. Either they will release your arm, or if they are the nose-scratching type, do it for you.

If your legs need to be in stirrups for the procedure, they will be moved after you are anesthetized. Operating room stirrups are not like office stirrups. They are cushioned footrests that cradle your feet and the back of the calves. Obviously, no effort is needed on your part to keep your legs in the proper position.

GENERAL ANESTHESIA

Once you enter the room, things happen pretty fast. The anesthesiologist will be keeping you busy, and if you are having general anesthesia, you will be asleep within five to ten minutes. Sometimes the anesthesiologist will put a mask over your nose and mouth in order to give you extra oxygen. If it smells funny, it's plastic, not drugs. The drugs that put you to sleep go into your IV and it feels just like drifting off to sleep at night. It's not unusual to feel a slight burning in your arm as the medication goes in.

What Happens After You Go to Sleep?

As soon as you go to sleep, everyone in the operating room goes into action. A catheter is placed in your bladder in order to keep it empty during the operation. It also allows close surveillance of urine output, which both the anesthesiologist and surgeon need to know.

It is usually at this point that the anesthesiologist, surgeon, and circulating nurse positions you for surgery. This is done very carefully since good positioning maximizes the surgeon's ability to operate and minimizes potential injury to you. Years ago, little attention was paid to surgical positioning, and many patients did fine from the surgery but had an injury to a nerve or joint resulting from inappropriate positioning. An anesthetized patient can't tell someone that his or her knee hurts in a certain position, or that something is pressing where it shouldn't. Now there is awareness of the importance of careful positioning in order to protect nerves and joints, and injuries from incorrect positioning are extremely rare.

Shaving is kept to a minimum and generally involves removing hair between your belly button and pubic bone. Resist temptation and do not shave yourself the morning or day before surgery (see chapter 15).

If a laparoscopic hysterectomy is planned, sometimes the abdomen is shaved in the event that the procedure needs to be converted from a laparoscopic to an open case.

Your vagina is scrubbed inside and out with betadyne, an antiseptic. The entire abdomen, from your breastbone to your thighs, is scrubbed with soap and then painted with betadyne.

You are then completely draped with sterile sheets with a small opening where the surgery will occur. A curtain is placed at the level of your shoulders so that the anesthesiologist (who, unlike the surgeon and the assistants, is not scrubbed) is separated from the sterile field. This curtain also functions as a barrier so that if you have a regional anesthetic, you can't watch your own surgery.

Waking Up

The anesthesiologist is constantly aware of what the surgeons are doing and roughly how long the surgery will take. They will often ask the surgeons for an estimate, knowing that it is just an estimate, so they can time their drugs appropriately. Don't worry if the estimate is wrong; you will not wake up before the surgery is over. The anesthesiologist knows better than to reverse the drugs before the surgeon is clearly finishing. You will not remember the waking up process, and you will not remember being transferred to the recovery room. The operating room personnel are expert at moving you safely from the operating table to the gurney, even if you are very large. There are also devices to aid in the process.

REGIONAL ANESTHESIA

If you chose to have a regional anesthetic, your experience will have some significant differences. A regional anesthetic is placed while you are sitting on the operating table, or while you're lying on your side. Some anesthesiologists will place an epidural while you are in the holding area to save time once you enter the operating room since an epidural takes a little time to achieve its full effect. Spinal anesthetics are always placed in the operating room since they work immediately.

What You Will Hear and Be Aware of During Surgery

Since you will be awake, you will obviously be aware of noises and conversation during surgery. However, you may not remember a whole lot, since you will receive sedation to make the time go faster, along with drugs that have an amnestic effect—in other words, drugs that make you forget. If you are alert, you will hear suctioning noises, buzzing noises, machines that beep, alarms may go off . . . all normal. Your surgeon will not converse with you, so if you have a question, ask the anesthesiologist or nurse anesthetist.

It may surprise you that a lot of the conversation during surgery is quite ordinary and not necessarily related to the surgery. If you hear the staff discussing a recent movie or play, it doesn't mean that they are not paying attention. On the contrary, it means that things are going very smoothly and they can talk while they operate. It is also not unusual for the surgeon to point things out to a medical student and ask him or her questions. Sometimes they are not even talking about you, so if you hear the words "ovarian cancer," they don't neccessarily pertain to you.

What if there is unexpected cancer? Everyone in the operating room is very aware that you are awake, and no one will say anything that would be disturbing to you within your earshot. Often music is playing so you can't even hear what the surgeons are talking about. If you would like your own music and headphones to shut out operating room noises and conversation, that's fine, just bring them with you and make sure your batteries are fresh.

Odds and Ends

One common fear is that as soon as you go to sleep, your surgeon goes out to lunch. Today's hospital regulations would never allow a surgeon to leave the operating room for frivolous purposes, but there are valid circumstances in which your surgeon might leave for a short time.

Surgeons have to use the bathroom like everyone else, and if a surgery goes longer than two or three hours, well, sometimes you just have to go. Surgeons do take bathroom breaks, but only if things are stable (no bleeding, etc.) and if there is an assistant. A bathroom break usually takes about five minutes and everyone simply waits for the surgeon to return.

If something unexpected happens during surgery, such as discovery of an unexpected cancer, the surgeon may leave to inform the patient's family members. Again, the surgeon never leaves you unattended and never leaves if things are not perfectly stable.

Another fear: what if your surgeon becomes ill or dies during your surgery? (Some people do worry about this.) There is *always* someone capable of picking up where your surgeon left off, available to step in and take over. It is an extraordinarily rare occurrence, but every hospital has a contingency plan.

As long as you're worrying about unlikely occurrences . . . what if there is a fire in the hospital? Every hospital has a fire plan in which the operating rooms can be blocked off from the rest of the hospital. If the fire is *in* the operating room, there is a protocol in place to safely move you to another area of the hospital while you are asleep. Power outage? Every hospital has emergency generators that are regularly tested for just that purpose. Nuclear weapon attack? It doesn't really matter, does it? Be glad you'll be under anesthesia.

RECOVERY ROOM

All surgeons know that it is a complete waste of time to tell their patients anything about their surgery while they are in the recovery room. You would have no recollection of the conversation five minutes later. Drugs that you received during surgery cause a temporary amnesia. Those, along with whatever pain medication you get, make the hour or two you spend in the recovery room a blur that most people never remember.

The exception is if you had a regional anesthesia rather than a general. In that case, you will be awake, alert, and have total memory of the experience. You also may have to stay a little longer to allow your anesthetic to wear off.

What Your Visitors and Family Should Expect

Once you leave the holding area, your visitors are given an estimated time of when they should return to the waiting room to wait for the surgeon. It's a good idea to get there a little early since sometimes surgery takes less time than expected. If the surgeon goes out to talk to the patient's family and no one is there, she or he will be starting another case and may not be available to speak to them for hours. The surgery may also take longer than expected, which does not mean that something went wrong. Sometimes it just takes longer. Once the surgeon has come out and talked with your family, it is usually a few hours until you leave recovery and go to your room. Tell your surgeon exactly who will be there, whom she can talk to, and how much detail you want them to know. Sometimes well-meaning friends or relatives show up to keep a visitor company and suddenly get to hear details of your surgery, which are none of their business.

Visitors cannot go to the recovery room so there is no reason for them to hang around after they have spoken to the surgeon. Some hospitals allow them to wait in the room on the gynecologic floor, but that varies from hospital to hospital.

THE REST OF THE DAY

Pain Control

Pain control has come a long way. It's rare to have someone say that the pain after surgery was anything other than tolerable. Most people comment that they had significantly less pain than expected. A number of options are available.

▼ **Patient-controlled analgesia.** Patient Controlled Analgesia (PCA) is exactly what it sounds like—pain medication you self-administer. Traditionally, if pain medication was requested, the patient would call for a nurse, request pain medication, wait for the nurse to return with an injection, and then wait for it to take effect. Depending on the availability of the nurse, the time from request to pain relief could be anywhere from twenty minutes to an hour, or longer. If PCA is used, a machine that administers pain medication is attached to the patient's IV line. If pain medication is desired, you simply press a button and a dose of pain medication goes directly into your IV, with rapid results. No waiting for the nurse and no waiting for an intramuscular injection to take effect. The machine is calibrated for your weight so that if you push the button too many times, nothing will happen. No matter how hard you try, you can't give yourself an overdose. Studies have shown that patients who get PCA not only have quicker pain relief, but better pain relief, using less medicine than the traditional way.

▼ **Epidural narcotic.** If you had an epidural catheter placed prior to your surgery, the anesthesiologist will usually inject a narcotic into the epidural space before removing the catheter. This results in excellent pain relief for twenty-four hours following surgery, with the ability to get up and walk around.

▼ **Narcotics.** Some hospitals do not use PCA, or your surgeon or anesthesiologist may not feel that it is an appropriate option for you. In that case, you will most likely receive intramuscular injections of a narcotic on request, or on a particular schedule. Some people have a lot of nausea from narcotics or don't like the way they feel. Others love the floaty, pain-free sensation. Do not worry about becoming addicted from one or two days of narcotics for postoperative pain relief.

▼ **Nonsteroidal Anti-Inflammatories.** If you are eating and drinking the first day, you may do fine with a nonsteroidal anti-inflammatory drug (NSAID), such as ibuprofen or naproxen. The dosages given after surgery are significantly higher than what you take for cramps, and they work surprisingly well. Typically, however, most women request a narcotic in the immediate postoperative period and switch to NSAIDs the next day.

Getting Out of Bed

This is the major event of the day. The nurse will help you and once you have accomplished it, you will probably vow never to do it again. Truly, each time will be easier. Your nurse is not being cruel by making you get up. She is preventing blood clots and starting you on the road to the imminent discharge your insurance company insists on.

Eating

If you had an abdominal hysterectomy, you may not get anything to eat or drink the first day. You won't be particularly hungry, but you will feel like your mouth is the Sahara Desert and you would happily trade your first-born child for some water. Your gastrointestinal tract is essentially shut down as a result of anesthesia and bowel manipulation. Anything you put in your stomach would just sit there until you inevitably vomit. Vomiting is really unpleasant in general. Vomiting is beyond unpleasant if it happens with a fresh incision in your belly. You usually can get some ice chips or a sponge to dip in water and suck, which you will enjoy more than the most gourmet of meals. If you had a laparoscopic or vaginal procedure, you may be given clear liquids or even actual food if you aren't feeling nauseated.

Urinating

The bladder catheter that was placed during surgery will still be there when you get to your room. Most people aren't even aware of the catheter and are grateful that they don't have to get up to urinate. Some women can't stand the catheter and want it out as soon as they are awake. Sometimes it can come out soon after you leave the recovery room, but keep in mind that you will be urinating a lot since you received plenty of fluid during surgery through the IV. Sometimes it's easier to keep the catheter than to get up to go to the bathroom every hour or two.

Visitors

The only visitor you should have on the day of surgery is someone whom you can throw up in front of, and who won't care if you fall asleep mid-sentence. It should be someone who has already seen you snore and drool and has seen your behind. That should narrow it down to your mother, your significant other, and maybe your sister. Everyone else should stay home.

Chapter 17

Recovering from Surgery

Some women are so focused on the day of surgery itself that they forget to prepare for the time *after* their surgery. Recovery issues include not only the first few days in the hospital, but what to expect in the weeks and months to follow.

HOSPITAL STAY

How long you stay in the hospital is dependent on a number of factors, including which procedure was done, how difficult it was, and, yes, what your insurance company allows. In general, a laparoscopic procedure usually requires only an overnight stay. An abdominal procedure usually requires a three- to four-day stay. Even if you are only spending a short time in the hospital, it helps to have an idea what to expect.

There are a number of bizarre things about hospital life. The people who work in hospitals are so used to these daily rituals that they don't consider them to be the least bit strange. For example, everyone seems to be obsessed with your bodily fluids and functions. Virtually every stranger who enters your room feels compelled to ask you about your urination, passage of gas, bowel movements, or any episodes of vomiting you may have had. Sometimes they even want to see it!

There is also no real day and night. Just when you're drifting off to sleep, the night nurse may pop in to see how you're doing, take your temperature, and yes, ask about your bowel function. It's not unusual for a nurse to walk into your bathroom while you're on the toilet and start a conversation at 2:00 A.M. as if you were sitting in your living room.

Morning is really busy. Between the hours of 5:00 and 8:00 A.M., you will be inundated with a constant stream of visitors. The medical student, resident, your doctor, the nurse, housekeeping, perhaps a dietician, and the volunteer selling newspapers all make an appearance. Just when you think you are never going to get any rest, everyone disappears and you wonder if anyone even knows you are still in the hospital. It's not unusual that the next person you see after the morning rush is the person who delivers your lunch. Speaking of lunch. . . .

Hospital Food

After surgery you may not get anything to eat or drink until your bowel kicks into action. You'll know that's happening because your stomach will gurgle, you will pass flatus (as opposed to belching), and you will be hungry as opposed to thirsty. When you proudly announce these accomplishments to all interested parties, you will be rewarded with actual food. Be careful what you wish for.

Hospital food is generally terrible, there is no getting around it. The best trick is not to eat the food. Once you are on a regular diet, you can order out from a nearby restaurant. The nurses are a great source of menus, of course; they know better than to eat hospital food. Beg friends to bring you things to eat. It will make them happy that there is something they can do for you. There are those who believe that bad hospital food is part of the overall plot by your insurance company to get you home more quickly. It works.

Seeing Your Surgeon in the Hospital

If all is going well, you won't see a lot of your surgeon after surgery. Surgeons generally see postoperative patients early in the morning before going to their office or operating room. Some also return in the afternoon, but that's often not the case, particularly if their offices are not attached to the hospital and you are doing well. It's hard to be prepared with questions at 6:00 A.M. before you've had time to gather your thoughts, but that is generally when your surgeon will be by. Jot down things when you are thinking about it. While you may not see him or her throughout the day, your surgeon is in contact with your nurse, particularly if there are any problems.

If you feel that you need to talk to your physician during the day, the first step is to let your nurse know there is an issue. She may call your physician for you, or ask the resident to stop by first. It's not that anyone is trying to keep you from dealing with your doctor, but if you think your incision looks like it might be infected, it makes a lot more sense to have the resident take a look since he or she is usually readily available. The resident can then call your physician and describe what is going on. That's one of the advantages of a teaching hospital; there is always someone around. Of course, you can always call your doctor directly, the same way you would if you were calling from home, but your doctor will most likely talk to your nurse and the resident first to see what the problem is.

Going Home

As a general rule, insurance companies want you out of the hospital as soon as possible. If nothing is being done for you in the hospital that can't be done at home, they want you home. Transfusions, intravenous antibiotics, and inability to eat are reasons to stay in the hospital. Difficulty getting in and out of bed and the fact that you have three children, a traveling husband, and two dogs waiting for you at home are not.

Your insurance company will try and sound like the good guy and tell you reassuringly that you can stay "as long as you need to." The problem is who defines your need? Not your doctor. Not you. Even if your doctor thinks you would benefit from an additional day in the hospital, it will not be granted unless the stay can be justified by specific criteria set by your insurance company. What if you feel you are not ready to go home, but you are not certified for additional nights?

No one will actually kick you out of the hospital; your insurance company just won't pay for it. A day in the hospital can run in the neighborhood of one thousand dollars or more; in a luxury hotel, this will get you a beautiful suite, gourmet meals, massage, and in-room movies. In the hospital, it gets you scratchy sheets, bad food, and possibly a roommate. If you have to pay for an extra day anyway, sometimes your best bet *is* checking into the nearest hotel.

As ridiculous as it sounds, many women who aren't quite ready to go home and face the three kids, two dogs, and pile of laundry, but aren't sick enough to justify staying in the hospital, can take a few interim days in a nice hotel. There's a lot to be said for having someone else bring your meals, change your sheets, and bring you a newspaper. It's also a good idea for the woman who lives alone and doesn't really have anyone to help out for the first few days after surgery.

If you have traveled far from home to have your surgery, a hotel stay also keeps you closer to your doctor if you have any problems or need to be seen. Obviously, your insurance company is not going to pay your hotel bill, but they're not going to pay for a few extra days in the hospital, either. It may be worth the extra expense. Most hospitals actually have special rates at nearby hotels, so it may not be as expensive as you think.

There are some non-financial reasons why you should get out of the hospital as soon as possible. One of the risks of staying in the hospital is that time in the hospital is directly related to the probability of getting an infection. Face it, hospitals are filled with sick people. Those sick people have all kinds of germs, some of them pretty nasty. Even if the hospital takes every precaution (hand washing, isolation of infectious patients, etc.), staying in the hospital for a long time will increase the odds of acquiring an infection.

In the 1950s and 1960s, it wasn't unusual for someone to stay in the hospital for a week or more. She may not have even gotten out of bed for days. Recovery took much longer. A big reason for today's shorter recovery period is improvement in surgical techniques and anesthesia. An equally important factor is the fact that people get up and around far more quickly, resulting in an earlier discharge, fewer blood clots, lower infection rates, and quicker overall recovery. In other words, there are good reasons you are being encouraged to get out of bed long before you may feel ready.

Pain Control

Pain control is taken very seriously and there has been dramatic improvement in what is available and how well it works. The details of pain control immediately after surgery are covered in chapter 19. Usually within a day or two, pain is minimal and most women do fine with non-narcotic oral medications. Certainly some women will need to continue the narcotic, particularly if they have large abdominal incisions, but it's a good idea to use as little as possible. Many women take pain medication out of fear of pain, rather than actual pain, resulting in constipation and lethargy.

When trying to taper off pain medication, it's a good idea to alternate a nonsteroidal anti-inflammatory drug (NSAID) with the narcotic. Usually nighttime is when you may need something a little stronger in order to get some sleep.

Getting Wet

Once the intravenous line is out and you have been given the go-ahead, it's fine to get in the shower. Usually that will be one or two days after surgery. The real danger in showering is not that the incision might get wet, it's that you might pass out. Most people prefer warm showers to cold showers. Heat makes blood vessels dilate. Dilated blood vessels can make your blood pressure drop, particularly if your blood volume is low. Most women are at least a little anemic after surgery. A hot shower could easily cause you to faint, particularly if you're a little lightheaded from a narcotic painkiller. Once you get permission to shower, don't make the water too hot and don't stay in too long. This is not the time to bask in the warm water and sing the entire score of *Oklahoma!* Get in, wash, and get out. Make sure someone else is around in case you do feel faint.

If you have an abdominal incision, you will be given something to cover it so it doesn't get wet. If it does get wet, it is certainly not catastrophic. The skin is sealed closed within twenty-four hours. A wet incision will cause the strips of tape to come off, but you won't fall apart. If you have staples, they are stainless steel. You won't rust.

Tub baths are another story. Getting in and out of the tub is a little tricky. Tubs have the same issues as hot showers. Most surgeons recommend waiting two weeks before you attempt a tub bath. If you want to take a bath earlier, it may be fine, depending on your circumstances, but definitely ask.

Those lucky enough to have a bidet can use it as soon as they can negotiate it comfortably. Don't make the water too hot.

Don't even think about a sauna or hot tub for at least two weeks, and ask before you get in. After six weeks, there are generally no restrictions on pools, tubs, hot tubs, saunas, or any other vessel you may want to get into.

GOING HOME: THE FIRST FEW WEEKS

Going home is exhausting. Hopefully, no one has sent flowers to the hospital. If they have, leave them there, or have someone take them home the night before. Next time a friend or relative is in the hospital for a short stay, send flowers to their home. Baggy pants with an elastic waistband or a loose dress are essential since your belly will still be too swollen and uncomfortable to get into normal clothes.

Make sure you have any prescriptions you need. If the hospital pharmacy has not filled them, swing by your local pharmacy on the way home. You don't want to be without your pain pills after you negotiate a flight of stairs for the first time.

Speaking of stairs, you *can* climb a flight of stairs. If you have stairs that lead into your home, you *must* climb stairs. Just do them slowly and rest when you need to.

Once you get inside, you most likely be ready for a nap. This is normal. In fact, you will find that fatigue will be your limiting factor for about two weeks, sometimes longer. Even if all went well, even if you are not anemic, even if surgery was laparoscopic, the most common complaint is fatigue. You may get up in the morning feeling like you have enough energy to paint the garage; by afternoon, you absolutely must take a nap. It's a combination of healing and the effects of the anesthesia. Postoperative anemia is another reason for an overwhelming fatigue even if you otherwise feel fine. Don't fight it. Take a nap and know that you will back to your usual energy level in a few weeks.

It's normal to feel a little lower abdominal heaviness or pressure. If pressure is building throughout the day, it means you've been on your feet too long. Get off your feet. Listen to what your body is telling you.

Things You Should Not Do When You Get Home

▼ **Do not vacuum or do anything else to clean up the house.** Don't even think about it. Accept the fact that your family is incapable of cleaning up the way you do. Ignore the mess. Resort to dimming the lights and lighting candles if necessary.

▼ **Do not plan on getting anything productive done.** Picture albums you thought you would sort, work you have brought home—you won't do it, so don't expect to.

▼ **Do not weigh yourself.** Getting on a scale after surgery is a leading cause of postoperative depression. You *will* gain weight from the surgery. This is not real weight but is temporary, related to the huge amount of intravenous fluid you received in the hospital. You will sweat it off and pee it away. Promise. What about those huge fibroids? Didn't they weigh at least ten pounds? Sorry. Fibroids are bulky, but they are not heavy. Even removal of *really huge fibroids* results in no more than a two-pound weight loss. You may go down a pants size or two, but the scale will barely quiver.

Visitors

People are well meaning, but unless they have had major surgery them-selves, they have no clue. The last thing in the world you want when you get home from the hospital are constant visitors and phone calls. But that's exactly what always seems to happen. People should just drop food off at the door and leave, perhaps taking your children with them.

Feel free to lie. Use your doctor as an excuse. "My doc says no vis-itors for _____" fill in the blank. Have someone at home answer the phone to let people know that you are fine, but can't come to the phone. Don't promise that you'll call them back, otherwise you'll have to. This way, you can return calls to people you actually want to talk to, which is usually nobody. Answering machines are fine, but then you feel obligated to return the call. You can always unplug the phone for a few hours' rest, but you are just postponing the inevitable, since they will try again later.

THINGS TO WATCH FOR:
WHAT'S NORMAL, WHAT'S NOT

Fever

If you think you have a fever, don't rely on how you feel. Take your tem-perature. This may seem obvious, but it is astonishing the number of times a patient calls to report a fever when they have not even taken their temperature. It's easy to get fooled since you may be warm from a hot flash (if your ovaries were removed), or you may wake up in a pool of perspiration from sweating off the extra fluid you accumulated in the hospital. Buy a thermometer before surgery so that no one has to do the 2:00 A.M. run to the drugstore. Call your physician if your temperature is over 100 degrees, unless you have been told otherwise.

In addition to fever, it is important to watch for other indications of infection. The most common infections after gynecological surgery are urinary tract infections and wound (incision) infections.

Urination

It's normal to urinate a lot. It is also normal to have a slight pilling or drawing sensation in the lower abdomen when you urinate. If you have pain with urination, the urge to urinate without the ability to do so, or frequently urinate tiny amounts, you may have an infection. Blood in the urine is also a sign of infection, but that gets a little tricky since a little vaginal bleeding is normal and it's often hard to tell if the blood is in the urine or coming from the vagina. If your urine comes out red, it's in the urine. If it comes out yellow, but seems to be mixed with red, it's almost always vaginal blood.

Vaginal bleeding should be minimal. If it gets heavier or persists for more than a few days, call your doctor. Light spotting for a week or two is not unusual.

What Should Your Belly Look Like?

Slight abdominal swelling is normal and may last as long as six to eight weeks. If your belly is getting distended, hard, and tender, there may be a problem. Nausea and vomiting are also indications that something is amiss and your doctor should be notified.

Some degree of skin bruising is normal, especially after a laparoscopic procedure. The green/blue bruises will turn lovely shades of orange and yellow before they fade away, and the whole process might take weeks. If the bruises are expanding after you get home, call.

Vaginal Discharge

A little odor is normal. If your discharge is really smelly, green, or pus-like, it may indicate an infection in the back of the vagina (see chapter 18), so call your doctor. If you had your cervix removed, or other vaginal procedures were done with your hysterectomy, you probably have stitches inside your vagina. No, they don't have to be removed. They will simply dissolve away. It's not unusual to see the tan or blue threadlike remnants of these stitches on your underwear, or when you wipe, weeks after your surgery.

What About the Incision?

If you had a laparoscopic procedure, you will have four tiny incisions on your belly with a bandage on each one. Sometimes the bandages are removed in the hospital; sometimes they are left on. It is fine to take the bandage off the day after surgery unless you have been told otherwise. You may see a stitch or two or they may be invisible, depending on how they were placed. Most surgeons use dissolvable stitches, but if your doctor used the kind that have to be taken out, you will have to go to the office for removal. A little dried blood is not unusual. There should be no bright red, active bleeding from any incision.

If you had an abdominal incision, most likely you were sent home with your staples removed and a row of tape (Steri-Strips) across the incision line (see chapter 10). Steri-Strips can be removed four or five days after surgery. Sometimes Steri-Strips are intended to remain in place for two weeks, depending on how the closure was done. It's best to ask your surgeon what he or she recommends before you go home from the hospital.

It is normal for any incision to be a little tender, puffy, or numb. Every day, your incision should feel a little better. If the incision is getting more painful, that may be a sign of a problem. If the skin surrounding the incision is bright red, hard, and tender, you may have an infection. Call your surgeon sooner rather than later since the earlier an infection has been detected, the easier it is to treat. Drainage from the incision should also be reported.

Normally, the puffiness and tenderness are gone by two to three weeks. Numbness can last for months. Many women find that there is a numb patch near an incision. In some cases, it takes years until completely normal sensation returns.

Is There a Way to Improve the Appearance of Your Incision?

The final appearance of an incision has less to do with how the surgeon closed it and more to do with genetics and luck. However, there are things that can be done to influence the long-term appearance of an incision. Dr. Thomas Mustoe, Chairman of the Division of Plastic and Reconstructive Surgery at Northwestern Hospital in Chicago, recommends the following steps to optimize healing of an abdominal incision:

▼ Steri-Strips should be placed horizontally, completely covering the incision, and left on for two weeks.
▼ When Steri-Strips are removed, silicone gel sheeting (many brands are available without a prescription) can be placed; it's one of the few things that have been shown to reduce keloid formation.
▼ If you have had problems with healing in the past, triamcinolone cream (available by prescription) should be applied as long as the scar is pink.
▼ Steroid injections have also been found to prevent keloid formation and can be considered in women who are known to have problems with keloid formation.
▼ If you're not happy with the appearance of your incision, a plastic surgeon should be consulted six to eight weeks after surgery.

Two Weeks: The First Postoperative Visit

Once you leave the hospital, most physicians don't see you until roughly two weeks after surgery, if all is well. This visit is usually an incision check to make sure your incision is healing properly. Sometimes Steri-Strips are removed. A blood count may be done, especially if you were anemic when you left the hospital. Sometimes a speculum exam is necessary to check internal vaginal healing.

The main purpose of this checkup is to see how you're doing in general, and make sure that you are where you should be in the healing process. If all is well, a lot of physical restrictions will be lifted. Usually, driving is fine after two weeks. If you want to start exercising, be specific about what you want to do. When one person at two weeks asks her physician if she can exercise, she may be thinking about riding her exercise bike for ten minutes. Someone else may be planning a seven-mile run.

The two-week visit is also the time to see how things are going hormonally (if ovaries were removed) and to make adjustments. This is an appropriate time to change your estrogen dose if you're having symptoms that indicate that you need a little more estrogen.

This appointment is also your first opportunity since your hospitalization to ask questions about what happened during surgery. Certainly, you saw and talked to your doctor in the hospital, but a lot of people don't remember the details of that discussion. This is the time to ask any questions as far as what was found, what was done, and what you should expect. This is particularly relevant if the procedure you actually had was not the procedure you planned to have.

This is also a good time to discuss the final pathology report. It's not unusual for the biopsy results from your uterus and/or ovaries to get to your doctor days after you have left the hospital. Certainly, if anything serious, such as an unsuspected malignancy, was detected, you would already have been notified so you shouldn't be nervous about this report. Frequently, though, unanticipated benign findings may have been found, such as endometriosis or an ovarian cyst. If you are curious what your uterus weighed, that is usually included in the report. Inevitably, you will be disappointed.

SIX-WEEK VISIT

The six-week visit is generally the final visit. Expect a pelvic exam, which will be no more uncomfortable than the usual pelvic exam. If all is well, you will be told to resume all normal activities, including sex, exercise, and pretty much anything else you can think of. In general, you won't need a return visit until it is time for your annual gynecologic exam.

Speaking of annual gynecologic exam, do you still need to see your gynecologist after a hysterectomy? What is there to check for anyway? The answer is yes, absolutely, you do. If you still have a cervix, you need an annual Pap smear. If you still have ovaries, those need to be checked. If you have no uterus, cervix, or ovaries, you're still not off the hook.

Your gynecologist is the expert who will deal with hormone replacement or alternatives, if you choose not to take hormones. Your gynecologist will be the only physician who puts a speculum in your vagina to screen for vaginal cancer and look at your vulva to check for vulvar cancer. The bimanual exam (one hand on your belly and two fingers in your vagina) will detect masses in your pelvis from colon or other cancers. Dropped bladders, rectums, sexual dysfunction, sexually transmitted diseases, osteoporosis screening, and breast examinations are typical of the things a gynecologist deals with in the woman who has had a hysterectomy.

You're Recovered . . . But Are You?

Physical recovery from the surgery is one thing. Resuming normal activities like exercise, work, and sex are addressed in chapter 23. Then there is your psychological well-being. . .

Depression After Hysterectomy

In 1890, an article in a medical journal identified hysterectomy as the surgery most likely to cause psychosis. This is particularly interesting, since historically the uterus was intentionally removed in order to cure "hysteria." It's almost amusing how, throughout history, both the presence *and* absence of the uterus has been blamed for psychiatric illness in women.

Most recent popular books regarding hysterectomy indicate that a major postoperative depression is to be expected, and may in fact be lifelong. The reality is just the opposite. Not only is it unusual to be depressed, most women report a tremendous sense of relief that they no longer need to deal with pain, bleeding, or fear of cancer.

Feeling a transient sadness after surgery is not the same as a clinical depression that requires treatment. It is perfectly normal, and even somewhat expected, to feel a little blue after any major surgical procedure that results in fatigue and an inability to be totally functional. The general "out of sorts" feeling invariably passes by the time a women has resumed her normal activities and no longer feels fatigued. A true depression occurs in only a small number of women.

Over the last twenty years, numerous studies have been published indicating that the small number of women at risk for postoperative depression can usually be predicted before surgery. Studies also show that low-risk women are at no higher risk for depression after hysterectomy than after any other surgical procedure, such as appendectomy or tonsillectomy. So who then, is at high risk for post-hysterectomy depression?

The greatest predictor for a posthysterectomy depression is the woman who suffered from clinical depression before knowing that she needed surgery. In fact, the problem with most early studies, which demonstrated high rates of depression, is that they did not look at pre-hysterectomy symptoms of depression within the postoperative group. If those women had been eliminated from the study, the actual number of woman who became depressed as a result of the surgery would have been significantly lower.

Another interesting finding is that while hysterectomy does not lead to depression, women who are depressed may be more likely to end up with a hysterectomy. This, of course, results in an artificial inflation of women who seem to be depressed as a result of their surgery.

This does not mean that if you are depressed *about* having a hysterectomy that you will suffer from depression after your hysterectomy. One study that looked at depression after hysterectomy said that women who were anxious and depressed prior to hysterectomy, *specifically* about having a hysterectomy, actually had a lower rate of depression after surgery than before. Very often fear about surgery, fear of cancer, or concerns about sexuality after surgery created the depression—not to mention depression from chronic pain and heavy bleeding, which were eliminated *by* surgery. After surgery, when things were fine, no depression occurred.

When depression does occur, it often helps to understand where this overwhelming feeling of sadness originates. Depression after hysterectomy is intimately related to an overall sense of loss, whether it be loss of menstruation, childbearing potential (perceived or real), sexuality, or simply loss of one's uterus.

Loss of menstruation is, for most women, a major bonus of surgery. After all, many women have hysterectomies precisely so that they *can* stop menstruating. However, there are women who don't have problems with heavy or painful menses who have surgery for entirely different reasons. Some of those women actually find a comforting rhythm in their monthly menses or feel that it cleanses their body. The absence of that familiar cyclicity has been known to create depression in a small group of women.

For some women, the loss of the ability to have children is devastating. Usually, it is the young childless women who require a hysterectomy for cancer or postpartum hemorrhage who are at the greatest risk. There are some options for those women (see chapter 26), but certainly depression under those circumstances is expected and is totally understandable.

The more complicated, and unexpected, group are the women who mourn the loss of childbearing potential due to their hysterectomy, but who, in reality, were not able to conceive before their hysterectomy. The fertility issues of peri- or postmenopausal women, or the infertility from severe endometriosis or large fibroids did not result from hysterectomy; the infertility of these women was an issue before hysterectomy. In spite of that, many women experience a depression directly related to the definitive end of their ability to become pregnant. It's one thing to be told you can't conceive: the finality of having your uterus removed is the ultimate blow for some women. Even women who concede that pregnancy would have been an impossibility report a sadness after their surgery. This is especially true of women who never had a child due to infertility or social circumstances.

Loss of sexuality as a cause of posthysterectomy depression has also been described, but it is relatively uncommon in informed women who have a clear understanding of what was actually removed and how little it actually has to do with their sexuality. There are women who think that a portion of their vagina was removed, making intercourse impossible. Many issues with decreases in sexual attractiveness are culturally related. In reality, study after study has shown that hysterectomy rarely effects sexual function, and in a significant percentage of women, even improves it (see chapter 25).

Loss of the uterus is a more intangible loss. Most women are unaware of their uterus, and if one's uterus could magically be removed without one's knowledge, in truth, women would not even know it was gone. But that is not the case. Women who undergo hysterectomy know that their uterus has been removed, and sometimes experience an inexplicable, even to them, sense of loss. Dr. Nehama Dresner, Associate Professor of Clinical Psychiatry and Obstetrics and Gynecology at Northwestern University Medical School in Chicago, and an expert in women's health issues, defines this loss of the uterus for some women as a loss of competency and self-worth. She explains, "For some women, anatomy can define and determine a woman's sense of femininity and attractiveness, as well as her sexuality and means of self-expression." Thus, a hysterectomy may threaten a woman's very identity.

Other factors that have been identified to increase the risk of postoperative depression include:

▼ Previous psychiatric problems
▼ Conflicts about ending childbearing
▼ History of sexual abuse
▼ Emergency or undesired surgery
▼ Age at time of surgery
▼ Poor social support
▼ Pre- and perioperative marital problems
▼ Low socioeconomic status
▼ Low educational level
▼ Removal of ovaries at the time of hysterectomy, creating surgical menopause

Clearly, many of the above categories include women who have misconceptions, fears, or who simply don't know what exactly happened to them and what they can expect to be like after. The best way to minimize the risk of preventable postoperative depression is to gather as much information as possible to understand what the surgery entails and what to expect after. Education and emotional support are essential to a good recovery. Informed consent, meaning that you understand what is to be done and all of your questions have been answered, is critical. It is also important that a woman chooses hysterectomy as her best option and feels emotionally ready to go through it. Obviously, that is not the case if there is cancer or an emergency hysterectomy, which is why those circumstances lead to an increased rate of depression.

It's important to recognize the signs of depression so that you can distinguish them from normal postoperative reactions. Being sad about not being able to become pregnant is an appropriate response to a significant loss. It is not the same as a severe clinical depression, which requires help. Let your doctor know if you:

- ▼ Can't sleep
- ▼ Have a loss of appetite
- ▼ Feel hopeless
- ▼ Have a loss of interest and energy
- ▼ Feel persistently sad or tearful
- ▼ Are unable to enjoy things
- ▼ Isolate yourself
- ▼ Think about killing yourself

No matter what the depression stems from, it needs to be addressed, and sooner rather than later. Your gynecologist should be able to refer you to a psychiatrist experienced in depression. If he or she is unable to refer you, or if you are hesitant to bring it up, the physician referral service of the hospital where you had your hysterectomy should be able to help you find an appropriate person.

Chapter 18

Complications and How to Reduce Your Risk

The only surgeons who don't get complications are surgeons who don't operate. Any surgeon that says he or she has never had a complication is probably lacking in credibility and may not be a surgeon you want to choose. Every preoperative discussion should include a discussion of potential complications, the likelihood of a complication, and what the consequence of a complication might be. There is no way to mention every possible untoward event that might occur, nor would you want to hear every potential possibility, since the likelihood of most of them would be miniscule. A general discussion of the more common complications follows.

Surgical complications fall into three general categories: infection, bleeding, and injury to surrounding structures. Certainly there are complications that are not within those categories, but they are either uncommon or not serious. Life-threatening complications occur in .06 percent of women who have hysterectomies. Half of those complications occur in women who undergo surgery due to cancer or a pregnancy-related hemorrhage. Three percent of women who have scheduled hysterectomies for benign disease will experience a complication that extends recovery.

263

INFECTION

Postoperative infection is by far the most common complication that occurs after hysterectomy and is seen in 9 percent of women who have surgery. Prophylactic antibiotics are usually administered at the time of surgery in order to minimize the risk of infection, but in spite of that, infections can and do occur. Surgeons take every possible precaution to prevent infection, which is what sterile technique is all about.

Fever is not always an indication of infection. Some studies have shown that up to 30 percent of women have slight transient increases in temperature during the first twenty-four hours after hysterectomy. There is no need to start antibiotics based on fever alone. Over 50 percent of women who have a fever are not infected and do not require antibiotics.

Infection from hysterectomy is usually divided by location and depends on the type of hysterectomy that was performed. For example, if the cervix was not removed, there is no vaginal cuff; therefore, there is no risk of a cuff infection. Typically, wound infections only complicate abdominal hysterectomies, although it is possible for one of the tiny laparoscopic incisions to have an infection. Common infection sites include the lung, the urinary tract, the pelvis, the incision, or the back of the vagina.

Women frequently ask what they can do to decrease the risk of infection. The number one thing, of course, is to spend as little time in the hospital as possible. Hospitals are nasty, germ-ridden places filled with bacteria from other sick people. It's not the hospital's fault; they can't help it that sick people hang out there. If you have the choice between staying the extra day or going home to your own relatively germ-free house, go home, if at all practical.

In addition, there are a few choices that may also decrease your risk. One thing that decreases the infection rate is to not remove the cervix, which serves as a barrier between the vagina and the pelvis (see chapter 19). It follows that laparoscopic subtotal hysterectomy has the lowest risk of infection and vaginal hysterectomy has the highest. Make sure hospital personnel wash their hands or wear gloves when they come in the room to do things for you. It is well known that hand-washing is the number one thing doctors and nurses can do to decrease hospital infections. It's no surprise that nurses are really fastidious about hand-washing; physicians are the worst.

Pneumonia

Pneumonia, or lung infection, generally occurs two to three days following surgery. Women who develop pneumonia have fever, cough, and sometimes chest pain and shortness of breath. While it is possible to suspect pneumonia based on symptoms, a definitive diagnosis must be confirmed on a chest X ray or chest CT scan. Sometimes women are surprisingly asymptomatic, so if you have a fever that is unexplained after surgery, a chest X ray will probably be done even if you don't have a cough.

Pneumonia occurs most commonly in women who have a history of lung disease like emphysema. General anesthesia, surgery lasting more than three hours, and smoking also predispose to pneumonia. Strategies to decrease the risk of pneumonia are discussed in chapter 15. Hospital-acquired (nosocomial) pneumonia is almost always bacterial as opposed to viral and therefore is responsive to antibiotics. It can prolong a hospitalization for many days.

Urinary Tract Infections

Urinary tract infections are one of the most common infections. One to five percent of women acquires a urinary tract infection following hysterectomy. This is not surprising since every hysterectomy requires some manipulation of the bladder and at least one catheter insertion. Sometimes there are no symptoms other than fever and an abnormal urinalysis. Other times, the classic symptoms of pain with urination, frequent urination, blood in the urine, and inability to urinate are present. If untreated, a kidney infection may result, in which there is high fever and back pain. If any of the above symptoms occur after leaving the hospital, a urinary tract infection is likely. It's important to contact your doctor to get started on antibiotics and ideally do a urine culture.

Pelvic Abscess

An abscess is a collection of bacteria and pus at one of the surgical sites in the pelvis. Women with a pelvic abscess have fever, cramping, and sometimes a foul-smelling vaginal discharge. Visualization of the abscess on ultrasound, CT scan, or magnetic resonance imaging (MRI) confirms the diagnosis. Treatment is usually prolonged antibiotics. Drainage is sometimes necessary and guidance from interventional radiology will help to accomplish it. Rarely, surgery may be needed to drain the abscess.

Cuff Infection

The vaginal cuff is the area at the back of the vagina where the cervix was detached. The back of the vagina is stitched closed, forming what is known as "the cuff." The cuff can become infected or an abscess can form, resulting in a foul-smelling vaginal discharge and fever. Like a pelvic abscess, treatment involves prolonged antibiotics and sometimes surgical drainage.

Wound Infection

Wound infection doesn't occur unless there is a wound. While a laparoscopic incision can become infected, it is extremely rare. Wound infection occurs in 3 to 4 percent of abdominal hysterectomies. Signs to watch for are redness around the incision, increasing incisional pain, and/or fever. In addition to being red, the area around the incision can become quite hard (indurated) and tender. Eventually, if the infection progresses, the incision will drain a purulent fluid and the skin edges will separate (see wound dehiscence, below).

Wound infections occur most commonly three to ten days after surgery. If you even think you have the beginning of a wound infection, call your surgeon. Early identification and treatment of an infection can prevent it from becoming severe.

If the infection becomes severe, in addition to antibiotics, the skin may need to be opened up in order to allow pus to drain. In a severe infection, the skin edges will likely separate spontaneously. After the wound is opened, it needs to be cleaned and packed with gauze on a regular basis. While an open incision takes longer to heal and is more uncomfortable, ultimately, it will heal just as well as an uninfected incision.

Scrubbing the abdomen using sterile techniques and the intraoperative administration of antibiotics dramatically reduce the rate of wound infection, but they happen anyway. There is little you can do to prevent a wound infection, but the earlier you see the signs and start antibiotics, the greater chance it will heal without opening up.

Pelvic Vein Thrombophlebitis

Sometimes there is a fever without explanation that persists despite antibiotics and culturing everything you can think of. The culprit may be a condition in which there is a blood clot in one of the veins in the pelvis known as pelvic or ovarian vein thrombophlebitis. Unlike typical infections, treatment is not only antibiotics, but also a course of heparin (a blood thinner) as well. This condition is difficult to diagnose and is essentially a diagnosis of exclusion. Sometimes a CT scan of the pelvis is helpful, but in many instances, the diagnosis is made because no other source of infection can be identified.

BLEEDING

The average blood loss during hysterectomy is actually minimal, in the neighborhood of 300 cc or less. Most women are not even aware of the slight anemia that results.

Most healthy women can tolerate a fairly significant blood loss without being in danger or requiring a transfusion. Women who start out anemic before surgery are at the greatest risk of having a symptomatic postoperative anemia. This is actually not an uncommon scenario since the reason many women have hysterectomies in the first place is because of a long history of heavy bleeding that has caused anemia.

Significant bleeding during surgery is rare, occurring in less than 1 percent of hysterectomies. Situations in which it would be more likely would be when a malignancy is present, peripartum (during or imme-diately after delivery), or if there are significant adhesions. Between 1 and 3 percent of hysterectomies involve excessive blood loss requiring transfusion as a life-saving procedure. This can occur during surgery or in the first day or two after surgery.

Bleeding after you have left the operating room occurs in less than 2 percent of hysterectomies and results from a blood vessel that doesn't bleed obviously during surgery, but gets "loose" from its suture and starts to bleed later. If there is continued blood loss after surgery, there will be signs, such as a continued drop in the blood count, a rise in the pulse rate, and a decreased urine output. There may also be excessive vaginal bleeding. On occasion, the bleeding blood vessel is at the back of the vagina and can be repaired vaginally. If the bleeding is intra-abdominal, the only way to know what is going on is to look inside, requiring a trip back to the operating room. If the blood loss is not too great, laparoscopy is an option, in hopes that the bleeding can be con-trolled through the scope. If blood loss is significant, an incision may be mandatory.

You can't decrease your risk of bleeding before or after your surgery. You *can* decrease your risk of anemia. As soon as you know you will need a hysterectomy, start iron supplementation. If you are anemic from heavy bleeding, seriously consider one of the strategies (see chapter 8) to alleviate the cause of the bleeding, even if it is only temporary. Many women are discharged home on the day of, or the day after, their sur-gery, which means you won't be in the hospital if you have delayed bleeding. Call your doctor *immediately* if you have heavy, bright-red vaginal bleeding, feel lightheaded when standing, notice your belly get-ting more distended rather than less distended, or if you pass out.

What to Expect If You Have Excessive Blood Loss

During the 1980s, physicians realized that transfusions were potentially risky, resulting in the trend towards avoiding transfusion in the absence of life-threatening blood loss. The medical profession learned that peo-ple did surprisingly well in spite of a low blood count. Most healthy women can tolerate a significant anemia as long as they minimize activity. Blood cells are regenerated amazingly quickly; within two or three weeks of surgery, even women with significant anemia are almost back to a normal blood count.

That doesn't mean you won't feel the effects of the blood loss; it just means that it isn't dangerous. You will be really, really tired—the kind of tired where you absolutely have to take a nap in the afternoon. It's also important not to stand up too quickly. If you are lying down, sit for a few minutes before you slowly stand up.

Driving should be avoided until your blood count is close to normal, as should hot showers and baths. You can take a shower—it just shouldn't be too long or too hot. Someone should also be available while you are in the shower in case you feel a little lightheaded.

It's also important to drink lots of water to expand your blood volume. Dehydration will cause a person who is anemic to be much more symptomatic. A lot of women think they should avoid drinking water after surgery since they are so puffy from all the fluids received in the hospital. Not true. You still need to drink, in spite of the fact that your legs and hands are swollen.

As soon as your stomach can handle it, start iron supplementation. If you can tolerate it, two or three pills a day is ideal. Red meat is also helpful if you are not a vegetarian. If you are, there are plenty of other iron-rich foods.

INJURY TO SURROUNDING STRUCTURES

In the same vicinity as the uterus, cervix, and ovaries are a number of other structures that need to be avoided during the course of a hysterectomy. Usually, that's not a problem. On occasion, adhesions, infection, cancer, endometriosis, or other factors present difficulties resulting in inadvertent injuries to other structures. The injury in and of itself is not really a problem: any structure that is injured can be repaired. It may make the surgery and recovery a little longer, but it is rare that an injury to a surrounding structure creates a long-term problem unless the injury is not recognized and properly repaired.

Bowel Injuries

Injuries involving the bowel occur extremely rarely, with an incidence of 0.3 percent of hysterectomies. If the injury is in the small bowel, the hole is simply repaired. If a huge defect is present, sometimes a section of bowel may need to be removed and the cut ends attached to each other. This most commonly occurs in the event of a malignancy or severe endometriosis. A large bowel (colon) injury may rarely require a temporary colostomy, but only if the injury is extensive.

Some gynecologists, particularly gynecologic oncologists, are very comfortable repairing an injury to the bowel. If that is not the case, a general surgeon may be asked to step in.

Bladder Injuries

Inadvertent injury to the bladder occurs in 0.5 percent of hysterectomies. These are usually recognized since urine output and the presence of blood in the urine is constantly being monitored during and after surgery via a bladder catheter. The majority of bladder injuries are small holes that can be repaired easily. Many gynecologists are perfectly comfortable repairing small injuries to the bladder. Sometimes a urologist will be consulted.

While there are no long-term problems after a bladder injury, a catheter is usually required until the repaired area completely heals. Usually the catheter goes through the urethra. Other times, the catheter is placed above the pubic bone and goes directly into the bladder. Either way, urine drains through the catheter into a plastic bag that periodically needs to be emptied. If you need to go home with a catheter, you will be given a smaller bag that attaches around your leg. It's rare to require a catheter for more than a week, so there is no need to invest in a new baggy pants wardrobe. One creative woman placed her urine bag in a Neiman Marcus bag filled with colorful tissue and went for a stroll downtown.

Ureter Injuries

The ureter is the tube that connects the kidney to the bladder and passes quite close to the uterus. It is sometimes difficult to visualize during hysterectomy, particularly if there is endometriosis, scar tissue, or distorted anatomy. Ureteral injuries occur very rarely, and quite honestly, are not always recognized. Since most people have two functional kidneys, it is entirely possible to have a ureteral injury that goes unnoticed if the other kidney is normal. Most ureteral injuries *are* noticed; they occur if the ureter gets kinked, nicked, or cut during dissection of adjacent structures. A urologist is generally asked to consult and assist in the repair of a ureteral injury.

OTHER COMPLICATIONS INVOLVING THE INCISION

Seroma

A seroma is a collection of serum under the skin edge of an incision. Serum is a watery, clear, light yellow fluid excreted by healing tissues. It is more likely to occur in obese women, or in the case of extensive procedures, such as a hysterectomy that involves a bladder repair, abdominoplasty, or cancer. A small seroma will almost always go away without any special treatment: the fluid will simply be absorbed. A larger seroma may need to be drained, or will drain itself by causing pressure under the incision line that ultimately causes the incision to open up. When this happens, the skin edges separate, the fluid comes out, and then the edges of the skin will, over time, completely close again.

You will know you have a seroma because the area under the incision will be hard and uncomfortable. Usually there is seepage of clear fluid through a small opening. Once the skin edges separate, copious amounts of fluid may drain.

While a seroma is a nuisance and will delay healing of the wound, it is not a dangerous situation. It is not an infection, but can increase the risk of infection since bacteria tend to multiply in stagnant seroma fluid.

In a woman at high risk for seroma formation, placement of a drain will decrease, but not eliminate, the possibility.

Hematoma

A hematoma is a collection of blood under the incision. When a surgeon closes the skin, he or she makes sure that there are no bleeding blood vessels under the skin. In spite of that, a small vessel will occasionally start to bleed after the skin is closed. If a hematoma is small and the bleeding stops on its own from pressure, there are no consequences and the blood will simply resorb. If there is a large amount of blood, a wound separation will result from the pressure of the accumulating blood. Frequently, when skin edges separate from a hematoma, the bleeding has already stopped and there is nothing further that needs to be done. If a vessel is still bleeding, the surgeon needs to identify and stop the source of the bleeding. This can sometimes be done at the bedside, but occasionally requires a quick trip back to the operating room.

Incisional Nerve Injury

Nerve injuries can occur from small nerves that are unavoidably cut at the time of incision, or from a retractor putting pressure on a nerve. Loss of skin sensation is an annoying result of small nerves being severed. Fortunately, there is enough sensation from adjacent skin areas that the numb, tingling feeling is almost always temporary. Very rarely, damage or entrapment of a nerve can cause pain, numbness, or weakness of lower extremities. These, too, are almost always temporary and spontaneously resolve. A painful neuroma occasionally results if a nerve has been cut and may need to be surgically resected.

Dehiscence

One of the great unspoken fears is that the incision will actually come apart if someone laughs, coughs, lifts, or climbs stairs. Separation of the skin edges is different from a true wound dehiscence in which there is separation of abdominal wall layers in addition to the skin. Sometimes the skin stays closed in a dehiscence but the layer above the muscle (the *fascia*) separates. Typically, the separation occurs one week after surgery, but can happen as early as four days, or as late as two weeks. Dehiscence occurs in 0.4 percent of abdominal hysterectomies.

Who gets a dehiscence? Any time abdominal wall pressure overcomes suture or tissue strength, tissues may separate. Therefore, the people at the highest risk of dehiscence are people who have poor tissue quality that is less likely to heal well. Diabetics, the extremely obese, alcoholics, the elderly, and patients with cancer or chronic illness are all at increased risk. Women who have had prior radiation or chronic steroid use are also at risk. Anyone at high risk for infection will also have weaker tissue. Smokers are at risk not only due to poor tissue, but due to the fact that coughing after surgery puts stress on the healing incision. Poor nutrition is often associated with many of the above risk factors and is directly responsible for poor tissue strength. The surgeon usually takes steps to strengthen the incision in high-risk patients in order to decrease the likelihood of tissue failure.

Usually a dehiscence is not a dramatic occurrence. Most occur four to eight days after surgery. Sometimes there is a popping sensation. More commonly, there is drainage from the skin incision, resulting in the skin edges opening up or the incision bulging. It is only when the surgeon gently probes the incision that a dehiscence is discovered.

If a dehiscence does occur, a short trip back to the operating room is required to close the fascia. If no infection is present, the skin will be closed as usual. A small "silent" defect in the fascia may result in the formation of an incisional hernia.

BLOOD CLOTS

The formation of blood clots is a risk of gynecologic surgery, but a relatively rare occurrence due to routine precautions. If a blood clot forms, it starts in the vein of a leg and is known as a deep vein thrombosis (DVT). It can travel to the lung, resulting in a pulmonary embolism, a serious and potentially fatal complication.

Who Is at Risk?

Anyone can develop a blood clot, but some women are at higher risk than others. Higher rates are seen in older women, smokers, women with prior history of blood clots, and women with cancer. The length of the surgery can also impact on the risk of DVT.

Low-risk women have a less than 1 percent risk of developing a DVT; the risk of a fatal pulmonary embolism is less than 0.01 percent. If no precautions are taken in a high-risk woman, the risk of deep vein thrombosis is 2.4 percent and the risk of fatal pulmonary embolism is 0.1 to 0.7 percent. Precautions lower these risks.

What Are the Symptoms?

A DVT generally causes pain and swelling in the calf. If the clot travels to the lung, chest pain, shortness of breath, and rapid heart beat are typical.

What Can Be Done to Reduce the Risk?

All women should have thromboembolic compression booties (inflatable leg wraps) placed during surgery (see chapter 16). In addition to compression boots, the best thing someone can do to prevent the formation of blood clots is to *get out of bed* and walk around as soon as possible after surgery. Ideally, everyone should take at least a few steps as soon as they are awake. It is usually a good idea to leave compression booties operational until you are fully up and about.

In addition to wearing compression booties and ambulating as soon as possible, high-risk women should receive a blood thinner that prevents the formation of large clots.

The Diagnosis

If there is a suspicion of a blood clot, a Doppler blood flow of the lower extremities is done in which sound waves are used to determine if blood is flowing properly. If there is concern that a pulmonary embolism has occurred, additional imaging studies are done to determine if there is a blood clot in the lung.

The Treatment?

Blood clots are treated with heparin, an intravenous blood thinner. After initial treatment, most women need to continue with long-term, oral anticoagulant therapy.

COMPLICATION ODDS AND ENDS

Slow Return of Bowel Function

A small minority—4.5 percent—of women have a delayed return of their gastrointestinal function. Days after surgery, they are still not passing gas, still experiencing nausea and vomiting, and still have a distended abdomen. In most cases, time will take care of the problem. Intravenous fluids must be maintained to prevent dehydration. Occasionally a naso-gastric tube must be inserted (through the nose and into the stomach) to decompress the stomach and prevent fluid from accumulating.

Women are more likely to experience delays if they have prolonged operations and lots of bowel adhesions requiring extensive bowel manipulation. It is particularly likely in cancer patients. Narcotic pain relievers are also responsible for slowing bowel function, so avoid nar-cotic pain relievers if you don't really need them. Women who have an epidural, as opposed to a general, anesthetic are also less likely to have a postoperative delay in function.

Slow Return of Bladder Function

Most women are able to urinate without difficulty within hours of the catheter's removal. Occasionally there is difficulty in voiding, requiring reinsertion of the catheter. This does not indicate that the bladder has been injured; it is usually a result of the swelling and inflammation that commonly occur during surgery. It is far more likely to occur in women who had a concomitant repair of their bladder for treatment of incontinence, but can occur even if no bladder surgery was done. Occasionally, a catheter is still required when you are otherwise ready to be discharged from the hospital. While it can be very distressing, it is always temporary and home catheter care is very manageable. You will pee eventually, usually within a week or two. Everyone does.

Adhesions

Adhesions are common; problems from adhesions are not. Since most adhesions are asymptomatic and don't show up on any imaging, such as X ray or ultrasound, there is no way to know if someone has adhesions unless they happen to have another operation or develop a problem from the adhesion. Studies show that between 60 to 90 percent of women are felt to have at least some degree of adhesions after gynecologic surgery. Less than 2 percent cause problems such as pain, infertility, or subsequent bowel obstruction.

A bowel obstruction is the most serious complication of an adhesion. It can occur weeks or years after surgery and is a result of a loop of bowel getting caught in scar tissue. Surgeons take many steps during surgery to decrease your risk of adhesion formation. There are far fewer adhesions following laparoscopic and vaginal procedures than abdominal hysterectomies. Ultimately, though, the only thing you can do to avoid adhesions is to avoid surgery.

Neurologic Injury

Nerve compression resulting in neurologic injury is now a rare event during surgery. These sorts of injuries used to be far more common than they are now due to an increased awareness of the importance of patient positioning. Meticulous attention is paid to the position you are placed in during surgery so that all vulnerable nerves are protected. Risk factors include a prolonged operating time, poor tissue that is vulnerable to injury, and extremely skinny patients. (The lack of personal padding makes nerves more vulnerable.) If injury does occur, transient weakness of a lower extremity results. Extraordinarily rarely, the problem is not transient.

Fistula Formation

A fistula is created when one structure connects to another structure that it does not usually connect to. There can be a fistula from the bladder to the vagina, bowel to the vagina, or ureter to vagina or pelvis. Most fistulas heal on their own, given enough time. Sometimes a surgical repair is necessary. Fistula formation is extremely rare and almost always occurs if there are dense adhesions or cancer. The diagnosis is suspected if there is passage of urine or stool through the vagina.

Death

The generally unspoken fear is the ultimate complication. In women under the age of forty, five of every ten thousand (0.05 percent) die, almost all from complications involving pregnancy. In women over the age of fifty, seventy-five of every 10,000 (0.75 percent) die, almost all from complications of late-stage cancers. Almost every death from hysterectomy is due to pregnancy-related massive hemorrhage or advanced cancer. The chance of a healthy woman dying as a result of a nonemergency hysterectomy for a benign problem is miniscule. It's not zero; it's just highly unlikely.

Part IV

Decisions Regarding Surgery

Chapter 19

The Cervix Decision

You've decided to go ahead with the hysterectomy. You've weighed the options, considered the alternatives, talked to surgeons, and set the date. You feel you've done your homework until a friend casually asks you, "Are you going to have your cervix removed when you have your hysterectomy?" Panic sets in . . . another thing to think about, yet another decision.

Before 1940, almost all hysterectomies were subtotal; the cervix was *rarely* removed along with the uterus. In the 1940s and 1950s, total hysterectomy (which includes the uterus and cervix) became the standard of care as a means of preventing cervical cancer. Today, the vast majority of hysterectomies still include removal of the cervix.

A study published in *Obstetrics and Gynecology* in August 2003 reported that only 18 percent of gynecologists even broached the topic of subtotal hysterectomy as an option, in spite of the fact that virtually all gynecologists felt that the subsequent risk of cervical cancer was negligible. Since screening techniques have reduced the incidence of invasive cervical cancer to less than 0.1 percent for low-risk women, it is appropriate for gynecologists (and patients) to question the routine removal of the cervix at the time of hysterectomy.

THE CERVIX

The cervix is the lower part of the uterus and functions as the "door" to the uterine cavity. It lets the sperm swim in, and menstrual blood flow out. During labor, it accomplishes the amazing feat of opening wide enough to allow a baby to exit the womb. The cervix is located at the back of the vagina and also functions as the separation between the vagina and the uterus.

Many experts feel that the cervix also plays a major role in sexual function and helps support other related pelvic structures, such as the bladder and the vagina. Unfortunately, there have been very few good studies examining the long-term consequences of preserving or removing the cervix. Now, new data are emerging as gynecologists reconsider the practice of automatically removing the cervix at the time of hysterectomy. There is no debate about removing the cervix in women who have cancer, or who are at high risk for developing cervical cancer. Unfortunately, other issues are not as clear-cut.

Does Sexual Function Change If the Cervix Is Removed?

This is a hard one. Sexual function is complicated and very difficult to study. Most investigations were small or not particularly well-designed, resulting in a lot of questionable information. One study, which appeared in *The New England Journal of Medicine* in October 2002, looked at sexuality in women following both types of hysterectomies. Two hundred and seventy-nine women had their uterus removed, but were not told the fate of their cervix. One year after surgery, the women were asked about frequency of intercourse, desire for intercourse, frequency of orgasm, vaginal lubrication, and frequency of multiple orgasms. No significant differences in sexual satisfaction were observed between the two groups (cervix in versus cervix out) and, since the women weren't told what kind of surgery they had, there was no bias.

Anecdotally, most women say that sex is the same or even better after hysterectomy, regardless if the procedure is subtotal or total. On occasion, removal of the cervix can lead to a shortened vagina, which may create some initial difficulty with intercourse, but is rarely a long-term problem.

Does Surgery Take a Lot Longer If the Cervix Is Removed?

On one hand, the length of time to remove a cervix has little relevance to an anesthetized patient. It is a fact, however, that the length of surgery influences infection rate, return of bowel function, and recovery from anesthesia. Studies have confirmed that women who have a sub-total hysterectomy have shorter surgery and a shorter hospital stay than do women who undergo removal of the cervix. In reality, removal of the cervix generally adds about fifteen to thirty minutes to the time of surgery, which is not significant in a healthy, stable patient.

Sometimes, if there are adhesions (scar tissue), the cervix can be quite difficult to remove and may take an hour or more. There are also circumstances when it is appropriate for a surgeon to leave the cervix in, even if during preoperative discussions you expressed a preference for removal.

Effect on Bladder Function

The bladder and the uterus have a very close relationship. In fact, the bladder is actually loosely attached to the front part of the uterus and cervix. During the course of a normal cesarian section or hysterectomy, the bladder is actually lifted away from the uterus in order to protect it from injury. One of the concerns after hysterectomy is that the bladder will not function the same way because it no longer has a uterus to rest on and support it. There is also the concern that the process of lifting the bladder off the uterus may compromise the bladder in some way, even if it is restored to its normal position. Theoretically, the alteration of the normal anatomy is less dramatic when the cervix is left in place, and should result in fewer problems with long-term bladder function. Again, there are few good studies that look at this issue, but to date, there is not one study that shows a difference in incontinence, urgency, or difficulty in emptying the bladder between women with or without a cervix.

Many people feel that by leaving the cervix in place, you avoid disrupting many of the structures that strengthen the vagina and support the bladder. This is particularly important for women who are concerned about prolapse (dropping) of the bladder and vagina. While theoretically this makes sense (don't cut things that are holding other things up), the long-term studies simply don't exist yet.

While some urogynecologists agree that preservation of the cervix can make a significant difference in subsequent bladder function and pelvic support, they feel that the cervix should be removed in surgery done for uterine prolapse since the support system has already been damaged and must be repaired.

Clearly, more studies are needed to determine the relationship of preservation or removal of the cervix and long-term bladder function. Currently, many experts recommend that the cervix be left in place unless there is a specific reason to remove it.

Complications of Cervix Removal

Complications of hysterectomy fall into three basic categories: infection, bleeding, and injury to surrounding structures.

Postoperative infection occurs in roughly 4 percent of women who have a hysterectomy. Infection can occur in various surgical sites including the incision (wound infection), pelvis (pelvic abscess), or back of the vagina (cuff infection). Infection in nonsurgical areas (such as pneumonia or urinary tract infections) can also occur from events that occur at the time of surgery, such as anesthesia or bladder catheters. Surgeons routinely do things to minimize infection, such as maintaining sterile technique and giving antibiotics, but even if everything is done correctly, infections occur. Not surprisingly, the rate of infection decreases when the cervix is left in place. Even though the vagina is always scrubbed with an antiseptic prior to hysterectomy (one of the many things that happens after you go to sleep), it is virtually impossible to totally free the vagina of bacteria. If those bacteria contaminate the surgical area, infection may result. Since the cervical barrier separates the "dirty" vagina from the pelvis, fewer infections occur if the cervix is left in place. Postoperative fevers are about three times lower in women who have subtotal hysterectomies and the infection rates are significantly lower.

The typical blood loss during an uncomplicated hysterectomy is quite minimal (usually less than eight ounces). It is rare to require a blood transfusion and while many women benefit from iron supplementation before and after surgery to facilitate the return to a normal blood count, most women are at normal levels weeks after surgery even without supplementation. There is generally less blood loss during an uncomplicated subtotal hysterectomy than a total hysterectomy (by around three ounces), but that makes little difference in the overall recovery rate.

The really significant decrease in complication rate is seen in the third category, injury to surrounding structures. The uterus, cervix, and vagina are intimately related to other pelvic structures such as the bowel, bladder, and ureters. More serious complications of hysterectomy that result in longer hospital stays, prolonged recovery, or further surgery involve injury to these structures. Intrinsic in any operation is the potential for injury, even if an experienced surgeon does everything correctly. During hysterectomy, injury to the bladder or ureter occurs less than 2 percent of the time, but almost all injuries occur during removal of the cervix since it is located so close to the ureter and bladder. This is especially a problem if there are other complicating factors, such as scar tissue from prior surgery, endometriosis, or infection. Many advocates of subtotal hysterectomy feel that injury to surrounding structures can be reduced dramatically by avoiding the extra dissection necessary to remove the cervix. More studies with large numbers need to be done, but this may be a valid argument against routine removal of the cervix.

Advantages of Keeping the Cervix

If there is no difference in sexual or bladder function, and preservation of her cervix puts a woman at continued risk for cervical cancer, possible future surgery, and need for annual Pap smears, why would anyone want to keep her cervix?

The decrease in complication rates associated with subtotal hysterectomy is certainly a compelling argument. In addition, surgery is shorter and recovery times quicker. Preservation of the cervix also makes it much more likely that someone can have a laparoscopic procedure, the ultimate in quick recovery. Many people feel that since so few good studies exist, there is no justification for removal of healthy tissue that may serve a benefit, as long as a women is willing to continue annual Pap smears.

Disadvantages of Keeping the Cervix

From a patient's point of view, the major disadvantage is probably the need to continue annual Pap smears. In reality, however, even if your cervix is removed, it doesn't mean you get to stop going to the gynecologist. In women who have no cervix, gynecologists still recommend annual exams to screen for vaginal cancer, ovarian cancer, breast cancer, and to address the myriad other gynecologic issues that continue to exist.

There is another possible disadvantage. Occasionally, a small amount of uterine tissue is left behind with the cervix. This can cause premenopausal women to continue to have cyclic spotting or bleeding. While the surgeon is almost always able to remove all uterine tissue, the only absolute guarantee that no uterine tissue remains is to remove the cervix. It is also theoretically possible for a woman to develop uterine cancer if even a small remnant of uterine tissue remains. It won't surprise any gynecologist if we start to hear reports of such cases as time goes on.

If a cervix does need to be removed at a later time, it is sometimes technically more difficult to do than at the time of hysterectomy, so it's important to make the right decision.

MAKING THE DECISION

Let's get back to the original dilemma. Leave the cervix? Remove the cervix? Sometimes the decision is made for you. If you are having a vaginal hysterectomy, the cervix is always removed. If you have cancer (cervical, uterine, ovarian, or tubal), your cervix must be removed as a life-saving procedure. It also makes no sense to leave a cervix in a woman who is at high risk for developing cervical cancer (women with a history of dysplasia, human papilloma virus, and heavy smokers). Some women (and you know who you are) can't seem to make it in for regular Pap smears and may be better served by removal of the cervix. Some women can't afford, or don't have access to, regular gynecologic care and simply don't get regular Pap smears. Some women would prefer not to have annual Pap smears and don't want to take any chance that they may develop cancer or need further gynecologic surgery. If you fall into one of the above groups, your cervix belongs with your uterus—in the pathology lab.

Sometimes your surgeon makes the decision for you at the time of surgery. One situation in which a surgeon may choose not to remove a cervix would be at the time of emergency hysterectomy following a cesarean section or vaginal birth. In a scenario like postpartum hemorrhage, there can be a dramatic blood loss and the goal is to make the surgery as short as possible to solve the immediate problem (removal of the bleeding uterus) as a life-saving procedure. Sometimes, especially in women with endometriosis or prior infection, scar tissue (adhesions) can limit exposure to the cervix and it is safer to not remove it.

Situations also exist in which the patient may have requested preservation of the cervix, but the surgeon must remove it anyway. That can occur if there is unexpected cancer, or if a fibroid has grown into the cervix in such a way that the only way to remove it is to remove the cervix. There are many scenarios where the decision can't be made until the time of surgery. Ultimately, you need to trust your surgeon's judgment.

It's important to let your surgeon know your preference and discuss what is most appropriate for you. Understand that things don't always go as planned and what seems best during a pre-op discussion is not always the best course of action in the operating room.

Chapter 20

The Ovary Decision

For many women, deciding the fate of their ovaries is a much more difficult dilemma than the fate of their cervix, or even their uterus. This is particularly true for the perimenopausal woman who is given multiple confusing, contradictory recommendations from "helpful" friends and talk-show hosts. It's no wonder that women agonize about this decision more than any other.

Actually, for some women, it is pretty clear-cut. Women under the age of forty-five usually keep their ovaries unless they have a situation in which there is a problem with an ovary, or their ovaries are contributing to their problem, as in the case of severe endometriosis. Women at increased genetic risk for ovarian cancer are also an exception (see chapter 21).

Most women who have completed menopause are comfortable with the concept of losing their ovaries, particularly if the specter of ovarian cancer is hanging over their heads. It is the woman in the forty-five to fifty-five age bracket who flip-flops back and forth, sometimes changing her mind on the gurney as she rolls into the operating room. The decision to deal with a surgical menopause at the same time as major surgery is understandably a difficult choice to make. However, before evaluating the pros and cons of ovary removal, the normal function of the pre-, peri-, and postmenopausal ovary need be considered.

THE PREMENOPAUSAL OVARY

A premenopausal ovary pumps out estrogen with no indication of slowing down and generally can be found in women under the age of forty-five. This ovary produces two types of estrogen: estradiol, and the weaker derivative, estrone. While most women are aware that ovaries produce estrogen, it is a less-known fact that ovaries produce androgens as well.

Androgens are sometimes thought of as male hormones since men make androgens in large amounts and have minimal amounts of estrogen. In fact, all women make androgens as an integral part of the female hormonal milieu. The levels are lower than in men, but they are definitely there, and *definitely* female.

The ovary produces two types of androgens: testosterone and androstenedione. Androgens, in combination with estrogen, contribute to libido and sexual response. They are responsible for increased sensitivity to sexual stimulation, sexual fantasies, arousal, enhanced capacity for orgasm, sexual energy, and a general sense of well-being. In short, androgens are what make women want sex and have great sex.

Fortunately for the thousands of women who have no ovaries, there is an androgen back-up. Most women are relieved to know that the ovary is not the only source of androgens; they are also produced in significant amounts by the adrenal glands, which sit on each kidney. There is a god.

THE POSTMENOPAUSAL OVARY

The postmenopausal ovary is essentially nonfunctional as far as estrogen production. However, postmenopausal woman still have some estrogen available since fat cells convert androstenediol (a hormone made in the adrenal gland) to estrogen, but the levels are nowhere near what they were before. The fact that fat cells are responsible for postmenopausal circulating estrogen explains why overweight women are at lower risk for osteoporosis and higher risk for uterine cancer. Interestingly, women who have their adrenal glands removed have lower estrogen levels than women who have their ovaries removed.

Even after estrogen production ceases, the ovary continues to produce androgens, since they are produced from a part of the ovary that still functions after menopause. Androgen levels gradually decline over the years starting at about age fifty, but unlike estrogen, the decline is gradual, not abrupt. And remember the back-up . . . the adrenal gland continues androgen production in spite of the aging ovary.

THE PERIMENOPAUSAL OVARY

The perimenopausal ovary makes the roller coaster at Great America look like a walk in the park. This perimenopausal ride can last a few months, or years. It's an experience that most women would just as soon skip. Hormonal fluctuations result in unpredictable bleeding patterns, exaggerated PMS symptoms, mood swings, insomnia, and hot flashes. The only thing that is predictable is that your period generally arrives the moment you get on a plane wearing white and carrying no tampons. Hot flashes usually disappear immediately after you've spent a month's salary at the local health food store for a year's supply of black cohosh and soy.

SURGICAL MENOPAUSE VERSUS
NATURAL MENOPAUSE

Before anyone knew anything about androgen production in the post-menopausal ovary, the issue of ovary removal was straightforward, particularly if someone was taking, or comfortable with, the idea of estrogen replacement. Since the ovary was felt to have no remaining function other than to potentially become cancerous, it was uniformly removed in women over the age of forty-five. Now that we know that the postmenopausal ovary does have some hormonal activity, the question is a little more complicated and removal is not automatic.

What, then, are the levels of androgens and estrogens in post-menopausal women who have oophorectomies (removal of their ovaries) versus those who don't? The following table illustrates post-menopausal hormone levels in women with and without their ovaries. Obviously, there is a wide range, particularly if someone is overweight, but these numbers give you an idea.

	Natural Menopause (Ovaries in)	Surgical Menopause (Ovaries out)
Estrone (pg/mL)	49 +/− 16	48 +/− 6
Estradiol	20 +/− 1	18 +/− 4
Testosterone (ng/dL)	30 +/− 4	12 +/− 2
Androstenedione	99 +/− 3	64 +/− 9
DHEA	197 +/− 43	126 +/− 36

Estrogen levels are essentially the same; it's the androgens that are significantly lower in the woman who has a surgical menopause. Herein lies the reason why many women choose to keep their ovaries.

How much androgen is needed for a healthy libido and a great sex life? That is probably one of the most complex questions in this whole dilemma. It would be nice if there were an exact critical amount of testosterone that was known to assure an intact sexual response. Unfortunately, sexuality is ridiculously complex and influenced by hormones, environment, and relationship issues, not to mention that all-encompassing catchall, "chemistry." It is known that women with very low testosterone levels often have healthy libidos and amazing sex lives, while women with high levels may be totally disinterested. Clearly, much more work needs to be done in this area since sexual dysfunction is an enormous problem, ovaries in or out.

Since there is now recognition among physicians and women that androgens are part of the normal hormonal milieu, androgen supplementation has become an important component of hormone replacement for the woman who has inadequate levels.

Removal of the Premenopausal Ovary

Why would anyone even consider removing a healthy ovary with years of normal estrogen and androgen production remaining? There are actually a number of situations in which premenopausal ovary removal is appropriate and should be seriously considered. There are also situations in which there is no choice but removal.

Endometriosis

Young women with endometriosis are unique in that the ovaries themselves may be normal, yet are responsible for creating the development of abnormal tissue. Women with endometriosis have endometrial glands in a variety of places outside the uterus that respond to hormonal stimulation. If you remove the uterus and preserve the ovaries, any endometriotic tissue located outside the uterus will continue to create problems. This is why a woman with endometriosis can have a hysterectomy and still suffer from painful cycles, pelvic pain, and discomfort during intercourse. She won't bleed and her pain will likely be better, but in some cases, hysterectomy alone doesn't totally eliminate the problem.

Risk of Ovarian Cancer

Many women are at increased risk for developing ovarian cancer based on genetic predisposition. Chapter 21 reviews the issues regarding prophylactic removal of ovaries in women at risk.

Benign Ovarian Pathology

It's not uncommon that a growth on the ovary is discovered at the time of hysterectomy, or that surgery is done because of the known presence of a growth that is either benign or questionably malignant. When that is the case, the surgeon has two options: remove the growth and preserve the ovary, or remove the entire ovary.

Surgically, it is far easier and quicker to remove the entire ovary than to dissect a large cyst or growth away from normal ovarian tissue. Therefore, unless there is a reason to save the ovary, it is usually more appropriate to remove the entire thing. The obvious exception is in a young woman, whether or not she is interested in pregnancy. No one would recommend ovary removal in a woman who is in her twenties or thirties, even if her other ovary looks perfectly normal. She has years of hormonal activity left, and it's unpredictable if the other ovary might develop a problem down the line requiring removal. If a woman is in her forties and has another ovary, it is reasonable to remove the abnormal one since her other ovary will provide normal hormonal levels. In fact, only one third of one ovary is needed to provide normal ovarian activity, including ovulation. If a woman is in her fifties, not only should the diseased ovary be removed, but it makes sense to remove the other ovary as well so you're not making a return trip to the operating room to check out the other side a few years later.

The downside to removing the cyst and leaving the ovary? It takes longer to do and once the cyst has been removed, you need to wait for the frozen pathology report before you conclude the operation. That can take anywhere from twenty minutes to one hour. In addition, there is more likely to be bleeding from the surgical site on the ovary or the need to go back at another time. This, of course, is all worth it if it is a young woman in whom ovarian preservation is critical. It doesn't make sense in the peri- or postmenopausal woman.

Cancer

In the event of ovarian cancer, both ovaries will be removed. In most cases, ovarian cancer is known or at least suspected before surgery. There certainly are times when it is found serendipitously at the time of surgery for an unrelated problem. Hormone replacement after removal of ovaries for cancer is usually not contraindicated, easing the transition into menopause.

Pelvic Abscess

Another scenario in which an ovary may need to be removed is in the case of pelvic inflammatory disease (PID) with a pelvic abscess. During the 1970s and 1980s, it was pretty much a given that even young women with PID were "cleaned out." They would inevitably end up losing their uterus, cervix, tubes, and both ovaries. The feeling was that the infection could not be eliminated unless all pelvic organs were removed, leaving the patient at risk for sepsis or death.

Today, the surgical treatment of pelvic abscess is not nearly so radical due to the availability of broad-spectrum antibiotics capable of killing the bacteria responsible for the infection. In addition, interventional radiologists are often able to drain the abscess nonsurgically, resulting in less frequent surgery. When surgery is necessary, it is less radical and ovarian preservation is frequently possible. Having said that, there are times when a pelvic abscess involves ovarian tissue and there is no way to save it, nor would it be functional if it was saved. Fortunately, this is a relatively rare occurrence.

Adhesions

Sometimes during a hysterectomy for benign reasons, such as endometriosis or fibroids, the surgeon encounters severe adhesions that have caused the ovaries to stick to the uterus or other pelvic organs. In most cases, it is possible to remove the adhesions and preserve the ovaries, if so desired. Sometimes it can't be done and the ovaries must be removed along with the uterus. Unless the patient has had a diagnostic laparoscopy, this usually can't be predicted in advance by ultrasound or pelvic examination.

REMOVAL OF THE POSTMENOPAUSAL OVARY

Few gynecologists recommend preservation of the postmenopausal ovary. While there is an awareness of the resulting decrease in androgen production, most gynecologists feel that the risk of ovarian cancer and the inability to detect it in its early stages are too dangerous to justify leaving the ovaries behind.

It is well-known that the majority of postmenopausal women have enough adrenal androgen production to ensure that sexual function does not suffer as a result of oophorectomy, particularly if estrogen is replaced. If estrogen supplementation alone is inadequate, the option of androgen supplementation is always there.

Removal of the Perimenopausal Ovary

The average age of menopause in the United States is fifty-one. Most women start to experience perimenopausal hormonal fluctuations by their late forties. There is wide variation in those numbers, but the majority of women no longer make estrogen from their ovaries by their mid-fifties. Most gynecologists use forty-five as the age in which they recommend removal of ovaries at the time of hysterectomy, even if the ovaries are healthy. Women who remove their ovaries are going to go through menopause and therefore need to make a decision about estrogen replacement therapy. It's a decision that will need to be made in any event; it just needs to be made sooner than nature intended.

Why Do It?

Oophorectomy (removal of ovaries) is recommended for one reason and one reason only—to avoid ovarian cancer. One out of seventy women is destined to develop ovarian cancer and there is essentially no way to detect ovarian cancer in its early stages. Most women who develop ovarian cancer are diagnosed when it has spread beyond the ovaries, resulting in a poor prognosis. Most gynecologists feel that in view of this, it makes sense to remove ovaries from women if there are only a few years of useful ovarian function left.

Another reason to consider oophorectomy is to avoid the need for removal later in life. Between 3 and 7 percent of women who retain their ovaries make a return trip to the operating room for removal of their ovaries after hysterectomy due to the development of cysts or other growths. Thirty percent of those women have cancer.

Why Not Do It?

There certainly is the point of view that healthy tissue should never be removed unless absolutely necessary, particularly if the reason for doing the hysterectomy in the first place had nothing to do with the ovaries. There is also little argument that the woman who goes through a surgical menopause has more symptoms than the woman who goes through a natural menopause, particularly if she declines estrogen replacement. There are also those who would argue that removal of the ovaries does not completely eliminate the development of ovarian cancer 100 percent since primary peritoneal cancer, or cancer from an ovarian remnant, are still possible.

The confusing issue is really androgen production. Until the last fifteen years, the feeling was that there really was no hormonal benefit to preserving the postmenopausal ovary. Since it is now known unequivocally that postmenopausal ovaries contribute hormones that influence libido and sexual response, that changes the balance. What's unpredictable is how much an impact there will truly be. The vast majority of women whose ovaries are removed report no difference in sexual response, probably due to the contribution of adrenal androgen production and the multiple other factors that contribute to human sexuality. Some women report a profound difference.

The woman who is comfortable with the idea of estrogen and androgen replacement during her menopausal years has a much easier decision to make than the woman who declines supplementation. Many women find that once they are comfortable with the idea of short-term replacement, as opposed to prolonged estrogen extension, they are able to part more easily with their ovaries (see chapter 24).

What Makes Sense for Ambivalent Perimenopausal Women?

There is no right answer for everyone. Sometimes it's helpful to measure hormone levels (FSH and LH) to see if perimenopause is soon to be menopause. The decision to remove ovaries might be easier if you know menopause is right around the corner, as opposed to years away.

Unfortunately, those levels bounce around quite a bit during the peri-menopausal years and are not accurate predictors of when ovarian function will cease completely.

Everyone has different fears about cancer, and some women truly are at greater risk than other women are. If a risk of cancer of one in seventy is acceptable to you, leaving your ovaries is reasonable. Read chapter 21, then consider if you would get on an airplane that you had been told had a one in seventy chance of crashing.

What to Expect

The woman who was menopausal before her hysterectomy should notice no immediate change after her ovaries are removed. Her estrogen levels are exactly what they were before surgery. Any change in sexual function won't be appreciated right away, since even the most sensual woman is usually not thinking about sex in the days or weeks following her surgery. If there is a change in libido and response, it is usually subtle. If it seems as if a switch has been turned off, androgen supplementation is appropriate. This issue is further explored in chapters 24 and 25.

The response of the perimenopausal woman to ovary removal is variable. Just as women experience a wide range of symptoms when they go through natural menopause, response to oophorectomy during perimenopause is also unpredictable. Some women have no symptoms and wouldn't know their ovaries were gone if they weren't told. Other women are hit with an abrupt onset of terrible hot flashes, insomnia, and mood swings followed by loss of libido and vaginal dryness, just as many women experience with a natural menopause.

If ovaries are removed from a young, premenopausal woman, most gynecologists strongly recommend estrogen supplementation to ease the severe symptoms that are pretty much inevitable. It makes sense to use an estrogen patch immediately after surgery so there is no down-time. Young women very often benefit from supplementation with a low-dose birth control pill that is started prior to surgery, so there is no transition. The exception is the young woman with breast cancer in

whom estrogen replacement is not advised. Alternatives to ease symptoms are available and are discussed in chapter 24.

What's Everyone Else Doing?

Of course, you would never think of making a decision based on what
other people do. As your mother used to ask you, "If everyone were
jumping out of the window, would you jump, too?" Anyway, this is what
everyone else is doing:

> ▼ 40 percent of women under age 45 remove their
> ovaries.
> ▼ 75 percent of women between the ages of 45 and
> 55 remove their ovaries.
> ▼ 65 percent of women older than 55 remove their
> ovaries.

One explanation for the relatively large number of woman over the
age of sixty-five who retain their ovaries is that many of these procedures are done vaginally since prolapse is a much more common indication for hysterectomy than fibroids or bleeding. Oophorectomy at the
time of vaginal hysterectomy can be technically challenging, especially
if the ovaries are high in the pelvis and difficult to reach. In experienced
hands, ovaries can be removed vaginally about 80 percent of the time.
Since removal of the ovaries can be technically difficult during a vaginal
procedure in a postmenopausal woman, it may not have been an option,
even if desired or requested.

It will be interesting to see what happens to these statistics when
there is a reliable method for early detection of ovarian cancer. Until that
time, the fate of one's ovaries remains one of the hardest decisions many
women must make.

Chapter 21

Women at Genetic Risk for Ovarian Cancer

M any women are frightened at the possibility of developing ovarian cancer. Women who have watched a mother or sister die from it are terrified. Once someone is aware that they are at genetic risk for ovarian cancer, they are generally also aware that current modalities for early detection are limited, and the mortality rate is high. It's no surprise that this terror prompts many women to remove their healthy ovaries to prevent the disease each year. The reality is that most cases of ovarian cancer are not hereditary, and relatively few women are appropriate candidates for prophylactic surgery.

One out of seventy women will develop ovarian cancer in her lifetime. It is the seventh most common cancer in women and the most common cause of death among women who develop gynecologic cancers. Contrary to what most people think, only 5 to 10 percent of ovarian cancer is hereditary. However, if a woman is a carrier of one of the genes associated with ovarian cancer, her risk is strikingly higher than the risk of the general population.

WHO IS AT RISK?

In the early 1990s, BRCA1 (breast cancer gene 1) and BRCA2 (breast cancer gene 2) were identified as gene mutations responsible for the majority of hereditary breast and ovarian cancer. Genes, of course, are the parts of each cell that contain the hereditary information one gets from each parent. A mutation is a misspelling of the gene that changes the function of that gene. If the mutation occurs in BRCA1 or BRCA2, there is an increased susceptibility to certain cancers, specifically breast and ovarian.

Women with BRCA1 mutations appear to have a 20 to 40 percent risk of developing ovarian cancer during their lifetime, as opposed to the 1.4 to 1.8 percent lifetime risk seen in the general population. Women with a BRCA2 mutation have a 15 to 25 percent risk of developing ovarian cancer. So, if someone does carry a mutation of the BRCA gene, we are talking a *significant* chance of developing cancer.

Certain groups of people are at increased risk for carrying the gene. Ashkenazi Jews are one group that has been identified as particularly high-risk, with 2.5 percent of the population carrying BRCA mutations. Ashkenazi Jews are Jews that come from Eastern Europe, as opposed to Sephardic Jews, who come from Spain, Portugal, Turkey, and the Mediterranean countries. Most American Jews are of Ashkenazi descent.

Who Should Be Screened for BRCA Mutations?

The presence of a BRCA mutation can be detected in a blood sample. Not everyone needs to be tested for the presence of this mutation, but there are certain risk factors that should prompt a discussion. Family history is the primary tool in determining the likelihood for hereditary cancer, but this can be harder to get from your relatives than you think. "Great Aunt Tilly died from (whisper) female trouble," Grandma Rose had problems "down there," or the very specific, "Cancer . . . all over!" It's not unusual to hear two entirely different family histories from sisters, leading one to wonder if they grew up in separate adoptive families. Be that as it may, your first step is to get as much information as possible about the not-too-distant relatives. If your first-degree (mother, sisters, daughters) or second-degree relatives (grandmothers, aunts) did not have ovarian cancer; you don't need to know if your relatives who came over on the Mayflower did. A three-generation family tree is optimal when evaluating a family for concern of hereditary cancer. This typically includes medical history on all first-degree relatives (parents, siblings, and children), second-degree relatives (nieces, nephews, aunts, uncles, and grandparents), and third-degree relatives (cousins, great-aunts, and great-uncles). Keep in mind that paternal ancestry is also a factor and women who have paternal aunts with ovarian cancer may also be at risk.

If you have breast cancer that developed before age fifty, you are at higher risk than someone who was diagnosed postmenopausally. If you have a first-degree relative who is BRCA-positive, screening should be considered. Screening is also appropriate if you have two or more first-degree relatives with ovarian or breast cancer.

Ideally, the best person to do counseling and screening is a medical geneticist who can delve into your family's history, determine your risk, and then explain the results of screening tests. If your doctor does not know a medical geneticist, call your nearest university hospital. They will almost always have a medical genetics department, or be able to refer you to one. A list of cancer risk genetic counselors can also be found on the National Society of Genetic Counselors Web site, www.nsgc.org.

At What Age Is Screening Appropriate?

For some women, the answer is never. Some people just don't want to know and wouldn't alter their care. Most women, though, don't know what they will do until they have the information. In general, even if you don't desire prophylactic surgery, you can reduce your risk of developing ovarian cancer, so it may be worth knowing, even if you don't think you would consider ovary removal. Occasionally, someone who is not at genetic risk requests testing (often women who watched a friend die from ovarian cancer). These women are almost always neg-ative and sleep a lot better at night knowing it. Peace of mind is worth a lot and, in the woman who is dysfunctional due to worry, testing may be appropriate.

If one does remove ovaries to prevent cancer, the most appropriate time is when pregnancy is no longer desired, but before cancer can occur. Hereditary cancers occur at a younger age than sporadic ovarian cancer, usually around ten years earlier. Therefore, many feel that the right age for prophylactic oophorectomy is age thirty-five. It would be unusual for someone to develop ovarian cancer before that age, and hopefully childbearing is complete. Obviously, that's not the case for many women, but in a statistically ideal world, age thirty-five is the point in which the most ovarian cancers can be prevented by surgical intervention. If someone has delayed pregnancy beyond age thirty-five, surgery should be scheduled as soon as childbearing is complete.

MENOPAUSE AT THIRTY-FIVE?

You may be thinking that it might be better to risk ovarian cancer than to go through menopause so young. However, when ovaries are removed at that young an age, hormone replacement is almost *always* recommended since it's not the hormones that create the risk, but the ovarian tissue. Even if someone is not a candidate for long-term hor-mone replacement, or is not planning on taking estrogen, the issues are different when a woman loses her ovaries at age thirty-five or forty than at age fifty. Most experts agree that hormone replacement is safe and appropriate in this scenario and that young women who have prophy-lactic surgery shouldn't have to go through menopause (see chapter 24). The decision about long-term hormone replacement therapy still needs be made when a woman reaches the typical age at which her ovaries would have wound down naturally, usually about age fifty.

While some young women are still concerned about the risk of tak-ing hormone replacement therapy at a young age, no data suggest that young women who take estrogen and progesterone are at higher risk for developing problems. We know a great deal about women in their thirties and forties who take hormones, since women in that age group often take birth control pills for contraception or control of irregular periods. Birth control pills actually contain four to five times more estrogen and progesterone than hormone replacement since the purpose of birth control pills is to *suppress* normal ovarian function and *prevent* ovulation, rather than to simply replace hormones that are no longer being manufactured. Even though birth control pills have a higher hormone level than hormone replacement therapy, they are still extremely low-risk in nonsmoking women.

One approach to the young woman who requires ovary removal is to start birth control pills during the years before surgery (which also decreases the risk of ovarian cancer) and then keep the pills going after the ovaries are removed. That way, a woman goes through *no* hormonal change as a result of surgery and can decrease her dosage gradually until she is at a comfortable replacement dose. At age fifty, she can then decide if she wants to continue hormone replacement therapy.

ARE THERE OTHER OPTIONS?

No question, removing your ovaries is a dramatic step to take. There are some easier alternatives one can take before surgery or instead of surgery to reduce risk.

It is an uncontroversial fact that taking birth control pills dramatically reduces the risk of developing ovarian cancer. Multiple studies have confirmed that women who take oral contraceptives for five years or longer have a significantly reduced risk of developing the disease. It's a mystery why pharmaceutical companies, who have made millions by advertising that birth control pills reduce acne, don't advertise that birth control pills reduce the risk of ovarian cancer. Pharmaceutical companies are profit-motivated, and there is a huge profit to be made by marketing pills to women thirty-five and older who may not even need contraception any more.

Other factors known to reduce risk include tubal ligation, having lots of children, and having had a hysterectomy, even if the ovaries were not removed. A lot of studies have looked at diet, but there is no solid evidence that avoidance or supplementation with any foods really makes a difference. There is also controversy about nongenetic factors that may increase risk. It is known that women who have had no pregnancies are at increased risk due to years of uninterrupted ovulation. Some data suggest that women who have taken fertility drugs may be at higher risk, but the studies are not definitive and are complicated by the fact that women who take fertility drugs are often the same women who don't achieve pregnancy.

What About Screening?

Anyone who spends any time on the Internet, particularly if they get a lot of e-mail from "helpful" people, has received the message touting the benefits of testing women to see if they have elevated levels of the tumor marker cancer antigen 125 (CA125), and suggesting that every woman should demand this test from her doctor. A blood test that detects CA125 was developed to identify women with ovarian cancer at an early stage when a cure would be more likely. Unfortunately, CA125 screening in the general population has not resulted in favorable results or every gynecologist *would* do it routinely. CA125 is a substance that cancer cells shed and that is detectable in blood. The problem is that CA125 is also made by normal cells that become inflamed. Therefore, the false-positive rate is extremely high; the majority of women with a slightly elevated CA125 do not have ovarian cancer but have a nonmalignant condition such as endometriosis or fibroids. Unlike Pap smears that detect abnormalities years before there is cervical cancer, CA125 levels don't increase until the disease is well established.

There is currently no evidence that regular screening in individuals at average risk for ovarian cancer reduces the number of women diagnosed with ovarian cancer or the number of women who die from ovarian cancer. Having said that, and because currently there is nothing better to offer, most ovarian cancer screening programs recommend that women who are BRCA1- or BRCA2-positive have a CA125 test every six to twelve months beginning at age twenty-five.

It would be ideal if routine transvaginal ultrasound could detect ovarian cancer, but unfortunately stage 1 cancer, where the cancer is only in the ovary, is rarely detected in asymptomatic women. It is entirely possible to have advanced ovarian cancer and have your ovaries appear normal on ultrasound. Newer ultrasound technology, with Doppler blood flow and three-dimensional imaging, is certainly better, but has not made a significant difference in early detection. Like CA125, annual transvaginal ultrasound is recommended in the high-risk population, in lieu of anything better.

Until early detection improves, the only way to significantly decrease one's chance of advanced-stage ovarian cancer is to remove the ovaries before cancer cells start to grow.

WHAT IS INVOLVED IN REMOVING THE OVARIES?

Surgically, removal of the ovaries is usually quite simple. The entire procedure is almost always done laparoscopically as an outpatient. An incision (see Fig. 21-1) is made through the belly button and two tiny incisions (about a quarter of an inch long) are made in the lower abdomen (these barely show after healing).

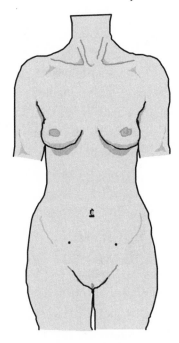

A laparoscope is placed through the belly button incision, enabling the surgeon to see the ovaries and other pelvic organs. The two smaller incisions are then used to introduce the instruments that cut the ovaries away from their connections. A baggy with a drawstring is then inserted through a port and the ovaries are dropped in the baggy and the bag pulled shut. That way, if there is microscopic cancer and the ovaries leak fluid on the way out, no cancer cells will be spread

Figure 21-1. Abdomen with incision placement.

or left behind. The baggy with the ovary in it is removed through the belly button incision and the tissue sent to pathology for analysis.

In experienced hands, the whole procedure takes less than an hour. Most women are home within two to three hours and feel entirely normal within a week.

SHOULD ANYTHING ELSE BE REMOVED?

This is where the controversy comes in. Women at risk for ovarian cancer are also at increased risk for fallopian tube cancer, which is much rarer, but just as bad. Removing the fallopian tubes at the time of ovary removal makes good sense. The problem is that the tubes actually burrow into the uterine wall (see chapter 2) so that the only way to remove the whole tube is to remove the uterus as well.

In addition, the same women at risk for ovarian cancer are at increased risk for breast cancer, which means that they may be taking a drug such as tamoxifen to reduce their risk of developing that disease. Women who take tamoxifen are at increased risk for developing uterine cancer or for having abnormal uterine bleeding, which will require evaluation. An argument could therefore be made for removing the uterus and tubes along with the ovaries if the surgery is to be truly prophylactic.

The cervix is not at risk and need not be removed (see chapter 19), so the entire procedure can still be done laparoscopically. In this scenario, the uterus is usually small, meaning that the surgery is not appreciably longer and the recovery still quick. Once a woman removes her ovaries, she has already made the decision not to become pregnant, making hysterectomy a reasonable choice.

SO, THERE'S *NO* RISK OF OVARIAN CANCER IF THE OVARIES ARE REMOVED?

One would think. Unfortunately there's primary peritoneal cancer, which is an "ovarian-like" cancer involving the lining of the pelvis. This cancer can develop even in women whose ovaries have been removed, and like ovarian cancer, it is usually detected at a late stage with high mortality. The same women who are at risk for ovarian cancer are at risk for primary peritoneal cancer. Some physicians feel that early rather than late removal of the ovaries can reduce the risk since peritoneal cancer may originate from existing microscopic disease if the ovaries are removed too late.

THE BOTTOM LINE

Even in women who are not at risk for ovarian cancer, most gynecologists encourage their patients to have their ovaries removed if they are perimenopausal or postmenopausal at the time of hysterectomy. The irrefutable frustrating fact is that one in seventy women will develop ovarian cancer, yet there is currently no good way to detect the disease early, and too many women die a death that could have been prevented. Women who are at increased risk should certainly have their ovaries removed if they are having a hysterectomy for another reason, and should consider screening and early surgery if they are BRCA1- or BRCA2-positive.

A WORD ABOUT INSURANCE

It would be nice if insurance companies were in the business of assuring that people get the best care possible, but the reality is that insurance companies exist to make money. Many women are reluctant to be tested, for if they are found to be genetically at risk, they may also find themselves uninsured. One strategy is to be tested anonymously so that only a number, which the testing facility gives you, identifies you. That way, the results never make it on to your permanent medical record. (This is how HIV testing is often done.) Once results *are* on your medical file, they cannot be removed, even at your request. That would constitute fraud on the part of the doctor who deletes the information. Your best bet is if you have a relative with breast or ovarian cancer, you can have *them* tested. Their insurance company already knows they have cancer so their status won't be affected. If they are negative, you are no longer high-risk. This is only an option, however, if that person is alive.

If you test positive and choose to have surgery, you'll need to have the insurance company pay for the surgery, which means you need to tell them something. If possible, try and find out in advance if your insurability will be affected. Sometimes another reason can be used to justify the procedure, such as an ovarian cyst or fibroids. This shouldn't be an issue, but it is the reality of health care in America.

Chapter 22

Time for That Tummy Tuck? Plastic and Associated Procedures

It's no coincidence that your friend who had a hysterectomy a few months ago actually looks, well, different. Younger, actually, more rested. Of course, she says that the few weeks off work did her a world of good, not to mention that she's not anemic from those nasty fibroids anymore. The truth is, she may have taken advantage of the down time from her surgery to have a few other things taken care of—like her face, breasts, and protruding belly. For many women, a medically indicated operation is the ideal time to sneak in some bonus surgery.

Very few women are thrilled about having to have a hysterectomy. Even though intellectually you know it's the right thing to do and will benefit you in the long run, it's a complex decision that is often psychologically difficult. Having a hysterectomy, more than any other type of surgery, stirs up all kinds of troublesome emotions . . . getting older, end of potential fertility, and for some, the beginning of menopause. Planning a cosmetic procedure that you've always secretly wanted is a way to turn things around. You may be losing your uterus, but at least you're gaining a flat stomach and perky breasts.

Even women who feel somewhat guilty about being vain are able to justify it: if they have to have major surgery, why not get something positive out of it? It's not uncommon for a woman who never even considered plastic surgery, but who is depressed at the prospect of a hysterectomy, to actually get excited about the thin thighs she'll acquire and move her surgery months sooner than originally planned.

Other women always wanted to do something, but couldn't justify the time off work. Since they have no choice but to take time off work for their hysterectomy, it's an opportunity to have the cosmetic procedure they've always wanted. Most realize it's now or never. In addition, there are other advantages to combining a plastic procedure with a medically necessary operation.

Cost

Plastic surgery is expensive and generally not covered by insurance. Costs include surgeon's fees, anesthesia fees, operating room fees, the recovery room, drugs, and hospital stay. It adds up really quickly, particularly if it is all coming out of your pocket. It's no surprise that it's usually the rich and famous who can afford plastic surgery. But if a plastic surgery procedure is done at the same time as a hysterectomy that your insurance does cover, it means that the *only* out-of-pocket cost might be the surgeon's fee and possibly the extra operating-room time. You can knock thousands of dollars off the cost of a plastic procedure by doing it at the time of your hysterectomy. You should, of course, check out the fees with your insurance company before surgery to avoid an unpleasant surprise.

The other cost of having elective surgery is the lost revenue from time off work. Many women who would never have plastic surgery because they couldn't possibly justify taking a couple of weeks off for something as frivolous as a tummy tuck realize that they will be taking time off from their jobs anyway to recover from their hysterectomies. Combining the two procedures makes a financially prohibitive procedure very affordable. The timing makes a lot of sense.

PRIVACY

Many women are reluctant to have cosmetic surgery because they don't want to tell their family or friends. It's easy to keep your tummy tuck quiet when everyone knows that you're recovering from major surgery since everyone expects you to have a sore belly and take a few weeks off from work. A face-lift is a little harder to hide unless you simply don't have visitors for a week or so after surgery, which isn't a bad idea anyway. The difficult part is explaining why you can't have visitors, or, if they do show up, justifying wearing sunglasses and a big brimmed hat as normal apparel when recovering from abdominal surgery.

THE DOWNSIDE

Before you schedule your face-lift, abdominoplasty (tummy tuck), liposuction, breast augmentation, and oh, by the way, hysterectomy, there are some negatives to consider. Cosmetic surgery is still surgery, and every surgery has the potential for complications. By adding an additional procedure, you are also adding the potential for additional complications. Risks of cosmetic surgery fall into the same three categories as gynecologic surgery: bleeding, infection, and injury to surrounding structures. The plastic surgeon can tell you exactly what those risks are and how commonly they occur.

Anesthesia Issues

Obviously, additional procedures mean additional anesthesia time. Prolonged anesthesia time means, for some people, slower return of bowel function, higher risk of blood clots, and feeling the effects of the anesthesia a little longer. Sometimes plastic surgery can be done simultaneously to decrease total anesthesia time, but this is usually not practical unless the cosmetic surgeon is working on your face while the gynecologist is doing a vaginal hysterectomy. In addition, since the plastic portion is elective, it makes sense to finish the required surgery and then continue only if all is well. In general, though, unless operative time exceeds five hours, additional risk is minimal.

Some cosmetic procedures are best done using local rather than general anesthesia. Dr. Thomas Mustoe, Chief of the Division of Plastic Surgery at Northwestern Memorial Hospital in Chicago, feels that local anesthesia can be beneficial during blepharoplasty (cosmetic eye surgery) to get an optimum result since it is helpful to the surgeon if the patient's eye muscles are not paralyzed by anesthesia. If you were planning a general anesthesia, you may want to consider a regional anesthetic so that you'll be numb from the waist down, but awake and able to move your eyes. With certain gynecologic procedures, such as laparoscopy, regional anesthesia is not an option (see chapter 14). Even in the case of blepharoplasty, however, the benefit is probably modest and needn't influence the decision as to what anesthesia is used.

Pain

The pain experienced after combined surgery has the potential to be significantly greater. The gynecologist is always happy to blame all the post-op pain on the plastic surgeon, and vice versa. In reality, it depends on who is doing which procedure. A laparoscopic hysterectomy usually results in minimal pain, and is an outpatient or overnight procedure. Most people feel like nothing happened within a week or so. Adding an abdominoplasty, which requires a large abdominal incision, is going to make recovery significantly longer and more painful.

Abdominoplasty is actually the most frequently requested plastic procedure at the time of hysterectomy. Many women have loose sagging skin and a lax abdominal wall from pregnancy or large fluctuations in weight. An abdominoplasty removes excess abdominal skin and tightens the abdominal wall, resulting in dramatic changes in body contour. While most abdominoplasties are done for cosmetic reasons, a loose abdominal wall can sometimes create back pain by putting stress on the lower back. If that is the case, or if an abdominal hernia is repaired at the same time, insurance will sometimes cover the cost of the procedure. A full tummy tuck usually results in minimal additional blood loss, but adds two to four hours of operating time.

Not everyone is a good candidate for abdominoplasty. Smokers in particular are known to have a significantly higher complication rate than nonsmokers. In addition, the closer someone is to her ideal body weight, the better the cosmetic result.

If you're already having an abdominal hysterectomy, adding a tummy tuck is not going to dramatically change your pain or recovery time since you would have an abdominal incision in either case. There is no question, though, that the abdominoplasty will require a larger incision and result in post-op abdominal tightness that makes it difficult to stand up straight for a few days. That's simply the price you pay for a belly you can bounce a quarter off of.

Blood Loss

All surgical procedures have the potential for some blood loss. There are some gynecologic and cosmetic surgeries that are more likely than others to result in more than minimal bleeding. It may not be the best time to add elective surgery if you are starting out anemic or having a gynecologic procedure with the potential for significant blood loss. Both surgeons need to participate in the decision if the combined blood loss would pose a risk to you or result in a significant anemia. If there is unexpected excessive blood loss during the gynecologic procedure, the plastic surgery portion will be cancelled. Know that this is a possibility and is in your best interest.

Suddenly an Incision

Adding the plastic procedure may change a well-considered surgical plan. If a laparoscopic hysterectomy is scheduled and then you decide to do an abdominoplasty, it makes no sense to have the minimally invasive procedure if you are going to end up with a large abdominal incision anyway. Suddenly your one-week recovery turns into three to four weeks of down time. This may be acceptable to you; just be aware that many aspects of your surgery and recovery will change.

Choice of Surgeons

If you are dying to use a plastic surgeon who operates at a hospital across town from the hospital where your gynecologist has scheduled your hysterectomy, you either have to choose a new gynecologist or a new cosmetic surgeon. Don't assume that doctors can operate at any hospital; most doctors are on staff at only one or two hospitals.

Combined surgery also needs to be scheduled way in advance in order to make sure that both the gynecologist and plastic surgeon are available and can be at the same location. Usually the gynecologist's office will coordinate this for you, but they need plenty of time.

Caution! Your gynecologist may tell you he can do the liposuction, tummy tuck, etc., and it's not necessary to involve another surgeon. Unless your gynecologist also happens to be a board-certified plastic surgeon, *don't do it!* While some gynecologists dabble in liposuction, the result will be far superior if a true expert does it. It will most certainly be cheaper to have the gynecologist do it, but when you're considering a body-altering surgical procedure, it's not the time to bargain hunt. Just as you wouldn't pick the cheapest surgeon to do your hysterectomy, or ask your plastic surgeon to do your hysterectomy, you shouldn't look for a bargain plastic procedure if you really want the best result possible.

Your best bet is to have your gynecologist make a recommendation of someone with whom she frequently works. He or she wants you to be pleased with your result and will refer you to someone whose work they know and respect. Make an appointment to see that surgeon and discuss what your objectives are. You may go thinking that all you need is a little liposuction to give you a flat belly and learn that the kind of result you want can only be obtained with a full abdominoplasty. Look at pictures and if you feel you're being talked into more surgery than is necessary or than you want, get a second opinion. Remember that this is elective surgery.

Vaginal Vanity

The exception to the "get a *real* plastic surgeon" rule is in the case of vaginal plastics. That's right, vaginal plastics. Gynecologists are frequently asked to do all kinds of things to improve the appearance of external genitalia.

Labioplasty refers to plastic surgery of the labia minora and is usually done for women who perceive their labia to be too long. What's too long? The average labia measure less than three centimeters from base to tip, but obviously there's a huge range. Some women, when reassured that their labia are slightly longer than average, but perfectly normal, still desire "a trim" based on their idea of what is attractive. There are even women who are reluctant to let their partners see them since they think their labia are too floppy, and therefore avoid being sexually intimate.

Some women do have abnormal, excessive length to their labia, a condition referred to as labial hypertrophy. Labial hypertrophy is defined as labia that are longer than four centimeters and extend well beyond the labia majora. When measuring labia, in case you are so inclined, you should spread the labia outward (like a butterfly) and measure from the base to the tip of the triangle. Common complaints in women with long labia include vaginal irritation, discomfort during walking, sitting, or other activities. Women who requested labioplasty in one study gave the following reasons for desiring surgery:

▼ 87 percent—aesthetic dissatisfaction
▼ 64 percent—discomfort in clothing
▼ 26 percent—discomfort in playing sports
▼ 43 percent—uncomfortable sex

Most women who undergo labioplasty are very satisfied with the results and are glad they went through with it, even if it means a month of no sex, bike riding, or tight clothes. A bag of frozen peas placed over the vaginal area for the first twenty-four hours after surgery is essential.

The other frequently requested vaginal plastic procedure is a "vaginal tightening," or perineoplasty. Women who have had many children, large children, or vaginal tears at the time of delivery often are left with a relaxed or scarred introitus. Basically, a relaxed introitus is a large, gaping vaginal opening which, for some women, is aesthetically bothersome or less sexually satisfying. Repair of a relaxed introitus can be easily accomplished at the time of hysterectomy, but again, must be discussed in advance.

OTHER CONSIDERATIONS

One of the limitations to combining surgeries is the position you must be in for each procedure. A hysterectomy requires you to be lying on your back. Liposuction of the thighs requires you to be on your stomach. Certainly you can be turned over while under anesthesia, but depending on circumstances, this may not be feasible or a great idea.

Choice of anesthesia also impacts on the ability to combine certain procedures. If you are having a laparoscopic procedure, general anesthesia is required. The cosmetic surgeon may do something in which local anesthesia is preferable.

COMBINING MORE THAN
ONE INDICATED PROCEDURE

Plastics are not the only procedures done at the time of hysterectomy. Many times, surgeons team up to combine two nonelective surgeries. If you need a hysterectomy and also need your gallbladder removed, it can often be done at the same time. All the limitations discussed above still apply (choice of surgeon, anesthesia, recovery, blood loss, etc.), but frequently, combining two or more procedures is safe and reasonable. Bunions, gallbladder, bowel surgery, hernia repair, and bladder surgery are all procedures that can potentially be scheduled at the same time as your hysterectomy. Orthopedic surgeons are frequently reluctant to share a procedure out of fear of infection of their surgical spot. There are virtually no studies that show a higher infection rate, but since it is so rarely done, no one really knows. Joint infections are so catastrophic that it's probably not worth taking the chance.

Bladder Surgery

One of the more common procedures to be done along with a hysterectomy is surgery to correct incontinence. Stress incontinence, or the inability to hold urine when coughing, sneezing, laughing, or jumping, is common in both young and older women. Stress incontinence results from loss of support to the lower part of the bladder and urethra, often as a result of childbirth. Surgery to repair incontinence involves lifting the urethra and bladder into their proper position.

There are a variety of techniques to accomplish this. Depending on the problem, the type of hysterectomy, and the preference of the surgeon, operations to repair stress incontinence can be done abdominally, laparoscopically, or vaginally. It is a procedure most gynecologists do, sometimes in consultation with a urogynecologist or urologist. Procedures to correct stress incontinence are easily done at the time of hysterectomy, but require appropriate preoperative evaluation to ensure that a surgical repair is the right approach. There are other causes of incontinence, which are not surgically correctable, so it is essential to identify the correct cause of the problem so that an unnecessary and ineffective procedure won't be done. This is discussed in more detail in chapter 11.

Incidental Appendectomy?

Often patients assume that their appendix will be removed while "in the neighborhood." Appendectomies used to be done routinely at the time of abdominal hysterectomy in the 1950s and 1960s, so this is not a ridiculous assumption. This practice stopped in the 1970s since the overwhelming majority of the removed appendixes were totally normal. Insurance companies decided that this was an unindicated procedure and added the unnecessary cost of the additional surgeon's fee, operating room time, and pathology fee. They stopped paying for removal of a normal appendix at the time of other operations, and surgeons stopped offering it. Now, gynecologists routinely look at the appendix, but leave it there if it is normal. Most will be happy to take it out if you request it; you'll just have to pay for it.

Little Stuff

If you want a mole or skin tag removed, depending on location, your gynecologist can often easily remove it at the time of surgery, but it needs to be discussed and agreed on beforehand. A large unsightly mole right below your belly button will still be there when you wake up from your laparoscopy unless you specifically request removal.

There's no limit to possibilities. If there is another procedure you need, or are thinking about having, bring it up. But bring it up well in advance since the biggest hurdle in scheduling combined surgery is not the surgery itself, but the logistics of getting two surgeons in the same hospital, on the same day, at the same time.

Part V

Life After Hysterectomy

Chapter 23

Exercise and Other Activities

There is life after hysterectomy and eventually you will need (and want) to return to the normal routine of exercise, work, travel, and sex, not necessarily in that order. It is really interesting how there are always far more phone calls from people eager to get started on their exercise program than from people eager to resume their sex lives.

EXERCISE

Like sex, exercise patterns after hysterectomy have a lot to do with what your exercise patterns were like before hysterectomy. The woman who ran a marathon the week before surgery is in an entirely different category than the woman who joins health clubs but never actually goes. In addition, the timetable for exercise after hysterectomy depends on the route of hysterectomy.

Why the Delay?

Despite great intentions before surgery, few women are eager to exercise in the first weeks after hysterectomy. Even if they have minimal or no pain, most women are simply too fatigued to contemplate anything more strenuous than normal daily activities. There are always those women who are raring to go and can't understand why they can't start their regular exercise routine within a week or two of surgery. It really is in your best interest to hold off. Ultimately your recovery will be better and quicker.

What could happen if you do too much too soon? One common misconception is that abdominal muscles are cut at the time of surgery and need to heal before they are stressed. In general, muscles are not cut, they are separated during surgery, resulting in no decrease in their strength (see chapter 10). What was cut was the fascia, the abdominal wall layer that holds everything together. It takes a good six weeks for the fascia to heal and resume its normal strength. Exercising too vigorously too soon is inappropriate and can result in separation of the fascia, which will result in a hernia or worse (see chapter 18).

The other reason to hold off on exercise is to allow the internal surgical sites to heal. Internal bleeding can result if vigorous, particularly high-impact, exercise is started too early. High-impact jumping and running can also compromise the placement of structures. Specifically, if you had your bladder repaired, it is particularly important to not jar things until healing is complete, since it's important that your bladder heal in the new location. You will increase your chance of a recurrent dropped bladder or incontinence if you exercise too soon.

Another special circumstance is if you had a tummy tuck at the time of surgery (see chapter 22). Plastic surgeons recommend that you avoid sit-ups for a minimum of two months. Keep in mind that since your belly will be flat as a board from the tummy tuck anyway, sit-ups are superfluous.

Anemia is another reason to wait. If your blood count is low from surgery, you will fatigue easily or even faint if you overexert yourself. Taking supplemental iron will facilitate your ability to exercise sooner rather than later.

Once you do start to exercise, listen to your body! If you are out of breath, experiencing pain, or just don't feel well, stop what you are doing. Recovering from surgery is not the time to push yourself. This is the time to get things going again, but only if your body is ready. Your heart rate should be at about 60 percent of the maximum you used to achieve, and you should be able to talk without being out of breath. There will be plenty of time to push yourself to the max after you are fully recovered.

In general, following an uncomplicated hysterectomy, normal exercise routines can be reestablished in six to eight weeks or sooner. In the meantime, modified exercise is the key to maintaining muscle tone, weight control, and sanity.

Many women are disturbed to find that they gain weight following hysterectomy. The weight gain is not a direct effect of the surgery; it is the result of inactivity and interruption of a regular exercise routine. A six- or eight-week hiatus is not going to create more than a few extra pounds, which are easily lost when exercise is reinstated. If you were in good shape before, you will be in good shape after. If you weren't, this is a great time to get started with an exercise regime.

Before you start your regular exercise routine, there are exercises that can be done in the hospital to facilitate recovery and strengthen pelvic and abdominal musculature. The following are guidelines. Your doctor will tell you specifically if there's anything you should avoid.

THE PELVIC FLOOR AND ABDOMINAL WALL

Pelvic physical therapists work specifically with pre- and post-hysterectomy patients to strengthen pelvic-floor and abdominal-wall tissues, which surgery may have damaged or weakened. In a perfect world, pelvic physical therapists see patients before surgery to evaluate the abdominal wall and pelvic floor and teach exercises to be performed after surgery. At that time, the therapist performs a detailed musculoskelatal evaluation of the pelvis and related structures in order to design a comprehensive program to maximize recovery and strengthening postsurgery. Therapists use manual therapy, neuromuscular education, and therapeutic exercise before and after surgery to strengthen, tone, and retrain neuromuscular components that may have been damaged prior to, or by, surgery.

In the real world, experienced pelvic therapists are a scarce luxury, not even found in most major medical centers, much less in small community hospitals. Judith Florendo, of Florendo Physical Therapy in Chicago, suggests the following recommendations to optimize recovery.

You may think you know how to breathe, but in spite of your obvious ability to get air in and out of your lungs, you may not be breathing in a way that uses your muscles correctly. Even something as automatic and seemingly innocuous as improper breathing techniques can have a major impact on healing and strengthening. To determine if you are breathing "correctly," try the following breathing exercise:

▼ Place one hand on your respiratory diaphragm (just under your chest) and the other at your chest.
▼ Take a deep breath and note which hand rises first and most.
▼ If your diaphragm hand rises first, congratulations! You are filling your lungs properly and without increasing intra-abdominal pressure.
▼ If your chest hand rises first, you have a paradoxical breathing pattern that increases intra-abdominal strain and may even strain the supportive ligaments of the bladder and bowel.

Now that you know how to breathe, it's time to move on to more advanced techniques. Almost everyone has heard of Kegel exercises, tried Kegel exercises, and abandoned Kegel exercises as a total waste of time and effort (see chapter 7). It's actually not that Dr. Kegel's pelvic floor exercises are worthless; it's that the vast majority of women do them incorrectly and therefore get no benefit. If done incorrectly, they can even be potentially harmful if organ prolapse is a concern. When done correctly and consistently, Kegel exercises can aid in maintaining bowel and bladder continence, assisting in organ support, and enhancing sexual appreciation. Here's how to do them correctly:

▼ Lie in bed.

▼ Try to contract the muscles in your pelvis responsible for holding back gas or preventing urine from leaking. You should be able to do this whether you are inhaling or exhaling.

▼ Do not use larger buttock muscles, inner thigh muscles, or abdominal muscles.

▼ *Do not hold your breath.*

▼ While you are doing this, breathe normally in the diaphragmatic pattern previously described.

▼ Hold the muscle contractions for 5 to 10 seconds. In the beginning, you may only be able to contract the muscles for a second or so before they fatigue and relax on their own ("quick flicks").

▼ Between each contraction, allow the muscles to relax fully for 10 seconds.

▼ During the first few days after surgery, try to work up to 10 to 20 repetitions of "quick flicks."

▼ After a while, work up to 10 repetitions at a time, mixing quick flicks with long holds.

▼ Once you are good at this, do this exercise in different positions throughout the day, allowing 5 to 10 seconds between each squeeze.

▼ Between 40 and 50 repetitions each day is the goal for maximum benefit. (This is why you are taking time off work!)

▼ It is also desirable to get in the habit of performing pelvic floor muscle contractions with functional activities. In other words, every time you get up out of a chair, lift, sneeze, or cough, *squeeze* those pelvic floor muscles.

▼ Stopping the flow of urine midstream is useful to test if you are contracting your muscles properly; it should never be done as an actual exercise.

Aside from strengthening pelvic muscles, it is important to do exercises in the immediate postoperative period to improve general circulation and help with the general aches and pains of lying in bed for several hours at a time. Most of these exercises seem ridiculously simple, but really make a difference in helping circulation and alleviating the aches and pains of lying in bed for several hours at a time.

All of the following maneuvers can be done in bed following surgery. It's really important to keep your spine stable and not allow your lower back to arch or flatten with the leg movement.

- ▼ **Heel slides.** Start with your leg straight. Slide your heel up toward your buttock, bending the knee, and then slide it back down. Repeat with the other leg.
- ▼ **Hip abduction/adduction.** Start with straight legs. Slide one leg out to the side, and return to midline. Repeat with the other leg.
- ▼ **Pelvic rocking.** Lying on your back, try to flatten your lower back against the bed in a pelvic tilt, then relax it and allow the normal curve of your lumbar spine to return.
- ▼ **Active range of motion exercises.** Tighten and tense the larger buttock muscles and then relax them. Do ankle circles and pumps. Raise your arms overhead and stretch gently. Slide your arms out to your sides and up to your head like angel wings.

It's also important to not lie in the fetal position or with pillows under the knees if you are on your back for any protracted length of time or while sleeping. This will cause shortening of the hip flexor muscles and your incision might heal in a shortened or tight position. This can adversely affect your lower back in the long run.

Most important, *get out of bed.* Speaking of getting out of bed, unless there is a crane available to haul you up the first time, you need to know how to do it. Learning to get in and out of bed correctly will greatly reduce your pain. Forget the old jackknife approach that can painfully strain your abdominal muscles. Instead, gently roll to your side fully. When you are at the edge of the bed, let your feet and legs drop down off the side of the bed while, at the same time, you push up with your elbow. This allows you to come to a sitting position with less effort.

Eventually, you will want to get back into bed. Do the same procedure in reverse. This method allows your legs to act as a lever to maneuver your upper body.

What About the Abs?

As anxious as you might be to have your six-pack back, you need to take it easy. In the first few days and weeks, it is advised only to tense the lower abdominal muscles. Although muscles are not cut during the vast majority of hysterectomy procedures, avoid crunches and sit-ups. It's really important not to add to intra-abdominal pressure that can strain other supportive tissues and ultimately contribute to prolapse.

Even after full recovery, crunches and sit-ups are not the best way to tone your abdominal muscles or strengthen your core, which is why many women have a little pouch in the lower abdomen despite doing a ridiculous number of repetitions. The transversalis muscle is not recruited effectively with those exercises, and this muscle is actually the key to a flat belly.

The alternative to crunches? A much more subtle exercise, but one that will result in a much flatter tummy. This is how it works:

▼ While lying on your back, find the front prominence of your hipbones. Move your fingertips in towards the midline about an inch and down about an inch. This is the deepest layer of all the abdominal muscles and the most important.

▼ Imagine you are zipping up hip-hugger pants that are too tight and tense the muscles lightly under your fingertips. If the lower abdomen bulges, you are doing it wrong, so re-examine your technique.

▼ Another image is to envision the muscle trying to pull the two hip bones closer together.

▼ Done correctly, you won't see a whole lot happening, so don't suck in your whole belly. If you do, you likely are contracting your oblique muscles, which is exactly what you don't want to do!

▼ Do not flatten your lower back as in a pelvic tilt; the lower back should remain in a neutral position.

▼ Within a few days, try doing this exercise when you are sitting up semi-reclined or in a chair. After a while, this exercise can be done on your hands and knees for a greater level of difficulty.

If you can isolate and specifically strengthen the transversalis muscle as above, your eventual resumption of fitness, including more advanced abdominal or core exercises, will be that much better.

EXERCISE GUIDELINES

Once you're out of the hospital (and know where your transversalis muscle is), it's time to consider a little more activity. Jim Karas, exercise consultant on *Good Morning America* and author of *The Business Plan for the Body* and *Flip the Switch*, designs postoperative programs based on prior fitness levels. He divides women into three categories:

▼ Avid exerciser
▼ Infrequent exerciser
▼ What is exercise?

All three categories of exercisers need to address the three components of exercise.

First, there is cardiovascular exercise. This includes any activity, such as walking, running, cycling, or stair-climbing, that elevates your heart rate for a period of time. During cardiovascular exercise, and up to two to three hours thereafter, your body burns calories at an accelerated rate.

The second category is strength and resistance training. Strength training involves placing force against a muscle using free weights, machines, exercise tubing, or your own body weight. Strength training is the *only* style of exercise that builds lean muscle tissue and increases strength. After the age of twenty, the average woman loses about half a pound of muscle per year. Around the time of menopause, that number doubles.

The third component of a comprehensive exercise program is stretching. After you stress a muscle, there is muscle growth and repair. Stretching after exercise keeps your muscles long and lean.

AFTER ABDOMINAL HYSTERECTOMY

First Two Weeks

Getting dressed and just being up and around is plenty. It's totally normal to absolutely have to take a nap at 2:00 P.M., even if you haven't taken an afternoon nap since you were two. Don't even think of your normal exercise routine.

Weeks Two Through Six

It's fine to start pushing yourself a little. Walking is your best bet. Don't be surprised if you're ready to stop after three blocks. If you're feeling pretty good, walking farther is okay. If you're feeling lower abdominal pressure and cramping, you've done enough. Get off your feet. If you're really fit, long walks, gentle stationary cycling, elliptical trainers, and light upper-body weights are fine. Listen to your body. If it doesn't feel good, hold off. Avoid high-impact activities such as jumping, running, and tennis. Don't worry and don't feel guilty if you don't feel like doing much of anything. You will. Some people just need a little longer.

After Week Six

After your six-week visit, there are usually no specific limitations. Jumping, running, lifting weights, and stretching are all fine. If you haven't done anything since the surgery, ease into it. You'll be surprised how soon you'll be back at your presurgical fitness level, even if you start out slow. In the event of a bladder repair, you may need to avoid high-impact activities a little longer. Your doctor will give you specific guidelines.

AFTER VAGINAL OR LAPAROSCOPIC HYSTERECTOMY

Since there's no abdominal incision, you'll feel like doing a lot more, a lot sooner. The temptation is actually to do more than you should do since you'll feel like you can. While it's tempting to push yourself, keep in mind that internal surgical sites still need to heal. So, even though you will be tempted to run and jump, you will be better off in the long run if you avoid high-impact activity for four to six weeks.

If someone has had a complication, or is anemic as a result of surgery, the above timetable is not reflective of reality. The key points are modify and listen to your body. Don't forget to drink plenty of water, particularly if you are still anemic.

Jim Karas suggests implementing the following programs before surgery to be in the best shape possible. As soon as you get the go-ahead from your doctor, it will be that much easier to get back into your routine.

Pointers for the Avid Exerciser

Most avid exercisers perform predominantly cardiovascular exercises. This is an ideal time to emphasize (or begin) a strength-training program. You don't need to add additional time for this style of exercise. Just cut your aerobics by fifty percent and use that time for strength training.

Strength training is important for two reasons. Regardless of the route of your hysterectomy, you are going to have to protect your "core," which includes both your abdominals and lower back. By improving strength in the upper body, you will ease the stress on your core when performing routine activities, such as picking things up off the floor and carrying grocery bags. The second reason is to rebuild those calorie-burning muscles that stagnated during the sedentary weeks after surgery.

Pointers for Infrequent Exercisers and "What is Exercise?" Women

If they're honest with themselves, most infrequent exercisers will realize they're not all that different from those in the "What is exercise?" category. Contemplating or recovering from surgery is an ideal turning point in life to get fit and improve your exercise habits. Nothing could be better in terms of enhancing body image and promoting long-term health. Before a major surgical procedure is a great time to start a fitness routine. However, it's vital to start to start out gradually and get the advice of someone who can make sure that you don't injure yourself or push too hard, which will inevitably doom you to failure in spite of your good intentions.

To see the kind of results that are going to make a difference in building strength prior to surgery or speeding recovery, you need to make a commitment to a serious program. It's all about motivation followed by planning. Plan when you are going to exercise, hire a trainer (check out www.jimkaras.com, www.nasm.org, www.acefitness.org, or www.ideafit.com) and/or find an exercise partner to keep you faithfully on track with an exercise program. Consider buying a new pair of exercise shoes. The Reeboks you bought in the 1980s are probably ready for retirement!

DRIVING

In general, do not plan on driving a car for two weeks. There are a number of reasons for this. First of all, your reaction time with a sore belly will not be as fast as it usually is. In addition, if there were an impact, the steering wheel and seat belt would ram right into your fresh surgical site. Also, if you are even slightly anemic, it's possible to experience an unpredictable episode of lightheadedness. Finally, where are you going anyway? You're supposed to be home resting, not running around doing things. Certainly you can drive in an emergency. In general, you're better off as a passenger. If you are a passenger, wear your seat belt even if it is more comfortable not to.

Travel—How About That Postoperative Trip to the Caribbean?

Most surgeons recommend staying close to home for at least two weeks after surgery. Almost any significant complication that might occur will have occurred by that time. Once the two-week visit has occurred, it is generally fine to leave town. Many women take advantage of their time off from work to go lie around a pool somewhere. (Ask your doctor about going *in* the pool.) This is when you should get really chummy with your friend who has the beach house in Malibu. This is not the time to take that long-delayed trip to Bora Bora. While a complication is unlikely, things can happen in the first six weeks, and if you're not close to home, you at least want to be somewhere where there is reasonable medical care (not to imply that Bora Bora doesn't have reasonable medical care). After six weeks, the sky's the limit.

If you are away from home and have a problem, call your doctor and let him or her know what is going on. If it is necessary for you to go to a local emergency room, your surgeon can facilitate things by calling over there and telling them what kind of surgery you had and any specifics that they should know. In other words, just because you can't see your own doctor doesn't mean that he or she can't still be involved.

Work

There was a real estate broker who closed a million-dollar deal in her hospital room five hours after surgery, and a lawyer who had a fax machine installed in her hospital room so she could prepare for a trial she was planning one week after surgery. Most people, however, are not quite that motivated.

Eventually, you will need to return to work. What you do for a living and your motivation are the greatest determinants of when you will be ready to start doing it again. The bookkeeper who sits at a desk all day long and works two blocks from her home can probably be back on the job in two weeks. The professional tennis player needs a few more weeks before she can get back on the circuit. A woman who loves her job and is going batty at home is going to feel ready long before the woman who is going to take advantage of the six-week leave she has been given and would just as soon never return to work.

Most jobs grant a six-week disability leave after surgery. Many women, especially if they have abdominal hysterectomies and have physically strenuous jobs, really need the full six weeks. Most women who've had a laparoscopic procedure can probably go back after a couple of weeks. Fortunately, your human resources people have no clue what a laparoscopic hysterectomy is and will give you the whole six weeks if you want it.

If possible, easing back into a full work day is a good option. If you can start back with half days, it's helpful. Half days don't work if you arrive at nine and plan on leaving at one. The lure of doing just one more thing is inevitable and suddenly it's five o'clock. *Arrive* at one, and you truly will end up working a half-day.

Returning to work is also easier if you have the luxury of having someplace to rest. Lying down for thirty minutes after lunch will make all the difference in the world as far as getting through the day.

Frequently, women ask for an extension of their sick leave. Human resource departments have gotten a lot more strict, and a lot more savvy, about granting paid disability time. It's not enough for your physician to say that he or she thinks you would benefit from an additional week off. There needs to be a specific reason why that extra time is necessary. If there truly was a complication that delayed recovery, it is easy to justify additional days. If not, you may be out of luck since your physician can only say what is true and what can be documented.

Many women who are highly motivated to return to work tell their employer that they will only need a week or two off after surgery. That may be true, but you don't want to be compelled to go back if you're not feeling ready, or if your expectations are unrealistic. Request the maximum time off that your job will allow. They will be thrilled if you are able to return early—a much better scenario than if they expect you back in a week and you take two or three or four.

SEX

Now that you're back to work, driving, and exercising, it's time to think about sex.

What your doctor will tell you is, "No sex for six weeks." For what that *really* means, turn to chapter 25 for specifics.

Chapter 24

A Word
(or Two)
About Hormones

In 1948, a *Reader's Digest* article proclaimed, "The melancholy sickness that blights the happiness of some women at their change of life [can be] controlled by female hormones; yet most women have gone on suffering . . . But now at last they are ready to transfigure the stormy afternoon of life . . . into a time of serenity and vigor."

If it were only that simple! Clearly, a detailed discussion of the pros and cons of long-term hormone replacement is beyond the scope of this book, especially since much of the information would totally change minutes after publication. Hormone replacement after hysterectomy is a less complicated dilemma and involves only a decision about short-term use, as opposed to long-term commitment.

Women who do not remove their ovaries and women who have already gone through menopause, don't need to make a decision about estrogen replacement following their hysterectomies because their estrogen levels will not change. The only women who need to make a decision are those who will be going through a surgical menopause due to removal of functional ovaries at the time of their hysterectomy.

The concept of hormone *replacement* versus hormone *extension* is important. Hormone replacement refers to replacing estrogen during the years when a woman normally would be producing estrogen on her own. That is, if a women under the age of fifty (the average age of menopause) no longer produces estrogen either because of a surgical menopause or a premature menopause, any estrogen she takes is truly hormone replacement. When a woman over the age of fifty chooses to take estrogen, that actually is hormone *extension*, or estrogen supplementation beyond the years that she ordinarily would produce her own estrogen. Since 2002, results from the Women's Health Initiative (WHI), a research project to study the effects of hormones, have appeared in the news regularly, creating a great deal of concern regarding the safety of estrogen use. It is estrogen *extension* in the woman over fifty, however, as opposed to estrogen *replacement* in the under-fifty group, that is controversial. Unfortunately, the two are usually lumped together so that the forty-two-year-old who takes estrogen feels she is putting herself at the same risk, and has the same issues, as the fifty-two-year-old who takes estrogen supplements.

A woman who goes through a surgical menopause faces the same decisions that every woman does when she goes through a natural menopause. The difference is in the timing. Unfortunately, the timing coincides with a woman's recovery from major surgery, and *no one should have to go through menopause and major surgery at the same time.* Even if your preference is to not take long-term hormone replacement therapy, it may be a reasonable plan to take estrogen for at least a few months to ease what might be a difficult transition. The long-term decision can be made later.

How bad is it if you don't take replacement estrogen? That depends. Some woman have no symptoms when they transition into menopause, surgical or natural. Others are aware of some hot flashes and may notice some vaginal dryness or insomnia, but nothing dramatic. Others? Totally miserable would be an understatement. It's fairly unpredictable who's going to have a rough time, but in general, the more estrogen someone makes on her own, the more symptomatic she will be when you remove the source. A thirty-year-old who loses her ovaries is going to be more likely to have severe flashes than a forty-nine-year-old who is already winding down.

When discussing estrogen replacement after hysterectomy, it's important to note that estrogen alone is being replaced, as opposed to the usual combination of estrogen and progesterone that is given to most women taking supplemental hormones. The sole purpose of adding progesterone is to protect the lining of the uterus from developing uterine cancer. If the uterus has been removed, there is no reason to take progesterone. This makes replacement a whole lot easier since it's the progesterone that causes the bloating, depression, bleeding, and negative effects on lipids and cholesterol. In other words, progesterone is the bad guy for most women, and women who don't have a uterus don't need to take it.

Before you decide what you want to do, consider what we know about estrogen replacement and what's still controversial.

KNOWN BENEFITS OF ESTROGEN REPLACEMENT

Relief of Vasomotor Disturbances

No one argues that estrogen makes hot flashes disappear. For some women, hot flashes (or flushes) are more debilitating than for other women. Women who get warm a few times a day don't understand why some women need help to get through menopause. The woman who flashes twenty to thirty times a day, can't sleep, and can't get through a business meeting fully clothed coined the bumper-sticker phrase, "I'm out of estrogen and I've got a gun." Estrogen not only works, it works fast. Women who start estrogen replacement generally experience relief within twenty-four hours and continue to get improvement over the first few weeks of treatment.

Sleep

It is well-known that hormones have a profound effect on sleep and can dramatically alleviate the insomnia that plagues many menopausal women. The inability to sleep through the night is not only because of hot flashes. Estrogen and progesterone levels influence multiple factors that control sleep. Hormone replacement therapy (HRT) is known to improve rapid-eye movement (REM) sleep and sleep quality, even in women who have no problem with flashes.

Vaginal Dryness

Vaginal thinning and dryness resulting in painful intercourse, or the inability to have intercourse, is arguably the most distressing menopausal symptom to the woman who had a satisfying sex life before menopause. Not every woman experiences this problem, but for the ones who do, it can be devastating. Estrogen therapy, either systemic or local, keeps vaginal tissues moist and elastic.

Sexuality

In general, women on estrogen replacement have a much healthier libido than women not on estrogen. This is due, in part, to the fact that women on estrogen have fewer problems with vaginal dryness and therefore have more frequent sex, which in turn stimulates libido. They also aren't as tired and depressed. Even if dryness and insomnia are not a problem, libido can still be an issue. This is covered in great detail in chapter 25.

Bladder Function

Estrogen also influences bladder function. This is no surprise since the urinary tract is derived from the same embryologic source as the genital tract. Estrogen receptors are found in the bladder and urethra, as well as in the vagina. Therefore, in addition to maintaining healthy urinary tract tissues, estrogen strengthens vaginal tissues that support the bladder and the urethra and prevent them from dropping into an abnormal position (prolapse). This is why menopausal women on estrogen are less likely than other menopausal women to have problems with incontinence, bladder infections, frequent urination, and prolapse.

Skin

Women on estrogen have better skin. It's not your imagination that women on estrogen have fewer, shallower wrinkles, due to increased skin collagen. Certainly other factors such as sun, smoking, and genetics contribute to skin changes associated with aging, but estrogen plays a part as well. This is not to suggest that vanity is a valid reason to take estrogen; it's just a fact and explains why many women in the 1950s used estrogen face cream.

CONTROVERSIAL BENEFITS

There are a number of symptoms that women experience around the time they go through menopause which estrogen is likely to help, but its benefits have not been absolutely proven by large, prospective, randomized studies. In other words, ask any woman who takes estrogen if she is less depressed, thinks more clearly, and generally feels better, and you'll usually get an emphatic yes! It just hasn't been proven in the kinds of studies that evidence-based medicine demands.

Depression, Mood Swings

Depression is one of the more complicated symptoms of menopause. Are women depressed because low estrogen has changed their chemical balance in such a way that they experience a chemical depression? Or are women depressed when they go through menopause because of sleep deprivation and the sudden lack of libido that has destroyed a formerly terrific sex life? There is also the issue of the ten extra pounds that have magically appeared on your belly and thighs, despite the fact that your eating and exercise routine is exactly the same as it was ten years ago. In case you're still feeling a little happy, remember that your last child is about to leave for college, you were passed over for the promotion, and your husband is going through his own mid-life crisis.

It's really not fair that a major hormonal plunge occurs at the same time as a lot of less-than-pleasant life cycle changes. It's hard to know how much depression is a direct result of estrogen deprivation, as opposed to other issues. The change in hormones is certainly is a contributing factor and many women find that estrogen replacement helps lift the depression and obviates the need for antidepressants.

Cognitive Function

Many experts do not consider estrogen's effect on cognitive function to be controversial. Multiple studies have demonstrated that hormones all profoundly affect perception, attention span, memory, and ability to learn. Estrogen receptors have been identified in many areas of the brain involved in cognition, and increased blood flow to the brain is known to occur in women on estrogen. In addition, sleep disturbances caused by lack of estrogen significantly contribute to an inability to think clearly.

The WHI results, in which worse cognitive function was reported, may not be definitive, due to significant problems in the design of the study. Putting what the experts think aside, the "true" experts, menopausal women, usually are quite clear on one thing: they were able to think more clearly and remember more things before they went through menopause.

Arthritis

A lot of women who stop their estrogen don't notice hot flashes, insomnia, or vaginal dryness. What they do notice is joint pain, stiffness, decreased mobility, and a need to increase arthritis medications. While it is not as well-known as other problems of estrogen deficiency, many women notice a real difference in arthritic symptoms when they go through menopause or stop taking hormone replacements.

PRIMARY PREVENTION ISSUES

Estrogen was originally intended for, and in fact is only FDA-approved for, treatment of menopausal symptoms such as hot flashes, vaginal dryness, and insomnia. It was never approved for prevention of heart disease, Alzheimer's disease, or osteoporosis. Observational studies over the last twenty years have looked at the potential long-term benefits of estrogen replacement, generating the flurry of studies and controversy about estrogen. No one questions that estrogen is beneficial for prevention of menopausal symptoms; the controversy lies in using estrogen for the primary prevention of problems that ultimately influence life expectancy.

A Huly 2002 WHI study divided 16,608 women into two groups: half received estrogen and progesterone, and half received a placebo pill. The purpose of the study was to determine if long-term use of HRT influenced medical conditions that could affect longevity, such as heart disease, stroke, and breast cancer. The results of the study resulted in a huge amount of media attention, with subsequent panic and discontinuation of hormones for huge numbers of women.

In summary, 97.5 percent of women in the WHI study had no untoward events, but for each 10,000 women per year who used estrogen *and progesterone*, there were:

▼ 7 additional myocardial infarctions
▼ 8 additional strokes
▼ 8 additional breast cancers
▼ 18 additional blood clots
▼ 6 fewer colorectal cancers
▼ 5 fewer hip fractures
▼ No additional deaths

What is striking is that the absolute number of women who had problems from HRT was quite small. Also, in spite of the fact that there were multiple problems with the design of the study, the consequences were huge. Many women were also unaware that the results only applied to women taking estrogen and progesterone.

The study group that included women who took estrogen alone was not discontinued until March 2004. Preliminary results in the estrogen-only group reported a decrease in fracture risk. There was no increased risk of breast cancer or heart disease. There was an increased risk of stroke, similar to the estrogen-progesterone group. Women who have had a hysterectomy, of course, take estrogen alone.

Heart Disease

Heart disease is the number one killer of women. While most women perceive breast cancer to be their greatest health threat, it is ten times more likely that an American woman will die from heart disease than from breast cancer. Over the years, many observational studies suggested that HRT would decrease coronary disease in women and therefore prolong life. This made sense since estrogen is known to dilate blood vessels, resulting in an increased blood supply to the heart.

The WHI study suggested that women who take estrogen and progesterone are *not* reducing their risk of heart disease, and are actually increasing their cardiovascular risk. Some experts question the WHI results since a number of factors were not accounted for, such as the use of aspirin and statin drugs, which are known to alter the risk of heart attack. In addition, the average age of the woman starting HRT was sixty-three, when coronary artery disease may already have been present. Prempro (the drug used in the study), while widely prescribed, is not the only HRT combination available; it has been known for some time that other estrogen–progesterone preparations result in a healthier lipid profile. Since Prempro contains a progesterone known to have a negative influence on cholesterol and triglycerides, the findings may be very different in a group taking a different progesterone.

While the WHI data are important and answer many questions, it certainly is not definitive regarding the impact of estrogen on cardiovascular health. What is not controversial is that women who are overweight, don't exercise or eat right, and who smoke are increasing their risk of heart disease far more than they would by taking estrogen. The WHI study de-emphasized the importance of smoking cessation, weight management, and proper diet in the prevention of heart disease. Based on current data, women who are at risk for coronary heart disease shouldn't take estrogen to prevent heart disease, but the real question is, should women not at risk for heart disease avoid it?

Blood Clots

WHI data showed that certain women are at increased risk of having a blood clot resulting in a pulmonary embolism, stroke, or deep vein thrombosis in the first couple of years when they initiate estrogen use. Women who have an abnormal lipid profile (high cholesterol and/or triglycerides) fall into that group. We know that it is imperative that all women evaluate their cholesterol and triglyceride levels before initiating hormone therapy. Women who have taken HRT for years, or who have a normal lipid profile, are at minimal risk for developing blood clots.

Breast Cancer

While most woman die from heart disease, most women worry about breast cancer. The WHI study demonstrated an increased number of breast cancers in the estrogen–progesterone group compared with the placebo group, but the absolute number was quite small (8 of 10,000).

Many experts feel that the increase seen in breast cancer in the first five years of HRT use was not due to new breast cancers, but to hormonal stimulation of existing tumors. Since it takes roughly ten years for a malignant cell to become clinically detectable, this is a reasonable assumption. If the study had been continued, many experts believe that the number would have leveled off. Since the study was cut short, that data will never be available. The estrogen-alone group, in spite of the fact that they had an additional two years of exposure, did not demonstrate an increase in breast cancer.

Even if one accepts the premise that estrogen increases one's risk of developing breast cancer, it is a small factor. Most women are surprised to learn that over 80 percent of women who have breast cancer have never taken hormone replacement of any kind. In addition, the risk of developing breast cancer from HRT is lower than the risk associated with daily alcohol use or obesity. It's important to keep the influence of hormones on breast cancer in perspective. A lot of questions are still unanswered, and a lot of work needs to be done before the influence of hormone replacement on breast cancer is really understood.

Nuisance, But Not Dangerous

A number of issues come up for women who take estrogen. These, while bothersome and annoying, do not indicate a health-threatening problem.

Bleeding

Years ago, when HRT was first prescribed, it was done in a cyclic fashion so that monthly bleeding continued after menopause for many women. Now, HRT is given continuously so that no bleeding is expected. It's not unusual for recently menopausal women to have unexpected bleeding during the first six months of hormonal replacement. Any heavy or continuous bleeding needs to be evaluated. Woman who have had a hysterectomy should, of course, have no bleeding at all.

Breast Tenderness

Breast tenderness is a symptom women experience while taking estrogen, but it is not an indication that something is wrong. Any breast tenderness on both sides and not localized to a specific area is from hormones, rather than an abnormal growth. Most women find that the tenderness goes away over time, but some women have to dramatically reduce the dose or stop taking estrogen altogether. Many times, full and tender breasts are related to progesterone-stimulated fluid retention, which is not an issue for a woman with no uterus.

Fluid Retention

Fluid retention is essentially always due to progesterone. It's rare for a woman who is taking estrogen alone to have a problem. Many of the newer progesterones create far less fluid retention and are tolerated better.

MYTHS ABOUT HORMONE REPLACEMENT

Weight Gain

Nothing you read here will convince you that estrogen does *not* make you gain weight, but the sad truth is that it doesn't. Not one study has ever shown that estrogen replacement causes weight gain. Changing metabolism in the early fifties is what causes those five extra pounds a year to creep up on you, estrogen or no estrogen. If you exercise and eat the same way when you're fifty that you did when you were thirty, you will gain weight. It happens to the men, too. Women who go off their estrogen usually find that the arrow on the scale still doesn't budge. Sorry.

Progesterone can add an additional few pounds due to water retention, but women who have had a hysterectomy don't take progesterone.

Your Doctor Benefits Financially

There are always those who think that somehow your doctor reaps some financial benefit from prescribing hormones. Nothing could be further from the truth. Most doctors were not savvy enough, or wealthy enough, to invest in pharmaceutical companies when they were in medical school. That's the only way there can be any personal gain from prescribing any drug. Every woman on estrogen replacement generates multiple phone calls and lengthier visits, particularly when the newspaper headlines scream warnings about the potential dangers of estrogen. Time is money, and the amount of time needed to explain new studies and controversies about estrogen are a strong financial disincentive to prescribing it. The woman who comes in every year for her examination and doesn't take estrogen takes a lot less time than the woman who has three legal-size pages worth of questions about her HRT and calls every time a new study hits the front page of the newspaper.

How Hormone Replacement Is Given

Pills, Patches, Pellets

The majority of available estrogen replacements are taken in pill form on a daily basis or less often. Oral estrogens pass through the gastrointestinal tract and are metabolized by the liver. Many different preparations are available and include plant-derived, synthetic, and animal-derived products. The first commercially available and most widely used estrogen is Premarin, derived from the urine of pregnant horses (PREgnant MARes' urINe . . . get it?). Contrary to popular belief, there is no evidence to suggest, and no reason to believe that "natural" estrogens are any safer than a synthetic preparation, or any less likely to cause cancer. There is not one study that shows it makes any difference whether a product is plant-derived, animal-derived, or synthetic. All estrogens stimulate estrogen receptors in tissue and one product does not promote cancer more than another. Anyway, what's more natural than horse urine?

In the 1980s, transdermal estrogen patches were developed as an alternative means of delivering estrogen. The advantage to the patch is that the skin absorbs the estrogen and it goes directly into the bloodstream without having to pass through the gastrointestinal system. Primarily, this is a benefit for women who have liver or gallbladder disease. In addition, another advantage is that you only need to remember to use it once or twice a week. The disadvantage is that many women don't like to wear a patch; it can irritate sensitive skin and, in some cases, come off. Sometimes there is also a sticky residue, which leaves faint circles on your skin unless you get it all off. For women who still have their uterus and must take progesterone, there is only one that which has progesterone included. Everyone else has to take a pill in addition to using an estrogen patch. A major postoperative bonus to the patch is that it can be used by a patient who is unable to eat or drink and therefore can be started immediately after surgery.

There are multiple products available to deliver estrogen vaginally. Keep in mind that while there is some absorption into the bloodstream, the amount is minimal and the effects of vaginal estrogen are local, rather than systemic. For that reason, vaginal estrogen is not beneficial for hot flashes, insomnia, depression, osteoporosis, cognitive function, colon cancer, etc. It will help with vaginal lubrication and may also have a positive impact on bladder function. The details are discussed below.

Europeans are generally much more comfortable with the concept of hormone extension, and the use of long-term, slow-release products are common. Many European women use a slow-release gel applied to the arms, shoulders, thighs, and abdomen. Other women have a pellet implanted in the fatty tissue under the skin of the arm; the pellet releases estrogen for four to six months. Most of these products are not available in the United States and probably won't become available in the near future.

SURGICAL ISSUES

Is It Menopause or Is It the Hospital?

If you chose not to take estrogen after surgery, be prepared for what you might experience. Women after surgery frequently wake up two or three times a night to change their soaked pajamas. Before you slap on an estrogen patch, be aware that profuse sweating episodes in the weeks after surgery are not necessarily from menopausal changes. Every woman receives huge amounts of fluid during surgery; perspiring after surgery is your body's way to get rid of all that fluid. It's also possible that you have developed an infection and have a fever, so take your temperature if you think that's the case. It could also be due to flashes from estrogen deprivation, but you won't know for sure for a few days.

Insomnia? Nobody sleeps well in the hospital between the plastic pillows, scratchy sheets, and the stream of people coming into your room to do things. Not to mention, you will most likely not be pain-free. You won't know until you get home if your inability to sleep is hospital routine, pain, or menopause.

Depression? Few women are depressed after hysterectomy (see chapter 17), but a transient depression is not unusual at the time of any surgical procedure. Again, it may not be a menopausal symptom.

Have a Plan Before Surgery

If you chose to remove your ovaries at the time of your hysterectomy, discuss a plan with your physician prior to the day of surgery. You may want an estrogen patch placed immediately after surgery to avoid any symptoms. You may want to be given something for the first few weeks as you recover from the surgery, and then discuss a longer-term plan at a post-op visit. If you decide to not take anything, you may want a prescription on hand in case you change your mind. Plan ahead so you're not making an emergency Walgreen's visit at 2:00 A.M. your first night home.

ALTERNATIVES TO ERT

For whatever reason, you or your doctor has decided that estrogen replacement is just not for you. Fortunately, there are many non-hormonal alternatives to alleviate menopausal symptoms.

Vasomotor Symptoms

Hot flashes will most likely be your first and most dramatic symptom. Flannel pajamas are not a great idea. While in the hospital, your best bet is to wear the lovely gowns they give you. Why sweat up your own stuff when you might be changing two or three times a night? If you do choose to wear your own, light cotton is best. Once you get home, layering is helpful and sleeping in the buff is always a good strategy. A small battery-operated fan is a godsend.

If your flashes are beyond what a fan can alleviate, and if ripping off your clothes is not a practical back-to-work strategy, you need to explore other options.

One group of drugs that has been shown to decrease hot flashes is the selective serotonin reuptake inhibitors, also known as SSRIs. These drugs are intended and FDA-approved to be used solely as antidepressants, but were serendipitously found to significantly reduce hot flashes in menopausal women. Drugs such as fluoxitine (Prozac), paroxitene (Paxil), and venlafaxine (Effexor), have all been found to be helpful. Effexor is the most studied and seems to do the best job of reducing flashes. It has been used for years in women with breast cancer, with great success.

Other drugs, such as clonidine, bellergal, and methyl-dopa are frequently prescribed for hot-flash reduction, the results are variable and the side effects are unacceptable. A number of new drugs that work directly on temperature regulatory centers in the brain are currently under investigation and should be available in the next few years.

Other remedies are frequently suggested, usually in articles in women's magazines written by a twenty-something who has never had a hot flash in her life. Brilliant remedies such as "turn down the thermostat," "avoid spicy foods," and the ultimate cure-all, "Do yoga," pop up regularly. No comment is necessary.

The good news is that for the majority of women, hot flashes don't go on forever. While 75 to 85 percent of women experience this phenomenon, the vast majority only have to contend with it for six months to a year. By the five-year mark, 25 percent of women are still flashing, but usually less frequently. However, there are those unlucky women (about 15 percent) who deal with hot flashes indefinitely.

Herbs, Spices, and Wishful Thinking

Lots of alternative herbs and spices have been touted as giving relief for hot flashes. Unfortunately, most have been shown not to work beyond the initial placebo effect. The successful ones work because they have estrogen-like activity, which is exactly what women who are choosing alternatives are trying to avoid.

Keep in mind that the companies that produce alternatives to estrogen are just as profit-motivated as pharmaceutical companies. A multi-million dollar industry has evolved to promote "natural" products to a vulnerable population of women who are suffering and seeking safe, effective alternatives to estrogen. While women generally distrust the pharmaceutical industry, which is obligated to test and report all negative findings, the general population seems to have little problem placing their trust in information and promotional ads placed by companies that have no efficacy or safety standards. Just because something is "natural" doesn't mean it is safe. Just because the health food store clerk seems very knowledgeable doesn't mean it works.

Many women question why more studies haven't been done on herbal preparations. Studies are in progress, but they are extremely expensive and difficult, since a large number of patients and a long time frame is required. In addition, products used to treat hot flashes are particularly hard to study since the placebo effect is so large. Whether you give women soy, Chinese herbs, or broccoli and sugar pills, at least thirty percent will experience fewer hot flashes for at least a few weeks. Herbs and other botanicals are also difficult to study since there are great variations in absorption and metabolism.

The bottom line is, "let the buyer beware." There are only two appropriate criteria when deciding to use alternative products: is it safe, and does it really work? Too often, no one really knows. Since these products are neither food nor drug, FDA approval is not necessary and manufacturers are not held responsible for safety or efficacy. The only ones who consistently benefit are the companies that sell the products.

Phytoestrogens

Phytoestrogens are compounds that have estrogen-like activity, or are metabolized into compounds with estrogenic activity. They are classified into three groups: isoflavones, lignans, and coumestans. Isoflavones are the most common form and are found in over two hundred plants.

The most commonly used products that contain phytoestrogens are the many soy compounds that are available. Red clover (promensil) is another commonly used compound that contains phytoestrogens. Several trials demonstrate little or no efficacy when red clover is compared with placebo. Furthermore, phytoestrogens exhibit a weak estrogenic effect that may potentially stimulate breast cancer growth.

Black Cohosh

Black cohosh (Remifemin) is derived from the root of a plant used by native North American Indians. It is one of the most widely used alternative therapies for treatment of hot flashes and may be one of the few that actually works beyond the placebo effect. Some women experience unpleasant gastrointestinal symptoms when they take black cohosh, but for many women, black cohosh, while not eliminating hot flashes, makes them more tolerable.

Dong Quai

Dong quai is often used in combination with other therapies, and it has been shown to reduce the frequency of hot flashes in at least one study. This is one to use with caution, however; in studies using mice, breast cancer cells were stimulated. In addition, it is known to interfere with anticoagulant drugs and may cause excessive bleeding in certain situations.

Evening Primrose

Evening primrose is another plant that has been promoted to alleviate not only hot flashes, but other menopausal symptoms as well. There is yet to be a randomized, placebo-controlled evaluation of evening primrose. Any benefits are anecdotal and have not been confirmed by scientific study.

Wild Yam Cream

Manufacturers of wild yam cream state that this "natural progesterone" increases libido and alleviates other menopausal symptoms. What they don't tell you is that the human body is biochemically incapable of converting the progesterone in wild yams to a biologically active form of progesterone. It will have the same effect whether you put it on your skin or on your shelf.

There are dozens of other products that claim to alleviate hot flashes and other troublesome menopausal symptoms. Until appropriate studies prove safety and efficacy, alternative compounds should be taken with caution and upheld to the same standards as prescription medications.

Vaginal Dryness

Vaginal dryness is the menopausal symptom that has the biggest impact on a woman who had a healthy, satisfying sex life before menopause. Suddenly, sex is something to be avoided, and is so painful and unpleasant when it does happen that the natural response is to continue to avoid it. If someone is dry, rarely has intercourse, and anticipates pain when it does happen, it's just not going to happen. The pain–no libido–avoidance cycle is difficult to break, but the motivated woman can do it.

Vaginal Lubricants

Vaginal lubricants have come a long way since the advent of K-Y Jelly. Any water-soluble lubricant intended for vaginal use is safe. The key is to use it *before* you attempt intercourse, as opposed to after an unsuccessful attempt. If you try to have intercourse and things are dry, your vagina will clamp down and really dry up in an attempt to not let anything in. If you use lubricant automatically, it works much better. If you didn't need it, the worst that will happen is things will be too slippery. It's a risk worth taking to avoid pain. Put it on your partner's penis and on the outside of your vagina. Even if you are using vaginal estrogen, lubricant should be used as an adjunct. There are a number of great products available. Astroglide is one of the best. Saliva is readily available and also works. Vitamin E capsules are another "natural source" to make things more slippery.

Vaginal Moisturizers

Vaginal moisturizers are products intended to increase a woman's natural vaginal lubrication. They are not lubricants and shouldn't be used as such. These products are nonhormonal and are used in the vagina two or three times a week to increase the amount of lubrication your vaginal walls produce. Their advertisements inevitably include happy couples swimming alongside gushing waterfalls. Some women find them useful, but they are not nearly as popular as lubricants.

Vaseline Petroleum Jelly

The only role for Vaseline during sex is to apply to the bedroom doorknob to keep the children out. Do *not* put it in your vagina. It is not water-soluble and will stay in your vagina for eons, promoting infections and unpleasant discharge.

Vaginal Estrogen Therapy

Many women who choose to not take estrogen replacement are comfortable with the idea of using vaginal estrogen. Yes, vaginal estrogen is absorbed systemically, but the amounts are miniscule if used appropriately, and no study has detected an increased risk of breast cancer, coronary heart disease, or stroke. Even some women with breast cancer can use vaginal estrogen with the blessing of their oncologist. Just as the tiny amount of estrogen won't increase risk, it also won't be beneficial for hot flashes or osteoporosis. What it will do is enable you to have comfortable intercourse. It can also exert a local effect on the bladder to help alleviate urinary tract problems.

There are a number of different ways to deliver estrogen to vaginal tissues. The most common products are vaginal creams such as Premarin (conjugated estrogens) or Estrace (estradiol). Estrogen creams are inserted into the vagina using an applicator similar to that used for yeast infection medication. They should not be used at the time of intercourse. Estrogen cream is not a lubricant; it enables your body's natural lubrication. The disadvantage of creams is that they are somewhat messy and are absorbed into the bloodstream more than other vaginal estrogen delivery systems. The advantage is that many varieties are available and women can easily taper the amount to the smallest amount necessary to alleviate dryness.

Another option is a vaginal ring. There are a number of silastic, soft, flexible rings that supply estradiol in a slow, steady release. The ring remains in the vagina for three months, and neither the woman or her partner can detect it. The advantage is that it's not messy like creams and you don't need to think about it. The disadvantage is that you can't taper the dose since it stays in for three months. The overall dose is quite low, but some women like the option of tapering and don't like having something in their vaginas all the time.

Vaginal estradiol tablets are inserted deep into the vagina with an applicator two to seven times a week. Like the ring, you avoid the mess of the creams. After a two-week nightly "loading dose," most women find that using it once or twice a week is adequate. All the above products work well; it's a matter of personal preference.

Like weight loss, alleviating vaginal dryness is a two-step process: repair, followed by maintenance. If someone is totally unable to have intercourse due to dryness, vaginal estrogen should be used nightly for a minimum of two weeks. After the two-week initial treatment period, go ahead and have sex, but be sure to use a lubricant. If everything is fine, estrogen can then be tapered to every other night for the next couple of weeks. If intercourse is still comfortable, feel free to use estrogen only every third night. Every woman has a different minimum maintenance dose to ensure adequate vaginal lubrication. Some women require the use of vaginal estrogen three times a week; for others, once a week does it. Don't underestimate the importance of having intercourse on a regular basis once vaginal elasticity is restored. "Use it or lose it" is one of those phrases that is actually true. If no ready or able partner is available, a toy is a good substitute, both for your own pleasure and to keep things alive until a priapic prince comes along (see chapter 25).

LIBIDO

Libido is complex and while the loss of libido at the time of menopause may be directly from the shift in hormones, other factors frequently contribute as well. It's no surprise that if sex is uncomfortable, you won't want it and you won't think about it. Sometimes solving the lubrication problem is a major aid to enhancement of libido. Frequently, however, even if lubrication isn't an issue, sexual desire is diminished.

As was discussed in chapter 20, androgens (particularly testosterone) are integral to a healthy sexual response and many women benefit from testosterone supplementation after menopause. Testosterone is available in pill, cream, and lozenge form and has minimal side effects other than increased hair growth and acne in a small number of women. While testosterone is an essential ingredient to a healthy libido, it works in conjunction with estrogen as opposed to on its own, so taking testosterone without estrogen is rarely a solution. In addition, testosterone is metabolized to estrogen, so if someone is trying to avoid estrogen, testosterone is not the answer.

What about other libido-boosting drugs? While men have Viagra to improve sexuality, there are currently no FDA-approved drugs to increase libido in women. That should change shortly since pharmaceutical companies have finally realized that women want, and will pay for, medications to help with sexual response. There are a number of products under investigation that should be available soon.

INSOMNIA

For the woman with insomnia, a good night's sleep is a clear priority over the issue of libido or vaginal dryness. If hot flashes are the reason for insomnia, it makes sense to eliminate flashes using one of the alternatives previously discussed. In addition, alcohol, cigarettes, and caffeine all can disturb sleep and should be avoided.

If all else fails, many women turn to short-term sleeping aids. A number of prescription hypnotics are available, but should be used sparingly. Some women turn to over-the-counter antihistamines. They do work, but may result in grogginess the next day.

DEPRESSION

There are many antidepressants on the market, and popping some Prozac is a tempting quick fix. It is widely recognized that depression can be caused by chemical and hormonal factors, in addition to issues going on in your life, and sometimes an antidepressant is the correct approach. Keep in mind, however, that despite direct marketing to the consumer, the treatment of depression can be complex and is often best left to an expert. Your gynecologist is not necessarily the best person to treat your depression, but can refer you to a therapist or psychiatrist who is familiar with the available medications and can address contributing factors.

OSTEOPOROSIS

Each year, 1.3 million women suffer fractures as a result of osteoporosis. Thirty percent of women hospitalized for treatment of a hip fracture die. By age eighty, 50 percent of women have osteoporosis and are at significant risk of fracture if they fall. It's not just about bad posture.

Risk factors for osteoporosis include:

▼ Smoking
▼ Caffeine
▼ Fair skin
▼ Inflammatory bowel disease
▼ Low body weight
▼ Alcohol use
▼ Early menopause
▼ Sedentary lifestyle
▼ Family history
▼ Use of certain medications (diuretics, lithium, synthroid)

Fortunately, there are a lot of options other than estrogen available for prevention and treatment of osteoporosis. A calcium intake of 1,400 mg/day is known to be protective, and is best taken in divided doses. Vitamin D (400 IU daily) is an important adjunct as well. Twenty minutes of weight-bearing exercise a day increases bone mass.

There are three nonhormonal types of drugs available to build bone and decrease the risk of fracture: bisphosphanates, selective estrogen receptor modulators (SERM), and calcitonin.

Bisphosphanates

Two bisphosphanates (nonhormonal drugs) are currently available: alendronate (Fosamax) and risedronate (Actonel). Both reduce fracture rates significantly, are taken once a week, and are associated with gastrointestinal problems in a small percentage of women. Bisphosphonates are well-tolerated but are somewhat a nuisance to take. The pill must be swallowed first thing in the morning and then, for the next thirty minutes, not only must you not eat or drink anything, but you can't lie back down. Waiting half an hour for your coffee once a week is a small price to pay for strong bones.

Selective Estrogen Receptor Modulators (SERM)

Raloxifene (Evista) is not the only SERM, but is the best-known drug in this category. While raloxifene is not as effective as estrogen or the bisphosphanates in reducing fracture risk, it is effective in preventing osteoporosis. Many women are prescribed raloxifene as a safe estrogen substitute, but are not informed that there are no benefits beyond reducing risk of osteoporosis and fracture. It is important to know that raloxifene can increase hot flashes. It can also cause leg cramps and increase the risk of forming blood clots. The good news is that there is no stimulation of uterine tissue (as is seen in its cousin, tamoxifen, a drug commonly used to treat or prevent breast cancer) and there is the possibility that it may reduce the risk of breast cancer.

Calcitonin

Calcitonin, another nonhormonal alternative for treating osteoporosis, is a nasal spray generally used in women who are unable to tolerate bisphosphonates or SERM. It is the least effective of the three, but definitely reduces fracture risk enough to make it a worthwhile option. It also is helpful in reducing pain from fractures. Many women discontinue calcitonin because of nasal dryness or swelling of their nasal membranes.

DON'T BE AFRAID TO BE A CLOSET ESTROGEN USER

If you choose not to replace or extend estrogen, it's important to be aware of the changes that may occur as a result of lack of estrogen and the alternatives available to address them. Women's current life expectancy is well into the eighties, and since roughly one third of your life involves the part after you no longer make estrogen, the choice you make will have an impact on a significant portion of your life. Having said that, don't make yourself crazy about this decision. If you start, you can stop. If you choose not to start, you can change your mind later. It's not surgery.

Many women have weighed the pros and cons of estrogen replacement and have come to the realization that they have minimal symptoms, are fine with alternatives, or are willing to put up with whatever menopausal symptoms they might have. Other women come to the realization that they are much happier, feel better, and prefer to take estrogen, accepting that there may be a small or unknown risk.

The problem is peer pressure. Wherever you turn, whichever friend you confide in seems horrified at the risk you are taking, even if they know nothing about your particular circumstances. It's always interesting how the friend who chides you for your risky behavior may be taking herbs for which there is no available safety or efficacy information. She may even have a few truly high-risk habits of her own. It's not unusual that the friend who says you are putting yourself at risk for heart disease and that's why she stopped her estrogen, is also the friend who smokes, is fifty pounds overweight, and hasn't exercised in weeks.

If you don't feel like defending yourself, don't bother. This is between you and your doctor, and you do not need to justify to the immediate world your decision to do what you realize is right for you. Let it be your secret and keep your friends guessing why you sleep great, have a phenomenal sex life, and have a little smile all the time . . . let them think it's the black cohosh and soy.

Chapter 25

Sex After Hysterectomy

In a perfect world, every woman has a partner in her life who enables her to have earth-shattering orgasms, intimacy, and amazing sex on a regular basis. He also cooks, gives massages, and makes the bed. If that is the case in your home, things will most likely be exactly the same after your surgery since the most important thing that determines what sex after hysterectomy is like, is what sex before hysterectomy was like.

Virtually every woman expresses concerns, if not to her doctor, to her partner, or even herself about how hysterectomy will affect her sexual function, desire, and desirability. Unfortunately, studies have shown that only half of gynecologists initiate a discussion of sex and few patients (about 13 percent) are willing to bring it up themselves. That means a lot of women who worry about their postoperative sexuality do just that, worry.

Recent studies show that in the absence of oophorectomy, there are no significant adverse effects of hysterectomy on sexual function. However, many women report changes in sexual response after surgery. A lot of speculation exists concerning the loss of the cervix and its effect on the quality of orgasm, but again, there are little data to support this theory (see chapter 19).

A 1999 study published in *The New England Journal of Medicine* tracked over one thousand women during the two years after their surgeries and, unlike many earlier studies, evaluated sexual function both before and after hysterectomy. The results of the study were reassuring and validated what most gynecologists (but not most pre-op patients) knew all along. Seventy-seven percent of the women in the postoperative group were sexually active one year after surgery, in contrast to only seventy-one percent of the group the year before. This finding is not surprising, given that the study also demonstrated that the number of women who experienced pain during sex decreased from 19 percent to 4 percent. The quality and number of orgasms increased, as did overall libido. The bottom line is that frequency of sexual activity consistently increased and sexual dysfunction decreased.

Women who become menopausal as a result of surgery have an additional set of issues to deal with. If estrogen supplementation is not initiated, it is likely that mood disturbance, vaginal dryness, and a much higher risk of sexual dysfunction overall will ensue. There is no question that estrogen and androgen supplementation will absolutely increase libido, lubrication, and sexual response. Some women are fine without it, but for many women, the loss of hormones is a major blow to sexuality. These issues are further explored in chapters 24 and 25.

For the sake of discussion, let's assume that while your sex life may not have been like Madonna's, it was pretty good. Since you've now had a hysterectomy, you want it to be just as good, if not better. So what can you expect and, more important, what can you do if things are not going well?

What's Better?

Contraception is no longer an issue. There is no need to avoid sex because of bleeding or fear of bleeding, not to mention pain from endometriosis or discomfort from uterine prolapse. In short, women who had pain with intercourse because of a gynecologic problem invariably find that eliminating the cause of the pain allows intercourse to become pleasurable again. In addition, you no longer need to avoid every intimate touch or sexual overture out of fear that it might lead up to an expectation of (painful) intercourse.

RISKS OF SEXUALLY TRANSMITTED DISEASES

A lot of women think that once the uterus is gone, you can throw out the condoms as well. It is true that you can no longer get pregnant. Unfortunately, you are still vulnerable to any sexually transmitted disease (STD) transmitted to vulvar or vaginal tissues. That list includes, but is not limited to, human papilloma virus (genital warts), herpes, syphilis, HIV chancroid, and molluscum contagiosum. Gonorrhea and chlamydia like to live in the cervix, so if you still have yours, you are at risk for those infections as well. The consequences aren't the same, since there are no uterus or tubes to travel through, decreasing the possibility of a fulminent pelvic infection. Also keep in mind that gonorrhea, herpes, and (rarely) HIV can be transmitted orally, so if you are not in a monogamous relationship, you still need to be careful.

THE FIRST TIME

Not *the* first time, just the first time after surgery. If there are no postoperative complications, most women are told to abstain from intercourse until five to six weeks after surgery. Why the wait?

If your cervix was removed, the back of your vagina was sewn shut by a row of dissolvable stitches. If you have intercourse the day after surgery, the back of the vagina could actually be torn open, with catastrophic results. By week four or five, healing is almost complete, but intercourse at that time could still potentially cause some damage to healing tissues. There is also still a risk of potential infection, pain, and, very likely, bleeding. By six weeks, your gynecologist has checked the back of the vagina to ensure that the area is completely healed, strong, and free from infection. Intercourse before that exam should really be avoided.

If your cervix was not removed, there are no stitches in the back of the vagina. The concern is that the thrusting involved with intercourse could disrupt healing tissue in the pelvis and create damage or internal bleeding. The truth is that intercourse could probably be initiated a little sooner when the cervix is left in place, but most women are unwilling to be the first on their block to try it.

Fear of Flying

Once the six weeks is up and you have had your final check-up, most doctors give the go-ahead. The biggest hurdle to overcome is fear. Many women are understandably nervous about having intercourse, thinking that it might create a problem or that they will experience pain. Partners are also sometimes leery, which hardly makes for a wild sexual experience. If your doctor has given you the okay, it really will be fine, but you won't believe that until you try. Unfortunately, fear usually results in paucity of response that leads to. . .

Total Lack of Lubrication

Even if you never needed a lubricant before, this is a good time to have one available since it is likely that your natural lubrication will be diminished. In addition, if your ovaries were removed, you are even more likely to experience vaginal dryness. Better to be prepared and have things too slippery than dry and uncomfortable. Always use a water-soluble lubricant meant for vaginal use (see chapter 24 for more information about lubricants).

What If Surgery Included Work on the Vagina?

Women who have had a perineoplasty (reconstruction of the opening to the vagina) or labioplasty (plastic surgery of the labia), often need a little extra healing time before anything is put in the vagina. This is a group that should definitely wait until they get the go-ahead from their surgeon before they try anything. If you have sex too soon you can tear the area that has been stitched on the outside of the vagina, and, yes, it will be painful.

Once you do get the go-ahead, be gentle. Lubricate the outside of the vagina and take it slow. It's helpful if the woman is on top so she can control penetration and pull back if things are uncomfortable. It is normal for things to feel a little tight, but there shouldn't be any pain.

I'm Bleeding!

Don't panic. Spotting after intercourse is no cause for alarm. Sometimes there is an area in the back of the vagina that is a little raw and the contact creates spotting. If there is no pain, the spotting is minimal, and it disappears within a day, refrain from intercourse for an additional week, then try again. If the spotting still occurs, make an appointment to have the back of the vagina checked. Sometimes there is an area of granulation (early scar) tissue that is causing the problem. A dab of medication from your gynecologist is all that is needed to make it go away.

If the bleeding is more than spotting, but not as heavy as a period, it would be prudent to have the back of your vagina checked before you try again since there is probably an area that has not quite healed. This can wait until the next day.

If your bleeding is heavy (like a period), bright red, and/or accompanied by pain, you need medical attention as soon as possible, even if it means a visit to the emergency department. There may be a bleeding blood vessel and it is likely to continue bleeding unless something is done to stop it. This is extremely rare, especially if you've already seen your doctor and gotten the go-ahead.

Incision Pain

Women who have had an abdominal hysterectomy also have incision soreness and healing to contend with, especially if the incision was made down the middle of your belly as opposed to along the bikini line.

By six weeks after surgery, an abdominal incision is usually well healed, but sometimes there are some tender areas that can be uncomfortable if there is any pressure. Using a position where the woman is on top, or on her side, usually alleviates that problem. An L-shaped position with bodies at 90 degrees, legs interlocking, and the man's leg lowest on the bed frees both the man and women from bearing weight or putting pressure on an abdominal incision. It also helps to place a thin pillow between the two of you to protect and cushion your belly.

Is It Really No Sex for Six Weeks?

When your doctor says "no sex for six weeks," what he or she really means is "no intercourse" for six weeks. It's actually a misnomer since sex is not synonymous with intercourse. There are no restrictions on kissing, hugging, fondling, or stimulation of external genitalia. Never underestimate the value of foreplay. High school is not the only time that caressing and other erotic play are satisfying without being simply a prelude to intercourse as the grand finale. Couples often find that eliminating the goal of intercourse from a sexual repertoire actually results in greater intimacy and ability to explore new options.

Oral sex is perfectly fine after hysterectomy with a couple of caveats. If you have had any reconstructive vaginal surgery, such as perineoplasty or labioplasty, oral sex and any vaginal stimulation should be avoided. This does not seem to present a major problem since most woman are not particularly interested in oral sex while those tissues are healing.

After a few weeks, orgasms are fine. The restrictions are in how those orgasms are initiated. If nothing goes in the vagina, it's usually not a problem. For all we know, the increased blood flow to the genital region during orgasm enhances healing. That study has never been done . . . or at least, never published.

Sex Toys

There are women who have never entered the wonderful world of sex toys. Sex toys are not for lonely deviants; they are . . . well, for you. Vibrators, dildos, and erotica are a world that may open up at the time after surgery when you realize that intercourse is temporarily not possible or desired.

Why is this important after hysterectomy? First of all, after hysterectomy is a time to rediscover and re-explore your sexuality. The elimination of painful, heavy periods and painful intercourse allows you to move ahead to a new chapter in your life when pregnancy is no longer an issue and your body is something that can give you pleasure. In short, this is the time to have a sexual reawakening.

Sex toys fall into two basic categories: those that are inserted in the vagina (and sometimes rectum) and those that are used for external stimulation. They come in multiple lengths, diameters, materials, and colors. There are vibrating and nonvibrating varieties. Sex toys can be used alone or with your partner. It's all a matter of preference. They're not for everybody, but it is worth considering if you haven't before.

Toys to be inserted vaginally or rectally should not be used until you have been given the go-ahead for intercourse. At that point, even vibrating dildos are safe, unless you have been told otherwise. After about two weeks, there are no restrictions with external toys, such as vibrators used for clitoral stimulation, but as always, listen to your body and stop if there is any discomfort.

So where do you get these toys? No, you don't have to go to a questionable neighborhood wearing a disguise and dark glasses. Most major cities have perfectly respectable erotica stores intended for normal women to go and shop comfortably. In addition to toys, most of these stores have fabulous sexy underwear and great selections of erotic books and tapes. They also generally stock better lubricants than Walgreens. The staff is usually very happy to help and will go out of their way to make you comfortable. Go with your partner or a girlfriend. It's easier and more fun. You can always say you're buying a gift for "a friend."

If you don't live in a big city, or are on the shy side, there are some terrific Web sites where you can shop without wearing a disguise.

▼ G Boutique (Chicago, Illinois) www.boutiqueg.com
▼ Good Vibrations (San Francisco and Berkeley, California) www.goodvibes.com
▼ Toys in Babeland (New York, New York, and Seattle, Washington) www.babeland.com
▼ A Woman's Touch (Madison, Wisconsin)

▼ Grand Opening (West Hollywood, California, and Brookline, Massachusetts)

▼ Come as You Are (Toronto, Ontario, and Montreal, Quebec)

▼ Womyns' Ware (Vancouver, British Columbia)

▼ Eve's Garden (New York, New York)

▼ Drugstore.com

Problems

In spite of waiting the proper amount of time, using appropriate lubrication, and the glass (or two) of chardonnay, things don't always go well.

Dyspareunia

Dyspareunia is defined as painful intercourse. *Superficial dyspareunia* refers to pain on insertion. As the penis enters the vagina, tightness, dryness, or a tearing sensation essentially make your body scream STOP. *Deep dyspareunia* means that everything is fine at the beginning, but once he is inside you, any thrusting results in pain that can vary from discomfort to extreme agony.

Superficial dyspareunia after hysterectomy is usually caused by vaginal stitches that have not healed, vaginal dryness, or tightness from a vaginal opening that is too small. Dyspareunia can result in *vaginismus*, a condition in which the vaginal muscles contract so that intercourse is impossible.

If the pain is due to a vaginal repair that has not healed, you may simply need a little more time. Six weeks is a guideline, not an absolute, and some vaginas just need a little longer. Take a look and see what things look like. If there is a particular area that just doesn't look right, or is hard, red, irritated, or swollen, have your doctor take a look. If everything looks fine, give it another week or two, use some lubrication, and take it slow and easy.

If dryness is an issue, use lubrication automatically when you attempt intercourse as opposed to attempting intercourse without it and then only using it if you need it. Once pain starts, the vaginal muscles will clamp down and dry up beyond a lubricant's help. Slather the lubricant on you and your partner before you start. The worst that will happen is that it will be too slippery.

If lubrication still isn't adequate, consider vaginal estrogen as an adjunct (see chapter 24). Vaginal estrogen shouldn't be used as a lubricant when you are having intercourse, but as a supplement to lubricants. If you need estrogen, regular therapy will be necessary for at least a few weeks to build and soften tissue. Most women are then able to taper to a maintenance dose with use once or twice a week. A prescription is needed.

Vaginismus is more complicated. Vaginismus refers to a clamping down of vaginal muscles, making intercourse difficult if not impossible. It is rare to develop vaginismus after hysterectomy if it was not an issue before. This is a correctable problem that a therapist experienced in sexual dysfunction should address.

Deep internal pain during intercourse is generally not due to vaginal dryness. Generally, the pain is caused by the penis hitting something at the back of the vagina, or behind the vagina. There are a number of things that could create this problem, all generally solvable.

Infection at the back of the vagina or behind the vagina occurs rarely after hysterectomy, but can be a cause of discomfort during intercourse. Usually, a combination of antibiotics, time, and sometimes drainage of a pocket of pus (if there is an abscess) will solve the problem.

Occasionally, there is an adhesion (scar) in the back of the vagina where a band of tissue has formed around a healing area. You would have no way of knowing it's there until a finger or penis pushes on it, creating pain. The pain is usually sharp and occurs without warning. Your gynecologist can easily identify this condition and it is not difficult to take care of; sometimes, it can be done in the office.

If the problem is behind the vagina in the pelvis, things can be a little more complex. On occasion, adhesions form and cause structures such as ovaries, tubes, or loops of bowel to adhere to the back of the vagina. Scar tissue doesn't inevitably cause pain; in fact, a pelvic adhesion creating pain during intercourse is quite rare. When it does happen, it can be difficult to diagnose since scar tissue doesn't show up on pelvic exam, ultrasound, or other types of imaging tests.

Frequently, the only way to identify and resolve a pelvic-vaginal adhesion is with a laparoscopic procedure. While it is usually possible to remove the adhesion surgically, surgery is not always required to solve the problem. Not infrequently, over time and continued sexual activity (if you are able), the tissues soften up and the pain dissipates. Pelvic physical therapists are often able to work with tender trigger points from trapped nerves or adhesions to manipulate tissue and decrease inflammation.

Dry Despite Lubricants

Sometimes in spite of using a lubricant and estrogen, dryness is still an issue. This may be due to a major fear factor creating the lack of physical response. Your vagina is not stupid—if it anticipates pain, it responds by drying up in order to prevent anything from going in it. This can sometimes be a tough cycle to break; usually it is associated with a libido that is essentially nonexistent.

Loss of Libido

Libido is complex, affected not only by hormonal status, but also by psychological, physical, and relationship factors. Add the fear of pain during intercourse and you have a no-win situation. It doesn't help that it's been so long since you have felt sexual that part of your brain has shut down as well. You need to stimulate your mind as well as your body. You need to wake up the part of your brain that has been hibernating, and it's not going to happen automatically.

Women who have issues with libido need to make a conscious decision that they want to make things better and are willing to put the time and effort into doing so. If things were fine before surgery, it may be as simple as taking estrogen and possibly testosterone supplementation. For the woman who had libido issues long before her surgery, it probably won't be a quick fix.

Dr. Laura Berman, author of *For Women Only: A Revolutionary Guide to Overcoming Sexual Dysfunction and Reclaiming Your Sex Life* and an Associate Clinical Professor at Northwestern Medical School in Chicago, feels that it is also important to consider the impact of relationship health on libido. Many couples are struggling not only with the emotional stress of hysterectomy, but perhaps with cancer as well. Some couples come closer together; others drift apart as part of a defensive maneuver. For all couples, the partner's support, their level of communication, and how able she is to communicate her sexual needs are all central to a woman's sexual recovery and libido. If her partner is not responsive to her sexual needs and requests, or their communication is lacking in this area, she will avoid sex as a result, or at the very least won't enjoy it as much.

WHAT ABOUT ANDROGENS, VIAGRA, AND OTHER PHARMACEUTICALS?

If your ovaries were removed and things were fine before surgery, but now you feel like the libido light was switched off, this may be a result of testosterone deficiency. A testosterone supplement might restore things to how they were before (see chapter 20).

Pharmaceutical companies, being the profit-motivated entities that they are, are finally recognizing that there is *a lot* of money to be made in female sexual dysfunction. While Viagra is not currently approved for women, there are preliminary data that suggest that the increased blood flow to the genital area may increase female sexual responsiveness and orgasmic ability. More important, there is a tremendous amount of research and development in this area and new drugs to increase orgasmic potential and libido should be available in the not-too-distant future.

Tight Introitus

There *is* such a thing as a vagina that is too tight following reconstructive surgery. Obviously, during a surgical repair of a gaping or scarred vagina, the surgeon has to make a judgment call as to the appropriate size to make the opening. Fortunately, vaginal tissues are elastic and will accommodate pretty much any size penis. Sometimes, though, even with lubrication, intercourse after repair is impossible since the vaginal opening may be on the small side and the tissues won't stretch. This is definitely fixable, but will take a little effort on your part.

When dealing with tight, inelastic vaginal tissues, you are best off temporarily avoiding an actual penis. Dilators in various sizes are a great way to gradually get your vagina accustomed to having something in it and to gently stretch the area. Medical dilators in graduated sizes can be ordered through your physician, but are expensive and not always readily available. You are actually better off going the sex toy route and starting with a small, slender vibrator or dildo, and gradually working your way up. Pelvic physical therapists are also helpful in helping stretch tight, inelastic tissue.

Using lubrication, gently slide the vibrator in and let it sit as your vaginal tissues relax around it. When you are at the point that a particular size slides in without discomfort, it is time to go up to the next size. Don't force and don't rush it. Sometimes it takes a few weeks of inserting one size on a daily basis until you are ready to trade up. If things are not going well, vaginal estrogen cream will help increase the elasticity of the tissue.

Sometimes an attempt at intercourse will result in a crack or tear in the skin at the opening of the vagina. This is really painful if there is another attempt at intercourse before the skin has fully healed. The best thing to do is put a dab of 1-percent hydrocortisone cream on the area once or twice a day until the fissure is gone. While the hydrocortisone cream will help the tear go away, it can also make the tissue thin and vulnerable to future tears. Use it as long as you need it and then switch to estrogen cream to thicken and strengthen the tissue. Only then should you attempt intercourse again.

"It Just Isn't the Same"

Some women have no issue with pain or decreased libido after surgery, but report that things seem different, their orgasms less intense. Most women have orgasms that are clitoral and vaginal in nature, but some women are aware of uterine contractions when they climax. If the uterus is gone, that aspect of their orgasm will also disappear. Few women report this phenomenon, and the ones who do often anticipate the change since they were aware of it before surgery. So it is possible that at least for a few women, things will be different.

Severe sexual dysfunction issues after hysterectomy are rarely the result of a change in hormonal or anatomic factors, but were present before. Hysterectomy can bring long-standing psychological issues to the surface and they may manifest through depression and/or a loss of libido and sexual responsiveness. This is particularly true if there are issues on the part of the partner, or if there is no partner. It's also difficult to know which changes are directly related to surgery and which changes are related to changes in response and desire, which are sometimes a natural part of aging or menopause. This is a complex, harder problem to solve. A therapist or psychiatrist experienced in sexual dysfunction issues should be consulted if this is the case.

Special Circumstances

Lesbian Health

There are no problems exclusive to lesbian women following hysterectomy. Oral and digital stimulation are perfectly safe after a few weeks. The only caution is in the use of sex toys that are inserted into the vagina. Nothing should be inserted deep into the vagina until the final postoperative exam, unless the surgeon has approved. This is particularly the case if the cervix was removed and there are stitches in the back of the vagina.

Cancer

Women who are treated for cancer have additional issues beyond those related to their surgery. Depression and anxiety regarding their diagnosis can have a major impact on sexuality. In addition, the extreme fatigue, nausea, and hair loss chemotherapy causes do not exactly enhance one's sexuality or sense of well-being.

Women who undergo radiation therapy for treatment of cancer often have severe problems with loss of vaginal elasticity, dryness, and irritation. A program involving estrogen cream, lubricants, and dilators can reverse the effects, but may take time.

Some cancer operations, unlike hysterectomy for benign problems, require removal of the upper portion of the vagina. This can result in a noticeable shortening of the vagina, as opposed to a narrowing of the opening.

Shortened vaginas are not seen exclusively in women who undergo hysterectomy for treatment of cancer, although are the most likely group in which this condition occurs. Even during hysterectomy for benign disease, the vagina on occasion can become shortened, particularly if extensive repair was done for pelvic relaxation issues. The good news is that vaginal tissues are amazingly elastic since they are intended to accommodate a nine-pound baby, if need be. Certainly the average penis shouldn't present a problem. You may just need to exercise the tissue to get it to accommodate . . . whatever.

Graduated dilators or dildos are useful once again, this time with attention paid to length rather than diameter. It's important to not force things, but to use gentle pressure. Over time, the vagina will expand in order to allow comfortable insertion. When first initiating intercourse, it's usually better for the woman to be on top so she can control depth of penetration.

WHAT ABOUT THE MEN?

What about the other person involved in issues of sex and sexuality? Lest we forget, the man in your life (or the lack of a man in your life) obviously has an impact on sexuality after hysterectomy.

The male response to a partner's hysterectomy has been essentially ignored. During the last ten years, a few studies have been published looking at men's view of hysterectomy, but most are limited in their scope and involve very small numbers. For some reason, almost all have been published in Sweden, where there is apparently greater interest in male sexuality after hysterectomy.

One recent study demonstrated that most men are not particularly concerned about their own sex life changing after their wife's surgery. Men *are* concerned about potential complications or a possible diagnosis of cancer in their partner.

This lack of concern about a negative impact on sexuality is appropriate since the best predictor of postoperative sexuality for *both* men and women has consistently been found to be preoperative sexuality. The majority of men in these studies consistently express that their partner's surgery had a positive effect on their overall quality of life and sexuality. The experiences relayed by husbands of women who have had hysterectomies confirms this (see chapter 27).

One difference between men and women is that while men think they understand what is involved in the surgery, many actually have minimal comprehension as to what surgery entails compared with women. Never assume that guys understand female anatomy and know exactly what a hysterectomy is and what will be removed. There are a surprising number of men who think that hysterectomy also includes a part of the vagina, explaining their subsequent fear of intercourse and avoidance of intimacy. Education and reassurance are critical before initiating sexual activity.

While not common, there are cultures where men look at women who have had a hysterectomy as being less sexual, less womanly. Women in those cultures are understandably reluctant to have hysterectomies, even if they are suffering from pain or heavy bleeding, since they know a hysterectomy may result in the loss of a relationship or have a negative impact on their marriage.

In general, men are more concerned about the health and well-being of the women in their lives than the impact it may have on their own sexuality. Most partner issues after hysterectomy were there long before surgery and have nothing to do with any physical change in you. If you didn't tell him about your operation, he would not even perceive a difference.

Chapter 26

Pregnancy After Hysterectomy

U sing donor sperm or a donor egg to become pregnant is a concept that most people are familiar with. What the woman who has had a hysterectomy needs is a donor uterus. Advances in assisted reproductive technology have provided a way for women without a uterus to "borrow" someone else's, otherwise known as surrogacy.

In all fairness, this is not a new concept. Sarah, the wife of Abraham, gets credit as the first known woman to avail herself of a surrogate. When unable to bear a child at the somewhat advanced maternal age of ninety, she graciously provided her husband with her maid, Hagar, to bear a child for her (Genesis 16: 1–4).

For some women, the removal of their uterus is a devastating end to their dream of having a child. For the young woman with cancer who has no children, the woman with one child who ends up with a post-partum emergency hysterectomy, the forty-two-year-old with severe endometriosis who has dealt with years of infertility, or the thirty-nine-year-old who just hasn't met the right guy, hysterectomy represents the most final of closures to the possibility of pregnancy.

Adoption used to be the only option for women who desired children but had undergone a hysterectomy. For many women who have not started or completed their families, that is still an acceptable plan. For other women, advances in assisted reproductive techniques, along with a major shift in societal attitudes, have provided new, viable alternatives.

One of life's absolute certainties used to be that a pregnant woman was the mother of the baby she carried. No longer can one assume that to be the case, due to advanced reproductive techniques. Is the mother the woman who supplies the egg, the woman who carries the pregnancy and births the baby, or the woman who ultimately loves, nurtures, and cares for a child? As any adoptive parent can tell you, a biologic connection is not necessary to have an intense maternal bond.

Modern attitudes have accepted and embraced the concept that there are many ways to be a mother and many ways to have a family. While adoption is an option that all women unable to have biologic children should explore, some women desire an alternative in which her and/or her husband's genetic makeup is involved.

SURROGACY

In vitro fertilization (IVF) has been available since 1978. In IVF, an egg is fertilized with sperm outside a woman's body and the developing embryo is transferred into the waiting uterus. This technology has made many advanced reproductive techniques, such as surrogacy, a reality.

There are three types of surrogacy:

▼ **Traditional surrogacy** is when a woman other than the intended parent is artificially inseminated with the sperm of the intended father. The surrogate mother's own egg is used so that biologically, the baby is a result of the intended father and the birth mother. In other words, the traditional surrogate donates both her egg and her uterus. Immediately after birth, the intended mother adopts the baby and the surrogate relinquishes her parental rights. Traditional surrogacy is rarely done due to legal obstacles.

▼ **Gestational surrogacy** is when the surrogate mother carries an embryo resulting from an IVF pregnancy from the egg and sperm of the intended parents. The surrogate mother has no genetic tie to the baby, but serves as a hostess uterus. The surrogate in this case is often referred to as the "gestational carrier." The first gestational surrogacy procedure was reported in 1985 in a woman who had had a hysterectomy but still had functional ovaries. Today, it is the most commonly utilized form of surrogacy.

▼ **Donor egg/gestational surrogacy** is when a gestational carrier carries an embryo made from the egg of a third-party donor and the sperm of the intended father. This is done when the intended mother has poorly functioning ovaries or none at all. Again, the surrogate has no genetic tie to the baby but is simply a hostess.

Choices, Choices

If you choose surrogacy, there are multiple decisions you need to make. The source of the egg is the first issue. Most women prefer to use their own eggs, if possible. Two essential components are necessary to have that happen. First of all, you need to be willing to go through IVF. An IVF cycle means submitting your body to hormone injections to stimulate ovarian egg production, followed by intensive monitoring requiring multiple blood draws, ultrasounds, and finally egg retrieval. Second, for IVF to occur with your own eggs, you must have functional ovaries with eggs that are still capable of pregnancy.

If your ovaries were removed at the time of hysterectomy, or if your age precludes successful IVF, there is no choice but to use someone else's egg. It can be the surrogate's egg or a third-party donor's. It can be a known donor or an anonymous donor. The most important thing is it must be a young donor.

Step-by-Step Guide to Surrogate Gestational Carriers

If you use your own egg, hormone injections will be used to stimulate your ovaries to release more than the usual one or two eggs a month. The cysts that form on the ovaries at the time of ovulation are called follicles. Once ovulation induction begins, daily monitoring of blood levels and ultrasound are used to monitor progress. Once ovarian follicles have reached the appropriate size, the eggs are ready to be retrieved by inserting a needle through the vagina into the ovary. Multiple eggs are then aspirated from follicles. Ultrasonic guidance is used to guide the needle, and yes, some sort of anesthesia is also involved.

The eggs are immediately taken to an adjacent lab where they are placed alongside the sperm, allowing fertilization to occur. Ideally, at least ten to twelve eggs are harvested per cycle. Two or three days after conception, two to four normally developing embryos are transferred to the surrogate uterus. Since all those embryos are not used, "leftovers" can be frozen and used for subsequent cycles if the surrogate does not conceive. They can also be used for a sibling after a successful pregnancy. Frozen embryos do not have as high a success rate as fresh embryos, but the rates are reasonable enough that they are still worth saving for future use.

Who Is Not a Candidate to Use Her Own Eggs?

While hysterectomy is often seen as signaling the end of the childbearing years, the reality for many women is that even if their uterus had not been removed, they would be infertile. Until the 1970s, most women had children when they were in their twenties or early thirties. For a variety of reasons, it became common for women of the next generation to delay childbearing, with first attempts at pregnancy often occurring in a woman's late thirties or forties. Even though women are increasingly aware that fertility rates diminish rapidly after age thirty-five, there is still an unfortunate complacency about delaying childbirth, resulting in unprecedented rates of infertility.

The reality is that most babies born to women well over the age of forty result from IVF techniques using donor eggs from a young woman.

That's right. Most of those forty-something movie stars who delayed childbearing and then seemingly effortlessly conceived, bore, and delivered a child, are usually the recipients of advanced reproductive techniques utilizing IVF with the egg of a twenty-year-old donor.

So at what age is it no longer realistic to conceive with your own eggs? That depends.

AGE

Imagine a woman who is over forty years old with a perfectly normal uterus, normal ovaries, normal tubes, who is in great shape, and looks no older than thirty. What are her chances of conceiving spontaneously? What are her chances of conceiving with IVF? How many of those women will require a donor egg?

It is well known that increasing age impacts on fertility more than any other factor. While some women spontaneously conceive after the age of forty, fertility rates for most forty-year-olds are quite low. Follicle-stimulating hormone (FSH) levels are one indicator of fertility. FSH is a pituitary hormone that is an indicator of ovarian function. FSH levels are low in young women and rise with age. Long before someone stops producing estrogen and is officially menopausal, FSH levels fluctuate and rise slightly, and it is at that point that fertility is diminished. For some women, that occurs when they are thirty-seven years old. For others, conception is still possible at forty-five.

If someone is unable to conceive spontaneously (otherwise known as having intercourse at the appropriate time of the month and getting pregnant), what are the chances that they will be successful with advanced reproductive technology such as IVF?

Age alone is the most important variable that indicates the probability of success using assisted reproductive techniques. Studies consistently show that a forty-year-old with a low FSH has a smaller probability of a successful IVF pregnancy than a thirty-five-year-old with the same FSH level. In addition, almost *half* of pregnancies miscarry following embryo transfer in women over forty. The end result is that only 10 percent of women over the age of forty who use their own egg for an IVF cycle end up taking home a baby.

In other words, most pregnancies that occur after age forty are either spontaneous (not using fertility drugs) or utilize a donor egg. The first step in deciding if it is reasonable to use your own egg is to consult a fertility specialist to see how likely success will be. If you are given the disappointing news that your own eggs are no longer useful, keep in mind that that would have been the case if you had not had a hysterectomy.

Freezing Eggs

Many single women inquire about freezing eggs in order to increase the possibility of pregnancy with their own genetic material when their own eggs are no longer usable. While freezing embryos is very successful, cryopreservation of unfertilized eggs has a very poor success rate. While some pregnancies have resulted from frozen eggs, the salvage rate is low since few eggs are still viable after thawing.

Choosing a Surrogate Program

Before entrusting your eggs and the probability of conceiving to a surrogate program, be aware that all programs are not created equally. Success rates vary dramatically and not all IVF centers even offer gestational surrogacy programs. Your own gynecologist can usually recommend a program that has a good track record. Most university hospitals with a fellowship in reproductive endocrinology (fertility) have an IVF program. There are also agencies that can not only recommend a good program, but are also able to give legal and psychological support. RESOLVE (www.resolve.org), a nationwide network for infertile couples, is an excellent source for finding reliable programs. This is obviously a lucrative field and it is easy for vulnerable couples to be enticed by slick marketing and advertisements promising inflated success rates.

At a minimum, make sure that:

▼ The center is headed by a board-certified reproductive endocrinologist.

▼ Statistics are provided for success rates per cycle. Clinical pregnancy rates do not take miscarriage into account and are *not* the same thing as "take-home baby rates."

▼ When requesting statistics, specify that you would like to know rates for IVF procedures, egg donation, gestational surrogacy, and frozen embryo transfer rates.

▼ The laboratory is headed by an experienced andrologist/embryologist.

▼ Fee schedules are available.

In 1998, the United States Department of Health and Human Resources, the Centers for Disease Control, and RESOLVE conducted a study to track IVF success rates, defined as live births per retrieval cycle. They found that 20 percent of pregnancies ended in miscarriage and the chance of multiple birth was roughly 30 percent. Success rates diminished with egg age so that a forty-year-old woman using her own egg had only a 10 percent success rate. Donor eggs significantly increase take-home baby rates and are dependent on donor age.

If you decide to proceed with surrogacy, you will need to address many other issues that are beyond the scope of this book—from choosing a surrogate to potential medical complications. It is critical that you establish a relationship with a center that has a good track record and can be trusted.

LEGAL ISSUES

It is crucial that an attorney who is familiar with surrogacy law in your state is involved from the beginning. Legal issues regarding surrogacy are incredibly complex and touch on every possible contingency. The laws of the state in which the child will be born in the case of an out-of-town surrogate must also be considered. If the surrogate is married, maternity *and* paternity must be established and confirmed. There have been nightmare cases in which a surrogate has conceived spontaneously (with her own partner or husband) during an IVF cycle. There are issues regarding availability for implantation procedures, pregnancy, delivery, adoption, transfer of custody, confidentiality, compensation of medical expenses, legal expenses, lost wages, surrogate life insurance . . . the list goes on and on. Don't try and muddle through the legal issues without the guidance of someone who really knows what they are doing. It will be money well spent.

FINANCIAL MATTERS

The cost of surrogacy is high and goes well beyond the cost of medical care for the biologic mother. Multiple disciplines are involved and all must be compensated. IVF fees, embryology fees, surrogate screening, prenatal care, labor and delivery, and the gestational carrier's fee are standard. Legal costs, psychological evaluations, transportation for an out-of-state surrogate, and lost wages for the surrogate due to pregnancy complications also must be factored in and can be astronomical. A donor egg adds another few thousand dollars. Some couples think there is an advantage to buying a premium egg, sold on the Internet. It is much safer to go through a professional agency with well-screened surrogates and sound legal support. While insurance frequently covers many costs, unfortunately there is not equal access when it comes to advanced reproductive options.

INTO THE FUTURE?

We can transplant hearts, kidneys, livers, and corneas. Why not a uterus?

There has been little incentive for research dollars to go towards uterine transplantation. The majority of women who have a hysterectomy are well out of their childbearing years, so it is a relatively small group of women who would benefit. In addition, while someone cannot survive without kidneys, a heart, or a liver, a functional uterus is not essential to sustain life. Since the option of a gestational carrier does exist, the concept of "rent a uterus" essentially takes the place of transplanting a uterus.

Chapter 27

What I Have Learned from My Patients (and Their Husbands)

Who better than women who have had a hysterectomy to tell what it's really like? One of the first things I did when I decided to write this book was go to the group of people who would have this unique insight. I appreciate the fact that while I have taken care of hundreds of women who have had this surgery, I myself have not had that experience. I also realize that one woman's experience is not every woman's experience. It is through my patients that I gained information that can't be read in any medical journal or book. I am fortunate that insightful, articulate, and thoughtful women have entrusted me with their care. I am grateful that these women have taken the time to share their experiences so that others can benefit.

Women have always turned to other women, particularly in matters regarding menstruation, childbirth, or anything having to do with their reproductive organs. Unfortunately, when women try to turn to other women regarding hysterectomy, they may not have access to many women who have had surgery. When they turn to the Internet or books, it is sometimes hard to find the viewpoint of anyone other than the angry woman who is on a mission to keep other women from making the same mistake.

While some women certainly have had bad experiences and probably never should have had surgery in the first place, most women have found that their hysterectomies were empowering, liberating experiences. Having taken control of their bodies and chosen a way to get rid of the pain, bleeding, anemia, and sexual dysfunction, the majority of women who have had a hysterectomy say, when asked if they would do it again, "In a heartbeat!" It doesn't mean that it was always easy, pain-free, or devoid of complications. It doesn't mean that they don't have lots of thoughts and experiences to share with other women who are contemplating the same thing. It just means that, like most difficult decisions, if it was carefully thought out, the end result was positive.

I sent a questionnaire to women who had had hysterectomies and invited them to share their thoughts through a series of open-ended questions. I asked about sexuality, what they had wished someone had told them, and what they think others should know who are about to have a hysterectomy. The following are their words, essentially unedited. The negative experiences, the sadness, and the regret are included along with the good.

ON FEAR OF SURGERY

The woman who fears absolutely nothing about the surgical process may exist somewhere, but I have yet to have a patient who wasn't anxious about some aspect of the whole process. The trick in alleviating the fear is to identify the fear. For some women, it is fear of anesthesia; for others, it's fear of terrible pain. The fears that are the hardest to address are the fears of what things will be like long after surgery is over, for those are often nonspecific. Ultimately, it is fear that makes women endure medical conditions, since it is human nature to avoid what you believe to be worse than what you are currently experiencing.

Carla, 39 years old, had huge, bleeding, painful fibroids. She had a total abdominal hysterectomy (TAH) and bilateral salpingo-oophorectomy (BSO).

I had suffered with fibroid tumors for years because I feared having a hysterectomy. Finally, the symptoms were too difficult to continue to live with. I wish I had had my operation much earlier than I did. Women should research, read, and talk to others who have had the surgery. Also, get a second or third opinion until you are confident with the doctor and the surgery proposed. I had seen one doctor and been scared to death by my visit with her. The doctor who did my surgery explained all of the possible options for my condition, which the first doctor did not.

Lucille, 45 years old, suffered from fibroids, severe adenomyosis, and two failed hysteroscopic resections. She failed Lupron, married, and had one child, but failed multiple attempts at conceiving again. She originally was scheduled for a laparoscopic subtotal hysterectomy, but at the last minute decided to have a tummy tuck and switched to an abdominal subtotal hysterectomy.

It's amazing what women are willing to put up with to avoid surgery. My favorite hemmorhage story is when I was at work and it was after-hours. I was stuck on the phone with a complaining board member and I felt that warm feeling below, but I couldn't get up to go to the bathroom. When I did get up, I didn't have any supplies or anything where I was sitting but large manila envelopes, not very absorbent but you get the picture. I was also wearing khaki pants and I had to take them off and wash them because it looked like I just bludgeoned someone.

Phoebe, 47 years old, with fibroids, planned laparoscopic assisted vaginal hysterectomy (LAVH) and converted to abdominal TAH.

I was very anxious about the procedure since I live alone and feared being discharged before I was able to walk. As it turned out, I was able to get around by the time I went home from the hospital.

Betsy, a 48-year-old medical dietician with huge fibroids, delayed surgery for years despite severe anemia from almost constant heavy bleeding. She sought multiple opinions before finally proceeding with abdominal subtotal hysterectomy.

I did enough reading, research, and consultation with experts on my own to satisfy myself that hysterectomy was my only viable choice.

I would urge other women to do the same. Knowing all the available choices, risks, consequences, etc., doesn't make the decision any easier, but when the patient herself chooses and controls her destiny, it keeps her from feeling victimized.

Thalia, 41 years old and single, had large fibroids, and failed uterine artery embolization (UAE). She opted for subtotal hysterectomy.

I did a lot of online research and had read several testimonies from other women before my surgery regarding sexuality after a hysterectomy. I admit I was frightened that my sexuality would suffer. Being in my early forties, I am glad that I was able to have only a partial hysterectomy (uterus only) and have experienced no changes in one direction or the other regarding my sexuality. I am the same person I was before.

ON WHAT I WISH I HAD BEEN TOLD BEFORE SURGERY

Since all of my patients had had a lengthy preoperative discussion in which recovery, options, anesthesia, possible complications, and sexuality were discussed in detail, most felt that they had been well prepared and that there wasn't a whole lot they had not been informed about before surgery. This is obviously an atypical population of a group of women who had been given a lot of information.

Cindy, 45 years old, with bleeding and painful fibroids, had an abdominal subtotal hysterectomy.

All the negative press and women's books make you believe that a hysterectomy is not the right decision. More discussion about why there is so much negative press would be helpful and help women avoid some sleepless nights. I wish it had been easier to obtain supportive information on my decision.

Fern, a 46-year-old interior designer, had large fibroids and opted for a laparoscopic subtotal hysterectomy BSO.

I wish I had known how dramatic Lupron would be. I decided not to tell my kids (ages 11, 15, and 18) about my surgery until after a family ski trip. I didn't want them to worry about me during what was supposed to be relaxing family time. What a huge error in judgment! I was taking Lupron to reduce the fibroid size (which worked quite well); however, the effect on my mood was so intense that my kids spent the vacation wondering who came in their mother's place. I remember bursting into tears one morning after my son said he was too tired to ski with me. I was told, and expected, hot flashes and depression. I didn't expect that my children and husband would call me Attila the Hun behind my back and hide during my rages. When I told my kids about the Lupron and the hysterectomy after the trip, they were so relieved that there was a logical explanation for my behavior and that I was not seriously (or mentally) ill. It was all worth it to have a laparoscopic procedure, and of course, now I'm back to my usual charming self.

I'm still really angry at my old gynecologist. When I was told I needed a hysterectomy, I wasn't told that a laparoscopic procedure was even an option. I did my own research and found out that some doctors were doing them. When I called and asked if I could have one, I was told it was too dangerous and my fibroids were too large. I found out later that he didn't do laparoscopic hysterectomy and never recommended it.

Susan, 49 years old, with heavy bleeding from large fibroids and severe anemia, had TAH-BSO.

I'm sorry I waited so long for the surgery. I had endured ten years of terrible monthly pain, blood loss, and secondary anemia. I tried every alternative recommended to me by other gynecologists who thought that women should die with their uterus intact. Having a hysterectomy was not the end of the world or my femininity. I was losing between seven and ten days per month and my life revolved around my period. The surgery gave me back my life, and I wish I had been advised to do it from the beginning instead of being talked into trying alternatives.

Marilyn, 70 years old, with uterine prolapse, underwent total vaginal hysterectomy (TVH), BSO, and repair of cystocele and rectocele.

I wish I had known how much better I would feel. A prolapsed uterus is not pleasant.

Jan, 57 years old, with uterine cancer, had TAH, BSO, and lymph node dissection.

My hysterectomy was due to uterine cancer. It was caught early and chemotherapy was not necessary after the surgery, but radiation treatments were. I was told that the radiation would make my vagina sore for four to six weeks. In reality, there was discomfort for about four months after resuming intercourse. Had I known or been made aware that this could be the case, I would not have been as concerned when it occurred.

Thalia, 41 years old, had fibroids, failed UAE, and no children. She had a subtotal hysterectomy.

In my early twenties and thirties, if someone had taken the time to explain to me that an enlarged uterus and heavy bleeding could potentially indicate fibroid tumors, I certainly would have had further tests and perhaps taken less invasive steps to reduce the fibroids before having a hysterectomy. As it turns out, the information was given to me a bit too late to have many choices. I tried alternative treatments. Better information would have changed whether I had children or not.

Lana, a 44-year-old banker with fibroids, had a TAH-BSO.

I definitely did not feel at all myself due to the tremendous hormonal change. I did not start feeling good again until my dosage of estrogen was increased.

ON PAIN AND RECOVERY

There was a wide variation of experience reported. Pain and recovery depended on whether the surgery was done laparoscopically or with an incision. Many women reported feeling fatigued, but otherwise totally fine within two weeks. Then there was the woman who, at her annual visit (fifteen years after her hysterectomy), reported that she was "almost" better! "A piece of cake!" was the most common phrase that popped up on the responses.

Tracy, 42-year-old mother of a 1-year-old and a 3-year-old, had uterine prolapse and early cervical cancer. She underwent TVH and bladder repair.

Other women should know that their bodies will heal quickly but the surgery can be painful to recover from. Use the painkillers, rest a lot, and try to get back into exercising, walking, etc. Read or get as much information as possible before your surgery so you will know what to expect and then you won't be afraid of the unknown. Talking to people helps overcome the fear of having surgery.

Regina, 76 years old, with severe uterine prolapse, cystocele, and rectocele, had a TVH with repair of cystocele and rectocele.

The first night, I was not even able to get out of bed. Within a few weeks, I was able to get down on the floor and play with my five grand-kids and get right back off the floor without any help. Yes, they call me the teenage grandma.

Alice, a 52-year-old with recurrent cervical dysplasia, history of breast cancer, ovarian cyst, and elevated CA125 levels, had an LAVH and BSO. The ovarian cyst was found to be benign.

My first choice was laparoscopic surgery, which I was able to have. I was in and out of the hospital in twenty-seven hours. I went back to work in three days. I had *no* pain and just three little Band-Aids. This type of surgery is a blessing.

Sophia was 62 years old with vaginal prolapse, cystocele, and rectocele. She underwent TVH with repair of cystocele and rectocele.

I had a vaginal hysterectomy. No one told me that there would be *no pain* during recovery.

Scarlet, a 65-year-old woman with a double uterus and fibroids, came to Chicago from Las Vegas so that she could have a laparoscopic hysterectomy. She had a laparoscopic subtotal hysterectomy and BSO.

If you are not feeling good immediately, know that it is only a temporary thing. It only gets better. Be positive about the situation.

Erica was 46 years old with huge fibroids. She was married and had no children before her subtotal hysterectomy.

It was not as bad as other women described. I was up and walking right away! The whether was nice and I spent time outside. I spent the time planning a trip to Argentina and had my office staff bring home work to me. It is *so great* not to have a period. It's so much easier to travel and gives me more freedom.

Sara was 42 years old with a suspicious ovarian tumor, found to be benign. She had a subtotal hysterectomy and BSO.

The surgery itself was manageable. However, many younger women who are mothers of school-age children don't give themselves enough time to heal physically and jump right back into car-pooling and activity. If possible, allow yourself time to heal and don't expect so much of yourself. I tired easily.

Paula, 48 years old with heavy bleeding from fibroids, had a history of breast cancer. She was divorced, with one child, and had a subtotal hysterectomy and BSO.

I was told what to expect as far as recovery, but I didn't take that information to be "gospel." It was difficult for me to believe I would be as incapacitated as I was told I would be. In fact, I was. Women need to know that they need to be realistic and to give themselves ample time to recover. Even for someone in good shape, recovery is a gradual process. My recovery was six weeks to the day, exactly as I was told it would be.

Nancy, 56 years old with hyperplasia and endometriosis, had a TAH.

I have an extremely low pain tolerance. To begin with, I took a lot of Vicodan, but I didn't like the out-of-control feeling, so I used a large frozen gel pack meant for the back over the incision area the first night I was home. That was great, faster than Vicodan and with no side effects. The first couple of nights, I slept in a chair that tilted because it was easier to get up than it would have been from a bed while the incision was still painful.

Tonya, 46 years old, had fibroids, endometriosis, and a prior myomectomy. She underwent a subtotal hysterectomy and BSO.

The initial pain from the surgery and the weakness after is not as bad as you would think. The first few days, I couldn't believe how bad I felt. Then I got well so quickly, I was surprised. Each week, I felt ten times stronger than the week before. Since I had had a similar surgery five years before, I felt very prepared.

ON COMPLICATIONS

Jane, 52 years old, had a laparoscopic subtotal hysterectomy.

Shortly after I came home from the hospital, I had a bad bladder infection that added to my recovery time and caused additional pain. In addition, and probably more significant, my abdomen was very swollen and extremely black and blue. I was told this was very unusual and that my doctors had not seen that degree of postoperative discoloration before. While this eventually went away, I still have a slight swelling on the left side of my abdomen. Maybe it was unrealistic to think I would have a flatter abdomen after the hysterectomy than before, but I do not.

Sophia, 62 years old, had uterine prolapse, cystocele, and rectocele. She had a TVH with repair of cystocele and rectocele and needed a urethral sling procedure four months after hysterectomy to correct incontinence.

I was warned of possible relapse of some problems. In fact, the bladder problem became worse, resulting in more surgery four months later. Tissue failure also resulted in the partial return of a rectocele. Currently, I have no problem with incontinence.

Mona was 64 years old with fibroids, bladder cancer, and possible uterine cancer. She had an exploratory laparotomy and a TAH-BSO with lymph node dissection.

In addition to the hysterectomy, I was treated all year for bladder cancer, so I don't know what caused the continued problems with my recovery and changes in sexuality. I ended up with a bowel obstruction and had to return to the hospital, which was more difficult than the surgery itself. It was a long recovery. The positive part is that I don't have to worry about getting cancer in that part of my body.

Margo, 67 years old with large fibroids, had a TAH-BSO.

I wish I had been told that feeling numb at the incision forever was a possibility.

Marlene, 62 years old with huge fibroids, had TAH-BSO surgery complicated by a small tear in the bladder. This was repaired at the time of surgery, but required a catheter for two weeks.

Even though I had a complication with my bladder, it totally improved in two weeks and I felt just fine! Even though I had a complication, I'm glad I had the hysterectomy.

Rachel, 43 years old with severe endometriosis, fibroids, and multiple surgical procedures prior to hysterectomy, had a TAH-BSO.

In my case, scar tissue was still an issue for years after surgery, causing chronic pain and a small bowel obstruction. I'm sure this is due in part to the number of surgeries I had before my hysterectomy and my tendency towards bad scar tissue.

ASSOCIATED PROCEDURES

The majority of my patients who had plastic surgery at the time of their hysterectomy also had an abdominoplasty (tummy tuck). Many of them were good candidates for a laparoscopic procedure, but were so motivated to have the plastic procedure that they elected to have an abdominal hysterectomy instead. All conceded that their recovery was a little longer but definitely worth it.

Jan was 53 years old with recurrent carcinoma in situ of the cervix. She had a TAH-BSO and an abdominoplasty.

I had a tummy tuck performed at the same time as my other surgery. Although the recuperation may have been more difficult in the beginning, it was something very positive to keep focused on. After four pregnancies, including a twin pregnancy, it was a treat to myself to get rid of all that excess sagging skin. It really gave me something different to concentrate on rather than experiencing any feeling of loss. If a woman is in a position to have the tummy tuck at the same time, I would highly recommend it.

Liz, 41 years old with fibroids and a family history of ovarian cancer, had a LAVH-BSO.

I wish I had been told before my surgery that I could have had my abdominal mole removed during surgery. I would have given permission!

Susan, 55 years old with fibroids, ovarian cyst, and stress incontinence, underwent TAH-BSO, Burch urethropexy, and abdominoplasty.

Even though I had extra things done with the hysterectomy, it was "a piece of cake." Ten days later, I did a mile and a half walk! I was surprised how soon I recovered and could pretty much return to my normal activities. I would say it was no more than three weeks.

On Exercise

Most women reported that they were back to their normal exercise routine by eight weeks. Women who had laparoscopic procedures were back by four weeks.

Mona, 64 years old with bladder cancer and fibroids, had TAH, BSO, lymph node dissection.

I would like to have had instructions in how to get my body back in shape. The size and location of the incision were a surprise to me.

Sophia, 62 years old, had a TVH for prolapse.

I experienced about a ten-pound weight gain without any notable change in diet, which I assume is due to reduced exercise during recovery?

Cindy, 45 years old with fibroids and bleeding pain, had a sub-total hysterectomy complicated by severe adhesions.

I was exercising (low-impact aerobics) three to four weeks after surgery and already felt noticably better than before surgery. The fibroids had negatively affected my lung capacity. Being in good physical condition is important and helps in the recovery.

ON DEPRESSION, PSYCHOLOGICAL ISSUES, AND SADNESS

The majority of the women answered the question, "Was your hysterectomy psychologically more difficult than you expected?" with a simple and emphatic NO! without further explanation. Of course, many of the women had *a lot* to say. The women who seemed to have had the most difficult time after their hysterectomies were women who had never had children. This was the case even if they were well past childbearing age.

Grace, 61 years old, had a prolapse and underwent TVH, cystocele, and rectocele repair.

It wasn't really psychologically difficult. The one issue it brought forth was ackowledgment of the aging process. Prior to my own, hysterectomy meant "old lady" to me. I'm trying to fight that feeling now.

Sara, 42 years old, had an ovarian tumor, ultimately benign. She had a subtotal hysterectomy and BSO.

Actually, I was glad to be done with periods and problems. If I had not had my kids, I am sure it would have been more difficult as I had them at the high end of childbearing years and didn't give birth to my first child until I was 37 and had another at 38. I was very grateful to have them and did not miss my uterus.

Rachel, 43 years old with severe endometriosis and fibroids, had a TAH-BSO and immediate postsurgical hormone replacement.

My hysterectomy was not psychologically difficult at all. It was a relief in many ways. I was 42 and unmarried. Before my hysterectomy, the pressure was on to date only potential "father of my children" men. Now that there is no ticking clock, I can date whoever I want just for the fun of it, without the pressure of needing to have a baby soon. I found this to be very freeing.

Betsy, 48 years old with huge fibroids, had no children and was divorced. She had a subtotal hysterectomy and BSO.

There is something about the finality of a hysterectomy and the suddenness of the ensuing menopause that make it difficult, both physically and psychologically. Although I was 48 at the time of my hysterectomy, it was surprisingly difficult to lose the organ that could enable pregnancy. Being a divorced, childless woman, I feel my prime childbearing years slipped by without my making the choice *not* to have a child. Sins of omission cause the most regret. I don't really feel any loss of feminity due to my hysterectomy—just the loss of one of life's big experiences: motherhood.

Erica, 46 years old, had huge fibroids. She was married with no children and underwent a subtotal hysterectomy.

I did break down and cry occasionally. I realized there was little to no chance of having any children, but this confirmed it. I felt it represented a transition in my life to the next half.

Jane, 47 years old, had endometriosis, chronic pelvic pain, and severe adhesions. She underwent an LAVH-BSO.

My hysterectomy wasn't psychologically difficult for me. I felt relief and had more energy—I was more even. At first I felt sadness, perhaps because that part of my life was over. But I have two healthy children. I felt I was healthier so it was less difficult, not more. I felt free of the burden of monthly pain, suffering, mood swings, and fatigue. I could occupy my life with other things. The estrogen has made my moods more even and has helped the effects of menopause.

Kim, a 46-year-old with severe endometriosis, had an unexpected hysterectomy after her doctor discovered a large ovarian mass that was

inseparable from her uterus. She had a subtotal hysterectomy and BSO.

I did not expect the anger and loss I felt after the surgery. To be honest, at the beginning that anger and loss was directed at the hysterectomy and the fact that I did not expect it. Never having had a child meant a great loss to me, even though I was past childbearing years. It is hard to explain the sense of loss of opportunity and possibilities.

Francey, a 46-year-old with large fibroids, had a subtotal hysterectomy with BSO.

I wouldn't say it was psychologically difficult, but I wouldn't be true to my own feelings to say it didn't bother me. It's very bittersweet to have had my surgery in the same place I gave birth. Although I wasn't going to have more children, there is a mind game knowing you can't, especially when you are surrounded by babies and young happy couples. I'm empty, have no parts, and the only thing that makes me different from a man is a little pill.

Linda, 45 years old, was an adopted woman concerned about her lack of knowledge of her own family history. She had fibroids with rapid growth and bleeding and underwent a TVH-BSO.

It was psychologically uplifting. It was an excellent decision to have a vaginal hysterectomy. No pain, no real troublesome side effects, and I felt great afterwards. I do not have to deal with getting my period, PMS, etc. Plus, I don't have to worry about cancer in that area.

Thalia, a single 41-year-old, had fibroids and no children. She underwent a subtotal hysterectomy.

I thought I would be sentimental about not having my periods anymore. It has always been a part of my female experience since I was 11 years old. Although my periods were always heavy and messy, I thought they helped to define me as a woman. Since my hysterectomy, I have not missed them at all. It is a pleasure not to have to worry about cramps, not to buy sanitary products, and to never have to wonder if I will get my period during a beach vacation.

Jan, a 57-year-old with uterine cancer, had a TAH-BSO.

No, psychologically, it was not difficult. One interesting side effect, perhaps from the anesthesia or from age, was that the deeply relaxed state that I found myself in while recovering has lingered. I find myself, at a base emotional level, in a much calmer state than before my surgery.

Tracy, a 42-year-old mother of two, had a uterine prolapse one year after delivery and early cervical cancer. She underwent TVH and bladder repair.

The most difficult adjustment for me was when I went home from the hospital. I looked fine physically, but emotionally, I felt different, kind of detached. My ovaries are still intact so I go through the hormonal changes monthly. I don't have the cramps, but the PMS symptoms are sometimes intense. It has been seven years since my operation. I think about my surgery every day and realize how lucky I was to have had the vaginal hysterectomy that removed the cancerous cells in my cervix.

Sandy, 51 years old with uterine prolapse, had a TVH.

I never had any difficulties psychologically. I was so grateful that I came through the surgery. I am sure it helped that I was able to keep one of my ovaries and I received a low dose of estrogen.

Nancy, 56 years old with a precancerous uterine lining and endometriosis, had a TAH.

Since my uterus was never tied to my idea of being a woman, it wasn't difficult at all to give it up. Psychologically, I benefited far beyond my expectations. All my adult life, I had been plagued by PMS off the Richter scale. I used to describe it to my husband as feeling as though my blood was boiling through my veins and my skin was trying to split. I would warn him when I was PMS'ing, so he wouldn't feed into a fight that I might start. Within days after the hysterectomy, I felt as if my mind had opened and I felt normal for the first time in many, many years. That sense of well-being still stays with me now that I've gone through menopause. No HRT for me, thank you.

Eve, a 48-year-old with fibroids, had a subtotal hysterectomy with BSO.

My hysterectomy wasn't psychologically difficult at all—in fact, it was a relief. The burden of feeling so badly all the time and wondering if I might be making it all up disappeared because I was not pushed into surgery. I was totally ready, both mentally and physically.

Dana, 52 years old with huge fibroids, had a TAH-BSO.

In the beginning, I was a little depressed and I had some fatigue that I was not used to. With time, I felt much better. I did notice, however, that I have more sadness than I used to. I identify with TV or reading sad things and cry easier.

Coco, 51 years old with breast cancer, uterine prolapse, fibroids, and genetic risk of ovarian cancer, had a TAH-BSO and abdominoplasty.

Psychologically difficult? Not at all! I was very relieved not to have to worry about ongoing periods, anemia, and the feeling that having my ovaries and uterus was like sitting on a time bomb. It was one of the best things I ever did—both psychologically and physically. I have had no ill effects as a result and it has been ten years since my surgery.

Carla, 39 years old with no children and huge fibroids, had a TAH-BSO.

No, I was not depressed. In fact, I was so happy to be relieved of the pain and complications from the fibroid tumors, I felt I had been given a new start at life!

Naomi, 46 years old with bleeding fibroids and a longstanding history of depression requiring multiple antidepressants, had a laparoscopic subtotal hysterectomy.

I wish I had realized (considering my history of depression) that I might fall into a depression after surgery. I would warn other women who have a history of depression that they might get depressed. In my case, I fell into a depression about three days out of surgery and it lasted nine weeks! I believe it was the general anesthesia that set my brain chemistry awry, not the surgery itself. I'm fairly certain of this, since I had surgery without general anesthesia a year earlier and I had no trouble with depression at all.

Once the depression lifted I had no psychological difficulty at all. I don't feel any less a woman without a uterus and without periods. In all other ways, the surgery was a piece of cake. For me, it was the right decision.

Cindy, 45 years old with fibroids, had an abdominal subtotal hysterctomy.

The time before my hysterectomy was more psychologically difficult than I expected. I think you need to be emotionally ready before the surgery. This is not something that you can have second thoughts about.

On Sex

Without a doubt, the subject that resulted in the largest response was the topic of sex. Many women returned pages of typewritten commentary about their sex lives before and after surgery. Even women who responded to every other question with a yes or no answer had a lot to say on this subject. Fortunately, most of the comments were positive, but there certainly were women who felt there had been a negative change in their sexuality.

Monica, 45 years old with multiple fibroids, had a LAVH-BSO.

I'm much more comfortable, relaxed, and carefree, which leads to more spontaneous activity. I feel *more* feminine and sexy now, which my husband appreciates very much!

Betsy, 48 years old with huge fibroids, had a subtotal hysterectomy.

My mother assured me she detected no difference in sex before and after her hysterectomy, but who trusts her mother's views on sex? I was told that most orgasms were clitoral. Knowing my own physical sensations, I was fearful about the change I anticipated with the loss of my uterus. I was told that preserving my cervix would keep my nerves intact and might preserve sensation.

I'm certain that my best orgasms involved powerful rhythmic, uterine contractions, followed by waves of warmth that emanated from my lower abdomen to my limbs—a totally engaging and satisfying experience. Without a uterus, I am unable to reproduce these sensations. If I achieve some semblance of an orgasm, rare and difficult as it is these days, it is a shallow, dissatisfying experience, a true anticlimax.

In spite of these complaints, I would still have had the surgery as it was my only option to deal with unpredictable and unmanageable periods and anemia so low it hindered every aspect of my life.

Tonya, a single 46-year-old, had fibroids and endometriosis. She had a subtotal hysterectomy with BSO.

The orgasms don't seem to be as intense, but other than that, they're not much different. Also, even with taking estrogen, I find I occasionally need to use a lubricant.

Tracy, 42 years old, is married and has two children. She underwent TVH and bladder repair.

It took me time to get my sex drive back, maybe six months. I was and still am a little self-conscious, even though I have great sex now. It's also great not to have to worry about birth control issues.

Rachel, 42 years old, is single and has no children. She had severe endometriosis and fibroids, treated by TAH-BSO.

My sexual desire is not the same as before my surgery, and my sexual response is not as good. On the positive side, hysterectomy totally alleviated pain during intercourse, which obviously makes the whole experience more enjoyable.

Marcy, 46 years old, had a laparoscopic subtotal hysterectomy.

It has not affected my interest in sex. It's not quite seven weeks, but we are sexually active again and I find no difference in my level of desire or responsiveness.

Sophia, 62 years old with uterine prolapse, had a TVH with repair of rectocele and cystocele.

I'm not aware of any impact. I have continued using estrogen, which may have minimized any effect.

Nancy, 56 years old. Had uterine precancer, endometriosis, and a TAH.

My sexuality was absolutely affected. If women tell you that they have the best sex after a hysterectomy, then they must not have been having very good sex before it. Or perhaps I'm unique. I still can have an orgasm, but it's strictly clitoral, for obvious reasons, when previously, it was both clitoral and uterine. My orgasms were deep and long and now they're very surface by comparison. Worse is loss of drive. I have to go looking to see where I lost it.

Heather, 46 years old with four children and fibroids, had a subtotal hysterectomy with BSO.

Sex is no different, except now I can have sex more often. I was bleeding almost the entire month, which made intimacy difficult. My blood count was really low and I was drained. So the hysterectomy improved my health which, in turn, improved my sex life.

Grace, 61 years old, had prolapse, cystocele, rectocele, incontinence, and bleeding from uterine polyps. She had a TVH with repair of cystocele and rectocele.

Since I had been bleeding and had several D&Cs, my desire for intimacy was practically nil before the hysterectomy. Now I find the "old me" has returned and I am still interested in having a sexual relationship—the only problem now is finding a man of my age who is also interested—and can "rise" to the task!

Patty, 42 years old with twins delivered by cesarian section, had large symptomatic fibroids and was treated by LAVH.

It made life easier. With young twins, it was great not to have to think about birth control. My husband said I felt different inside to him at first, but he couldn't explain how.

Lill, 54 years old and married, had large fibroids, treated by TAH-BSO.

My diminished sexual appetite is aided by a combination of estrogen and testosterone. Sex is not painful. My libido is somewhat diminished.

Lori, 56 years old and single, has no children. Her fibroids were treated with LAVH-BSO.

My sexuality was not affected at all that I can tell—I still have a good sex life (at almost 65). Probably the fact that I've been on estrogen is part of this.

Francey, 46 years old, had large fibroids and was treated with a subtotal hysterectomy with BSO.

My desire has never been stronger. Unfortunately, my spouse is still the same middle-aged man. Perhaps someday, someone will invent a male hysterectomy patch. If a woman leaves the recovery room wearing a hormone patch, then we need to slap a kind of Viagra patch on the husbands. I guarantee the recovery time would be cut in half.

Dana, 52 years old with huge fibroids, had a TAH-BSO.

I did have some difficulty desiring sex with the realization that my body had changed. My husband and I have worked it out.

Julie, 54 years old with huge fibroids and heavy bleeding, had a subtotal hysterectomy with BSO.

It's hard for me to judge if it was the hysterectomy or general aging. I don't feel as sexual as in my younger years, but I truly feel it is the age thing most of the time.

Sara, 42 years old with an ovarian mass that was suspicious for cancer but found to be benign, had a subtotal hysterectomy with BSO.

I thought it would affect me more than it did. I never felt "less of a woman" or different. I don't think it was denial. Of course, I was started on estrogen immediately, so hormonally that was a plus. Before my surgery, my hormone levels were very low due to the type of ovarian tumor I had.

Amy, 47 years old with a family history of ovarian and breast cancer, had a laparoscopic subtotal hysterectomy with BSO.

Although I believe this varies from one woman to the next, uterine contractions during orgasm are obviously gone after your uterus is removed. Related to this, I highly recommend keeping your cervix if this is possible. Although it's been less than a year, I would like to note that sex is different, though equally good. In some ways, it was like having sex for the first time. You need to rediscover your body.

Carla, 39 years old with fibroids that caused pain and heavy bleeding, had a TAH.

My sexuality was improved. Before the surgery, sex was painful and I had a lack of interest. My fibroids had distended my abdomen to the size of a seven-month pregnancy. Afterward, sex was enjoyable, I had more energy throughout the day, and had more confidence.

Maureen, 46 years old with fibroids and a history of depression, had a laparoscopic subtotal hysterectomy.

I would say my sexuality is better than it was before the surgery. I am more orgasmic and more interested in sex!

ON NOT BELIEVING WHAT PEOPLE TELL YOU

Thalia, 41 years old, failed uterine artery embolization complicated by femoral artery aneurysm. She had a subtotal hysterectomy.

There always seems to be one person out there who, when she finds out you are about to have a hysterectomy, tells you that if it is not absolutely necessary, do not do it, because doctors are just eager to operate. It is not to say this has never happened in history, but I think that this is grossly untrue today and is an old fallacy. These busybodies can really scare women who are trying to make difficult decisions regarding their bodies. In my case, my surgery was not absolutely necessary, but it did alleviate a tremendous amount of discomfort and prevent future problems that could have been worse than what I was already experiencing. Nobody talked me into surgery. In the end, having the hysterectomy helped improve the quality of my life.

I would like women to know that not all hysterectomies are horrible surgical experiences. Because of my line of work as a hair colorist, I was able to speak with many women who had hysterectomies before me, and heard some pretty awful horror stories. It seems some women are competing for who had the worst experience and who was bedridden the longest. They really scared me. Also, if you go online, you will read some pretty frightening things. However, I was fortunate to have one dear friend who told me how smoothly her surgery went. She said it was not as painful as others had suggested and that she was able to stand up straight when she got out of bed the day after her operation. She said having a hysterectomy was one of the best things that had ever happened to her because it eliminated many of her physical problems. She returned to work not long after her operation. I used her as my role model, and attribute part of my quick recovery to the positive attitude she shared with me, and to having excellent medical care.

Nena, 49 years old with fibroids and constant pressure on her bladder, had a laparoscopic subtotal hysterectomy with BSO.

I didn't know laparoscopic hysterectomy was an option until I heard about it from a friend who had had one. I saw three doctors before I had my surgery and not one mentioned it as an option. When I asked about the possibility, I was told it was dangerous or that my fibroids were too big. When I finally found a doctor who would do it, I was told that I was an excellent candidate. I had a laparoscopic hysterectomy, I was home eight hours later, and two weeks after surgery, I felt like nothing had happened. *I'm so angry at those other doctors.* I almost had much bigger surgery than I needed. If they couldn't do the procedure, they should have at least told me that there were doctors who would do it. I shouldn't have had to find a doctor on my own. What about the women who don't know enough to ask?

Julie, 54 years old with huge fibroids, had a subtotal hysterectomy with BSO.

I had read about how "different" many women feel after a hysterectomy. I had three children and was not going to have more at age 55. I had fibroid tumors and was going through menopause. It was a relief to have the surgery. I had heavy bleeding for weeks at a time and multiple fibroids. I did feel "different," but only in a positive way!

Kathy, 52 years old, had mild uterine prolapse, fibroids, cysto-cele, and rectocele with years of heavy bleeding that continued even after menopause. She had a TVH, with cystocele and rectocele repair.

I had been told that endometrial ablation would solve my problem. Also, that the fibroids would disappear after I went through menopause. Neither was true for me. The hysterectomy solved my problems and I was very happy for that.

Judy, 47 years old with an ovarian cyst and heavy bleeding that caused severe anemia, had a laparoscopic subtotal hysterectomy with BSO.

You won't be any less of a woman, or an empty cavity, or any of those things they say. You will feel like a new person and be free from pain and bleeding. Unlike what I was told, everything is just fine. It hasn't affected my sexuality in a negative way at all.

WHAT THE MEN HAVE TO SAY

Throughout my research, it was striking to me how little had been written regarding men's experiences when the women in their lives, and generally their sexual partners, have a hysterectomy. A questionnaire was sent to the husbands of the women in the previous section to get their input into how their lives were affected and any changes they perceived in their wives. The results were very interesting.

Question # 1. Were you concerned prior to your wife's hysterectomy that sex would be different as a result of the surgery?

Only two men expressed any concern that the surgery would change their sex lives. Both of those men said afterwards that their sex life was the same, if not better. Women, on the other hand, were very concerned about possible impact on their sex lives.

Question #2. Did you discuss sexual concerns prior to surgery?

Since the men weren't concerned about sexual repercussions, it's not surprising that there were only a couple of men who said that it was even a topic of conversation before surgery.

Question #3. Do you feel that your sexual relationship has changed as a result of the surgery?

Twenty-five percent of the men said that it had changed for the better; the other 75 percent said it was essentially the same as before surgery. The one person who stated that intercourse occurred less often cited other relationship factors, not the hysterectomy, as the reason for the decline.

Question #4. Does your wife's vagina feel the same during intercourse?

Every single man who returned the questionnaire said that their wife's vagina felt exactly the same. The sample polled did not include anyone who had surgery for cancer, which sometimes results in a shortened vagina. There were, however, equal numbers of women who preserved their cervix, as opposed to those who did not.

The bottom line is that not one man felt that their sexual relationship had suffered as a result of the hysterectomy, and many felt it had improved. It's important to keep in mind that results were biased—not every husband returned the questionnaire, and it is entirely possible that it is the man who feels comfortable discussing sexuality and who has a good sexual relationship who tended to respond.

Jim: We always had a very active sex life up until several months before the surgery. When she learned that she would need the surgery, I was concerned that things would change. Our sexual relationship got much better since her worries about a possible cancer have been removed. It's important to be supportive and roll with the punches. A man cannot comprehend what a woman is going through, especially the emotional issues. Attend the presurgery conference. Also, buy her anything she wants!

Gary: The preoperative consultation was very informative and eliminated most of our questions and concerns. By hearing the options available and asking questions, we were both able to participate in making decisions regarding surgery. I thought that she would be less interested in having sex and would be less stimulated during sex. Thankfully, this was not the case; everything stayed pretty much the same.

Jon: At the time, the overriding concern was a possible cancer diagnosis. Sex was much lower on the priority list.

Paul: I anticipated that reconstructive surgery would improve sex.

Michael: I don't feel our relationship has really changed as a result of the surgery, but there was a period of adjustment. I would say it took six to twelve months for her to feel totally comfortable with intercourse again. I'm embarrassed to admit it, but it took me no time at all.

We do have sex less often, but I'm not sure it has a lot to do with the surgery. It is difficult to separate all the factors that affected the frequency of intercourse and our sexual relationship in general. My wife's surgery was ten months after our second child was born, which was a big transitional time for our family. So factors like busy or conflicting schedules, lack of sleep, childrearing, etc., all impacted our sexual relationship at the same time. It's also difficult qualifying frequency without factoring in quality. While the frequency is less, our quality of sex is as good as it's ever been.

Her vagina feels the same, maybe slightly different. Seven years after the surgery, I can't feel the difference, but I remember her feeling "tighter" for about a year after the surgery. I can't say that I view this as a negative result of the surgery.

Her response (which I view as excitement, orgasm, etc.) seems the same, but her frequency of desire is less. I'm not sure that had to do with the surgery, but then again maybe it did.

Ian: For my wife, there was something important about having a period. Hard to describe, but it connected her to her body somehow.

For example, she has difficulty predicting a PMS cycle, so she gets more troubled when she's feeling out of sorts because she can't take comfort in relating it to her period. She's sort of driving blindly through monthly hormonal changes.

Fred: A change in our sex lives was not a concern on my part. Our sexual relationship changed for the better. Before the surgery, she was dealing with the pain and bleeding of her period. There was a time before and after her period when I would not approach her for sex. Thinking back, her mood was so black, I would just try and keep a distance. Now, she doesn't have such big mood swings, which makes getting along easier.

Since the surgery, when she *is* in the mood, there is much more lubrication in the vagina. Although we only have intercourse once a week on average, she does seem to enjoy it more. I would say her response is better since the surgery.

It is great to see my wife not have the pain and heavy bleeding each month. This is a really good thing. My advice to other men: don't worry about your sex life going away. I feel mine has gotten better.

Daniel: After the physical healing was done, I thought our relationship would be instantly great. Gone were the mood swings, PMS, and yes, the actual scowl that came over her face. Instead, we entered a phase so bad, I almost left her after thirty years of marriage. In spite of the fact that her ovaries were not removed, her hormones seemed to be totally out of whack. I don't remember the exact timeline, but it was months after surgery. It got to the point where anything I said or did was wrong. She took everything as a personal attack on her. Example: she bought a new can opener, I kept using the old one—big fight. Stupid things like this.

There was a period of one or two months when we had little contact, verbal or otherwise, although we lived in the same house. I mentioned that maybe her hormones needed adjusting. That didn't go over good, either.

Things have returned to normal. There are still times when it doesn't take much to set her off, but I deal with it. Overall, things are pretty good now.

David: I was so concerned with the health of my wife that, quite frankly, I didn't think about any sexual repercussions. I don't think we even discussed it prior to surgery. Any problems related to frequency of sex have to do with timing and exhaustion more than anything. Since the surgery, our sexual relationship has actually been fantastic!

I feel lucky to have a healthy, sexy wife. Based on my experience, there was no real change in our relationship due to surgery.

Bill: Before surgery, I anticipated that my wife might be emotionally affected by the surgery. Without question, her worries and discomfort have significantly subsided. Before surgery, she was concerned about her health and well being, now she is relieved.

We actually have intercourse more frequently since the opportunity is less deterred due to periods and concerns regarding spotting and bleeding.

Ed: I was really concerned that sex would be different as a result of the hysterectomy even though I knew that she was not enjoying sex due to the painful periods, migraines, and the fibroids that were growing and causing problems.

Thankfully, there were no negative sexual side effects. Since the surgery, our sexual relationship is great—more spontaneous sex, more relaxed, more orgasms!

Al: My wife is happy to be rid of the monthly cramps and headaches and the sometimes unexpected and heavy periods. Once she got the HRT adjusted she began to sleep better and feel better overall. My advice to other men? If it is necessary, then just help her to accept it and get through it. She will still be "all woman" and the monthly pain and stress will be behind her (and you) for the rest of your lives!

Index

About the Author

Lauren Streicher, M.D., FACOG, is a practicing obstetrician gynecologist on staff at Northwestern Memorial Hospital in Chicago. She is on the faculty of Northwestern's affiliate medical school, the Feinberg School of Medicine.

Dr. Streicher is frequently interviewed regarding gynecological issues and has made over a hundred local and national television appearances, including *The McNeil Lehrer News Hour*, *Chicago Tonight*, and the Discovery Channel's *Birthday*. As a member of Chicago's Channel 2 (WBBM) Health Team, she made weekly appearances to discuss new obstetric and gynecologic research. She is recognized as an expert in her field by her peers and is consistently included (by physician vote) in *Chicago* magazine's list of top doctors. Her column, "Ask the Ob-Gyn," appears weekly in the *Chicago Sun-Times*.

When she is not writing, performing surgery, delivering babies, or driving her daughters to their various activities, Dr. Streicher can be found taking a ballet class, playing the piano, or rehearsing for amateur musicals.